SUMMARY OF AMERICAN CANCER SOCIETY RECOMMENDATIONS FOR EARLY DETECTION OF CANCER IN ASYMPTOMATIC PEOPLE AT AVERAGE RISK

Examination	Sex	Age	Periodicity
Sigmoidoscopy	M and F	Age 50 and older	1 examination every 3 to 5 years
Stool blood test	M and F	Age 50 and older	Every year
Digital rectal examination	M and F	Age 40 and older	Every year
Pap test and pelvic examination	F	Women who have been sexually active or have reached age 18 or older	Every year. After 3 or more satisfactory, consecutive, normal annual examinations, the Pap test may be performed less frequently at the discretion of the physician
Endometrial tissue sample	F	At menopause; women at high risk*	At menopause
Breast self-examination*	F	Age 20 and older	Every month
Clinical breast examination	F	20-39	Every 3 years
		Age 40 and older	Every year
Mammography	F	35-39	Baseline
		40-49	Every 1 to 2 years
		50 and over	Every year
Health counseling†	M and F	20-40	Every 3 years
Cancer checkup‡	M and F	Age 40 and older	Every year

*History of infertility, obesity, failure to ovulate, abnormal uterine bleeding, or estrogen therapy.
†To include counseling about tobacco control, sun exposure, diet and nutrition, risk factors, sexual practices, and environmental and other occupational exposures.
‡To include examination for cancers of the thyroid, testicles, prostate, ovaries, lymph nodes, oral cavity, and skin.

TNM STAGING SYSTEM

Tumor
T0	No evidence of primary tumor
Tis	Carcinoma in situ
T1, T2, T3, T4	Progressive increase in tumor size and involvement
Tx	Tumor cannot be assessed

Nodes
N0	Regional lymph nodes not demonstrably abnormal
N1, N2, N3	Increasing degrees of demonstrable abnormality of regional lymph nodes. (For many primary sites an "a" may be added (e.g., N1a) to indicate that metastasis to the node is not suspected; a "b" may be used (e.g., N1b) to indicate that metastasis to the node is suspected or proved.)
Nx	Regional lymph nodes cannot be assessed clinically

Metastasis
M0	No evidence of distant metastasis
M1, M2, M3	Ascending degrees of distant metastasis, including metastasis to distant lymph nodes

From the American Joint Committee for Cancer Staging and End Results Reporting: Clinical Staging System for Carcinoma of the Esophagus. *Cancer* March-April 1975, pp 25-51.

CANCER'S SEVEN WARNING SIGNALS

1. Change in bowel or bladder habits
2. A sore that does not heal
3. Unusual bleeding or discharge
4. Thickening or lump in breast or elsewhere
5. Indigestion or difficulty in swallowing
6. Obvious change in wart or mole
7. Nagging cough or hoarseness

If you have a warning signal, see your doctor.

GRADING OF TUMORS

G_x	Grade cannot be assessed
G_1	Well differentiated
G_2	Moderately well differentiated
G_3 and G_4	Poorly to very poorly differentiated

The more poorly differentiated a tumor is, the less it resembles normal cells and the poorer the prognosis. Grading systems vary according to the site of the disease.

CANCER NURSING

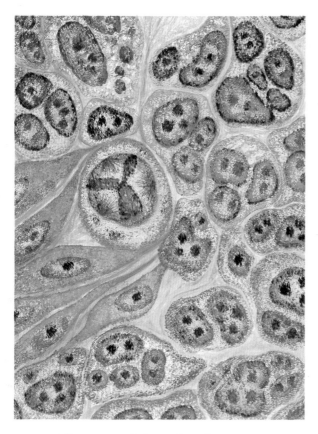

Cell in center with abnormal tripolar structure

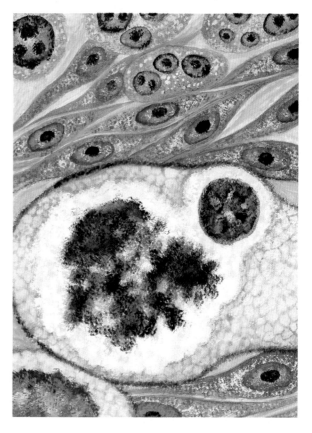

Giant multinucleate tumor cell

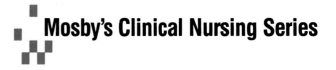

Mosby's Clinical Nursing Series

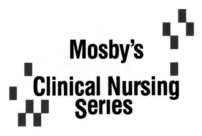

Mosby's Clinical Nursing Series

Cardiovascular Disorders

by Mary Canobbio

Respiratory Disorders

by Susan Wilson and June Thompson

Infectious Diseases

by Deanna Grimes

Orthopedic Disorders

by Leona Mourad

Renal Disorders

by Dorothy Brundage

Neurologic Disorders

by Esther Chipps, Norma Clanin, and Victor Campbell

Cancer Nursing

by Anne Belcher

Genitourinary Disorders

by Mikel Gray

Immunologic Disorders

by Christine Mudge-Grout

Gastrointestinal Disorders

by Dorothy Doughty and Debra Broadwell

CANCER NURSING

ANNE E. BELCHER, Ph.D., R.N.

Professor of Oncology Nursing, American Cancer Society;
Associate Professor, University of Maryland School of Nursing,
University of Maryland at Baltimore,
Baltimore, Maryland

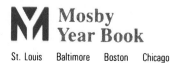
**Mosby
Year Book**

St. Louis   Baltimore   Boston   Chicago   London   Philadelphia   Sydney   Toronto

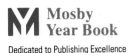

Mosby
Year Book
Dedicated to Publishing Excellence

Editor: Sally Adkisson
Project manager: Mark Spann
Production editors: Stephen C. Hetager, Christine O'Neil
Design: Liz Fett
Layout: Doris Hallas

ACKNOWLEDGMENTS

The author wishes to acknowledge the contributions of the
University of Maryland School of Nursing, the University of
Maryland Cancer Center, and the Departments of Radiation Oncology
and Radiology, University of Maryland at Baltimore.

Printed in the United States of America

Mosby–Year Book, Inc.
11830 Westline Industrial Drive
St. Louis, Missouri 63146

The authors and publisher have made a conscientious effort to ensure
that the drug information and recommended dosages in this book are
accurate and in accord with accepted standards at the time of
publication. However, pharmacology is a rapidly changing science,
so readers are advised to check the package insert provided by the
manufacturer before administering any drug.

Library of Congress Cataloging-in-Publication Data

Belcher, Anne E.
      Cancer nursing/Anne E. Belcher.
         p.   cm.—(Mosby's clinical nursing series)
      Includes bibliographical references and index.
      ISBN 0-8016-1809-6
      1. Cancer—Nursing.   I. Title.   II. Series.
      [DNLM: 1. Neoplasms—nursing.   2. Oncologic Nursing—methods.   WY
156 B427c]
      RC266.B35   1992
      610.73′698—dc20
      DNLM/DLC
      for Library of Congress   92-6002
                                                                                      CIP

92 93 94 95 96 CL/CD/VH 9 8 7 6 5 4 3 2

Contributors

Radiation Therapy Section contributed by
Roberta Strohl, R.N., M.N.
Clinical Nurse Specialist,
Department of Radiation Oncology,
University of Maryland at Baltimore,
Baltimore, Maryland

Chapter 16, Pharmacologic Management, contributed by
Katherine Stefos, Ph.D.
The University of Texas M.D. Anderson Cancer Center,
Division of Pharmacy,
Houston, Texas

Original illustrations by
George J. Wassilchenko
Tulsa, Oklahoma
and
Donald P. O'Connor
St. Peters, Missouri

Original photography by
Patrick Watson
Poughkeepsie, New York

Preface

Cancer Nursing is the seventh volume in *Mosby's Clinical Nursing Series*, a new kind of resource for practicing nurses. The *Series* is the result of the most elaborate market research ever undertaken by Mosby–Year Book, Inc. We first surveyed hundreds of working nurses to determine what kinds of resources practicing nurses want to meet their advanced information needs. We then approached clinical specialists, proven authors and experts, and asked them to develop a format that would meet the needs of nurses in practice. This format was presented to nine focus groups composed of working nurses and refined between each group. In the later stages we published a 32-page, full-color sample so that detailed changes could be made to improve physical layout and appearance, section by section and page by page. The result is a new genre of professional books for nursing professionals.

Cancer Nursing begins with a clear and concise discussion of the pathophysiology of cancer, which includes a variety of illustrations that depict sometimes difficult-to-visualize aspects of normal and abnormal cellular changes. These diagrams enable the reader to better understand normal and malignant cell division, cellular and humoral immunity, and cancer metastasis, to site only a few.

Chapter 2 is a pictorial guide to the nurse's assessment of the body systems affected by cancer. Clear, full-color photographs show proper position and technique in sharp detail, augmented by concise instructions, rationales, and tips. Also of interest is the discussion of the early detection of cancer, with emphasis on cancer detection in the elderly.

Chapter 3 presents the latest in diagnostic tests, using full-color photographs of equipment, techniques, monitors, and output. A consistent format for each procedure provides information about the purpose of the test, indications and contraindications, and nursing care associated with each test, including patient teaching.

Chapters 4 through 11 present the nursing care of patients experiencing site-specific cancers and the major surgical and other therapeutic interventions. The sites of cancer that are included reflect the major cancers in the United States today, as well as some less commonly occurring but challenging types. Chapter 4 focuses on lung cancer; Chapter 5 on breast cancer; Chapter 6 on colorectal and other gastrointestinal cancers; Chapter 7 on genitourinary cancers; Chapter 8 on gynecologic cancers; Chapter 9 on skin cancers; Chapter 10 on lymphomas; and Chapter 11 on head and neck

cancers. Information on pathophysiology answers questions nurses often have. Definitive diagnostic tests and the physician's treatment plan are also reviewed.

Chapter 12 focuses on metastatic disease and its management. Chapter 13 addresses oncologic emergencies, which are becoming increasingly common as patients with cancer are treated more aggressively and live longer. Chapter 14 describes cancer therapies—surgery, radiation, chemotherapy, bone marrow transplantation, and the biologic response modifiers. Supportive therapies such as colony-stimulating factors, blood and blood-component therapy, nutritional support, and pain management are also described.

The heart of the book is the nursing care, presented according to the nursing process. These pages are bordered in blue to make them easy to find and use on the unit. The nursing care is structured to integrate the five steps of the nursing process, centered around appropriate nursing diagnoses accepted by the North American Nursing Diagnosis Association (NANDA). The material can be used to develop individualized care plans quickly and accurately, and it meets the standards of nursing care required by the Joint Commission on the Accreditation of Healthcare Organizations (JCAHO). By facilitating the development of individualized and authoritative care plans, this book can actually save you time to spend on direct patient care.

In response to requests from scores of nurses participating in our research, a distinctive feature of this book is its use in patient teaching. Background information on diseases and medical interventions enables nurses to answer with authority questions patients often ask. The illustrations in the book, particularly those in the color atlas (Chapter 1) and the chapter on diagnostic procedures (Chapter 3), are specifically designed to support patient teaching. Chapter 15 consists of 18 patient teaching guides written to be copied, distributed to patients and their families, and used for self-care after discharge. In addition, patient teaching sections in each care plan provide nurses with checklists of concepts to teach, promoting this increasingly vital aspect of care.

The book concludes with a concise guide to cancer drugs, and, inside the back cover, a resource section directs you to organizations and other resources concerned with cancer care for nurses and patients.

We hope this book contributes to the advancement of professional nursing by serving as a first step toward a body of professional literature for nurses to call their own.

Contents

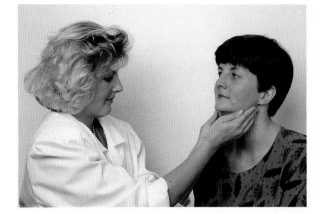

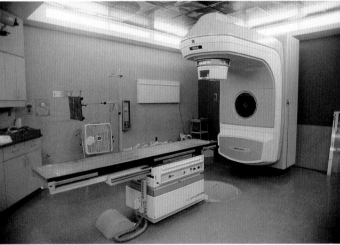

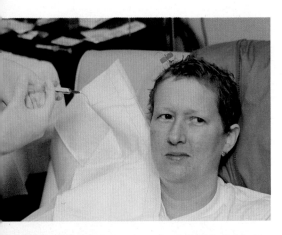

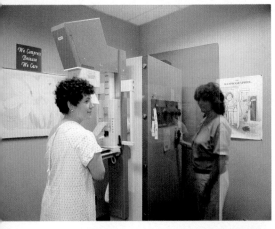

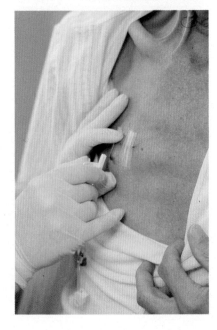

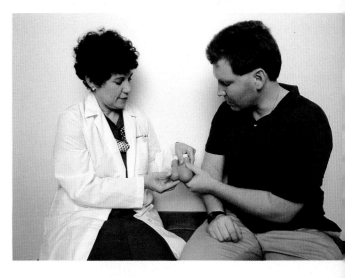

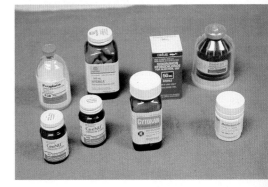

COLOR PLATES

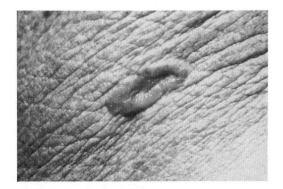

PLATE 1   Basal cell carcinoma.

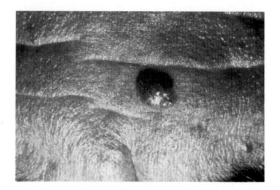

PLATE 2   Basal cell carcinoma.

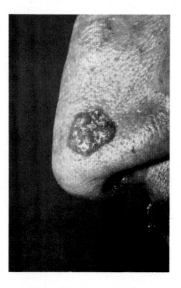

PLATE 3   Basal cell carcinoma.

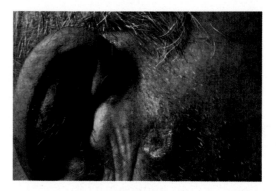

PLATE 4   Squamous cell carcinoma.

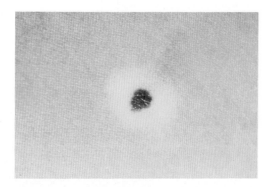

PLATE 5   Halo nevus.

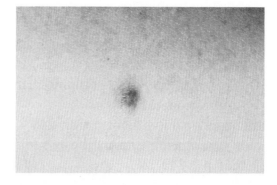

PLATE 6   Compound nevus.

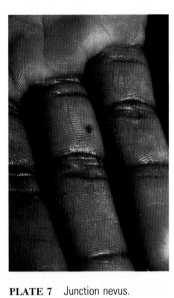

PLATE 7 Junction nevus.

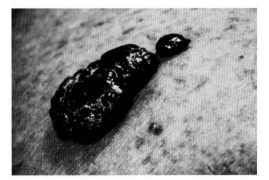

PLATE 8 Nodular melanoma.

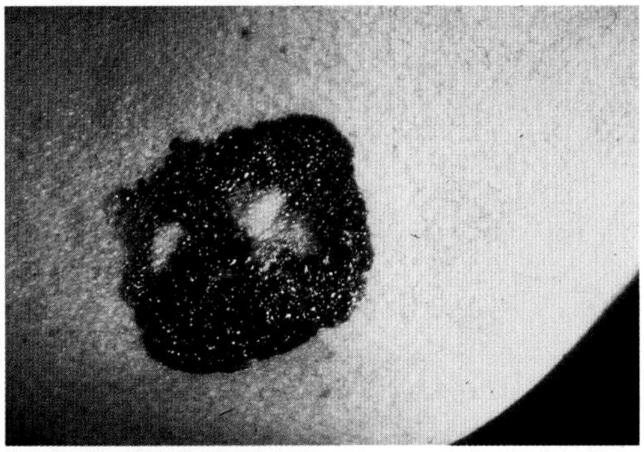

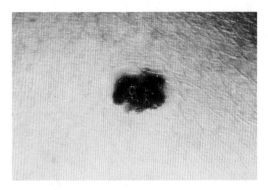

PLATE 9 Superficial spreading melanoma.

PLATE 10 Malignant melanoma.

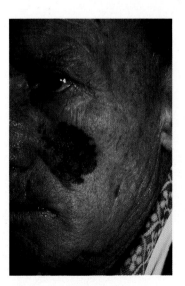

PLATE 11 Lentigo maligna.

Men	Incidence	Death
Lung	102,000	92,000
Kidney	15,000	6,100
Stomach	13,900	8,300
Pancreas	13,600	12,100
Colon/rectum	76,000	30,000
Bladder	36,000	6,500
Prostate	106,000	30,000
Leukemia/lymphoma	38,500	20,300
All others	45,200	19,200

Women	Incidence	Death
Lung	55,000	50.000
Breast	150,000	44,000
Stomach	9,300	5,400
Pancreas	14,500	12,900
Colon/rectum	79,000	30,900
Ovary	20,500	12,400
Uterus	46,500	10,000
Leukemia/lymphoma	32,300	17,600
All others	35,900	15,300

Color Atlas of Pathophysiology of Cancer

Cancer is the second most common cause of death in the United States, resulting in the deaths of about 514,000 people in 1991. New cases of cancer were diagnosed in 1.1 million people in this same year, not including the approximately 600,000 cases of basal and squamous cell skin cancer. The trend toward earlier diagnosis and treatment of certain cancers, as well as better overall health practices, has improved the outlook for people with cancer. Four out of 10 people diagnosed with cancer this year will be alive in 5 years.

Cancer is a universal disease that affects people without regard to race, gender, socioeconomic status, or culture. However, different forms of cancer strike specific age, ethnic, and gender groups with varying frequency and severity. For example, cancer morbidity and mortality increase rapidly with age; some researchers believe that anyone who lives long enough eventually will develop cancer. Socioeconomic factors are thought to explain many of the ethnic differences in cancer. Both the incidence and mortality of certain cancers are higher in African-Americans than in Caucasians. Although women are more likely than men to develop cancer, more men die of the disease. The sites in men that are associated with the greatest mortality are the lungs, prostate, and colon and rectum. In women the leading sites are the lungs, breasts, and colon and rectum (see opposite page).

CANCER ETIOLOGY

Although cancer is a universal disease, factors such as age, gender, and ethnicity play a role in the incidence of certain types of cancer (see previous page). Another factor associated with the differences in cancer incidence is heredity. Certain cancers, such as those of the stomach, breast, colon and rectum, uterus, and lung, occur in a familial pattern. It is not known whether this indicates that people inherit a specific susceptibility or that they share exposure to a carcinogenic factor. Certain diseases that are cancer precursors, such as multiple familial polyposis and Gardner's syndrome, seem to be hereditary.

MULTISTAGE THEORY OF CAUSATION

Cancer probably is caused by many interacting factors rather than by a single one, and it appears to develop in a multistep process. The currently accepted model includes initiation, transformation, and promotion (Figure 1-1). **Initiation** results when a carcinogen, such as ultraviolet radiation, is applied directly to a cell. If cells exposed to the initiating factor become progressively dedifferentiated, then **transformation** is said to have occurred. **Promotion** results from the application of one or more cocarcinogens to the cell, such as tobacco products or estrogens. This process takes place in the deoxyribonucleic acid (DNA) of the cell, creating a mutated gene that causes uncontrolled cell division and development of malignancy. Reversing factors, which inhibit the effects of promoting factors, have been discovered, and research into the use of these factors is called **chemoprevention.** Examples of reversing factors include certain drugs, such as actinomycin D, certain enzymes that protect the cells from peroxides, and such dietary factors as vitamins E, C, and A, beta-carotene, and indoles (found in brussels sprouts, cabbage, turnips, and broccoli).

POSSIBLE CAUSATIVE FACTORS

Some causative agents have been determined, and others are suspected. One factor predisposing to cancer is chronic irritation, such as frequent, prolonged exposure to sunlight or sustained alcohol consumption. Some benign lesions, such as leukoplakia of the oral cavity, colon and rectal polyps, and pigmented moles, may undergo malignant transformation. People whose cancer has already been diagnosed are at risk for later occurrence of the disease at the same or another site.

Environmental carcinogens that have been identi-

fied include cigarette smoke, asbestos, and vinyl chloride. Iatrogenic factors that have been implicated are radiation and drugs such as diethylstilbestrol (DES); certain cancer chemotherapeutic agents, such as cyclo-

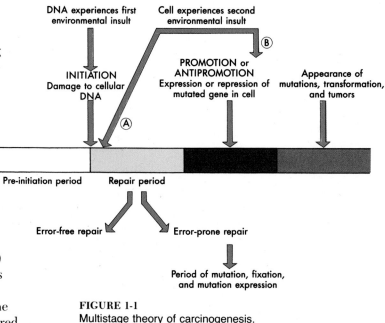

FIGURE 1-1
Multistage theory of carcinogenesis.

phosphamide; radioisotopes, such as phosphorus (^{32}P) and radium; and immunosuppressive drugs. Evidence continues to mount that dietary fat may be an important factor in colon cancer; further study is needed on the role of dietary fiber in preventing colon and other cancers. The American Cancer Society has developed guidelines for primary prevention that reflect research findings to date (see box).

Viruses associated with cancer include the adenoviruses, papovaviruses, herpes viruses, human T-cell lymphoma–leukemia virus (HTLV), Epstein-Barr virus (EBV), and hepatitis B virus. Age and immunocompetence may modify the effects of the viruses, in that the very young and old are more susceptible, and many viruses are oncogenic only if the host becomes infected prenatally or perinatally (see box on page 3).

CANCER PREVENTION

Avoid those factors that might lead to the development of cancer (primary prevention).

Smoking	Cigarette smoking is responsible for 85% of lung cancer cases among men and 75% among women—about 83% overall. Smoking accounts for about 30% of all cancer deaths. Those who smoke two or more packs of cigarettes a day have lung cancer mortality rates 15 to 25 times greater than nonsmokers.
Sunlight	Almost all of the more than 600,000 cases of basal and squamous cell skin cancer diagnosed each year in the United States are considered to be sun related. Epidemiologic evidence shows that sun exposure is a major factor in the development of melanoma and that the incidence increases for those living near the equator.
Alcohol	Oral cancer and cancers of the larynx, throat, esophagus, and liver occur more frequently among heavy drinkers of alcohol.
Smokeless tobacco	Use of chewing tobacco or snuff increases the risk of cancer of the mouth, larynx, throat, and esophagus and is highly habit-forming.
Estrogen	Estrogen treatment to control menopausal symptoms increases the risk of endometrial cancer. Use of estrogen by menopausal women needs to be carefully discussed by the woman and her physician.
Radiation	Excessive exposure to ionizing radiation can increase the risk of cancer. Most medical and dental x-rays are adjusted to deliver the lowest dose possible without sacrificing image quality. Excessive radon exposure in homes may increase the risk of lung cancer, especially in cigarette smokers. If levels are found to be too high, remedial action should be taken.
Occupational hazards	Exposure to several different industrial agents (e.g., nickel, chromate, asbestos, vinyl chloride) increases the risk of various cancers. The risk from asbestos is greatly increased when combined with cigarette smoking.
Nutrition	The risk of colon, breast, and uterine cancers increases in obese people. High-fat diets may contribute to the development of cancers of the breast, colon, and prostate. High-fiber foods might help reduce the risk of colon cancer. A varied diet containing plenty of vegetables and fruits rich in vitamins A and C may reduce the risk for a wide range of cancers. Salt-cured, smoked, and nitrite-cured foods have been linked to esophageal and stomach cancer. Heavy use of alcohol, especially when accompanied by cigarette smoking or chewing tobacco, increases the risk of cancers of the mouth, larynx, throat, esophagus, and liver.

From The American Cancer Society.[1]

ONCOGENES

Oncogenes are located on specific chromosomes and normally are expressed at significant levels only during embryogenesis; however, their expression may be altered by chromosome rearrangement, chemical carcinogens, radiation, or other factors. The resulting changes in expression may disrupt normal cell growth, gradually transforming normal cells into cancer cells.

NORMAL CELL STRUCTURE, DIVISION, AND DIFFERENTIATION

A normal cell is composed of the cell membrane, cytoplasm, cell organelles, and nucleus (Figure 1-2). The **cell membrane,** which is composed of protein and lipid substances, encloses the cytoplasm and is selectively permeable. Its functions are to maintain a consistent internal cellular environment, support and regulate enzyme systems, maintain specific metabolic processes, and participate in cellular recognition. The **cytoplasm** is a fine, granular substance that contains various cellular organelles, including the mitochondria, Golgi apparatus, and centrioles. The **mitochondria**

serve as the powerhouse of the cell and manufacture most of the adenosine triphosphate (ATP) needed for cellular energy. Each **Golgi apparatus** contains enzyme systems that encase manufactured substances in secretory vesicles; these vesicles float to the cell's interior surface, fuse their membranes with the cell membrane, and release their contents into the extracellular fluid. A centrosome is a specialized area of cytoplasm close to the nucleus. **Centrioles,** of which each centrosome has two, are actively involved in cell division.

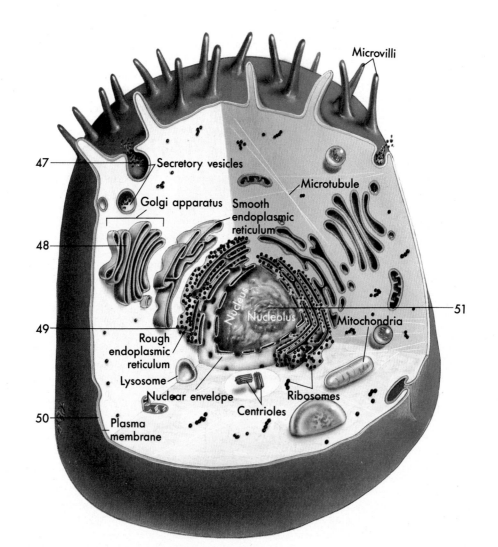

FIGURE 1-2
Normal cell showing major organelles. Although no single cell contains all these organelles, many cells contain a large number of them. (From Seeley et al.[52])

MITOSIS

Mitosis is a continuous process, but it is divided into five stages (see box) for clearer understanding of the characteristics of each phase (Figure 1-3).

THE STAGES OF MITOSIS

Prophase: Chromatic strands condense to form chromosomes, each of which is composed of two separate strands, called chromatids, that are joined at one point by a specialized region called the centromere. As prophase proceeds, one pair of centrioles moves to each side of the cell. Microtubules form near the centrioles and project in all directions. Some end blindly and are called astral fibers. Others, known as spindle fibers, project toward the equator and either overlap with fibers from other centrioles or attach to the centromeres of the chromosomes. At the end of prophase, the nuclear envelope degenerates and the nucleoli have disappeared.

Metaphase: The chromosomes align along the equator with spindle fibers from each pair of centrioles attached to their centromeres.

Anaphase: The centromeres separate, and each chromatid is now a chromosome. When the centromeres divide, the chromosome number doubles, producing two identical sets of 46. The two sets of chromosomes are pulled by the spindle fibers toward the poles of the cell. Along the equator of the cell, the cytoplasm becomes narrower as the cell membranes move toward one another.

Telophase: A new nuclear envelope develops from the endoplasmic reticulum, and the nucleoli reappear as distinct organelles. Spindle fibers disappear, and the chromosomes unravel to become less distinct chromatin threads. The nuclei of the two daughter cells assume the appearance of interphase nuclei. The process of mitosis is complete.

Interphase: The period between active cell divisions is called the interphase. During this period DNA and its associated proteins are seen as dispersed chromatin threads within the nucleus. When replication begins, the two strands of each DNA molecule separate and each serves as a template for production of a new strand of DNA. Each of the two new DNA molecules produced has one strand of nucleotides derived from the original DNA molecule and one newly synthesized strand. During interphase the centrioles within the centrosome also are duplicated.

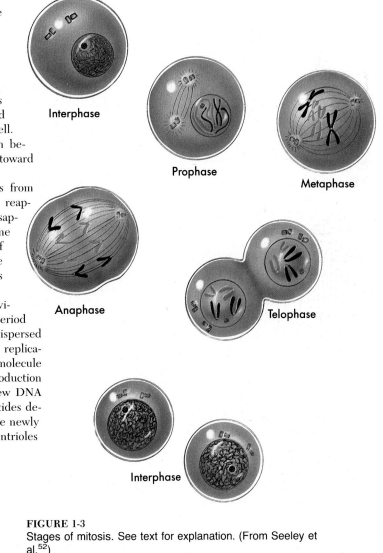

Interphase

Prophase

Metaphase

Anaphase

Telophase

Interphase

FIGURE 1-3
Stages of mitosis. See text for explanation. (From Seeley et al.[52])

CELL CYCLE

The cell cycle refers to the movement of a cell from a resting state (G_0) through mitosis. Cell cycle time, the time between successive episodes of mitosis for both normal and neoplastic cells, is 1 to 5 days (Figure 1-4). The physician uses this information to determine therapeutic protocols, which include agents that are both cell cycle specific and cell cycle nonspecific.

DIFFERENTIATION OF CELLS

Differentiation is the process by which cells attain specific structural and functional characteristics. A differentiated cell is one that does not divide again under normal circumstances, performs a selected function, and has a specific structure. Differentiated cells may be unipotent or pluripotent. A unipotent cell has only one structure and function (e.g., neurons and pancreatic cells). A pluripotent cell, or stem cell, can become more than one type of cell. Stem cells are found in the bone marrow, skin, and gastrointestinal tract.

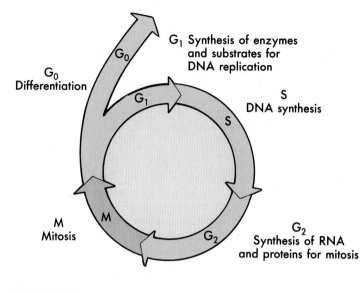

FIGURE 1-4
The cell cycle.

HEMATOLYMPHATIC SYSTEM

The hematolymphatic system is composed of blood and blood-forming organs, the bone marrow, spleen, liver, and the lymphatics.

BLOOD AND ITS COMPONENTS

Blood, which circulates continuously through the heart and vascular system, performs numerous vital functions:

- Transporting oxygen and absorbed nutrients to cells, and waste products, including carbon dioxide, to the kidneys, skin, and lungs
- Transporting hormones from their origin in the endocrine glands to other tissues
- Protecting the body from life-threatening microorganisms
- Regulating body temperature through heat transfer.

The major characteristics of blood include color (arterial blood is bright red; venous blood is dark red); viscosity (blood is three to four times thicker than water); acidity (the pH is 7.35 to 7.40); and volume (adults have approximately 70 to 75 ml/kg of body weight, or 5 to 6 liters).

The liquid portion of blood, plasma, is a suspension of colloid, electrolytes, proteins, and numerous other substances. The particulate matter includes red blood cells (erythrocytes), white blood cells (leukocytes), and platelets (thrombocytes). All of these cells are believed to be derived from a single stem cell (Figure 1-5).

Erythrocytes

There are approximately 5 million erythrocytes, or red blood cells (RBCs), per cubic millimeter of blood. The principal functions of these cells are:

- Transporting oxygen to the tissues (Oxygen attaches to hemoglobin, the iron-containing substance of the red blood cell.)
- Transporting carbon dioxide to the lungs
- Maintaining normal blood pH through a series of intracellular buffers

Red blood cells are produced in the red bone marrow, which is found in the ribs, sternum, skull, vertebrae, and bones of the hands, feet, and pelvis. The average life span of an erythrocyte is 115 to 130 days.

Normal hemoglobin amounts to 15 g/dl of blood. It is composed of a simple protein called globin and a

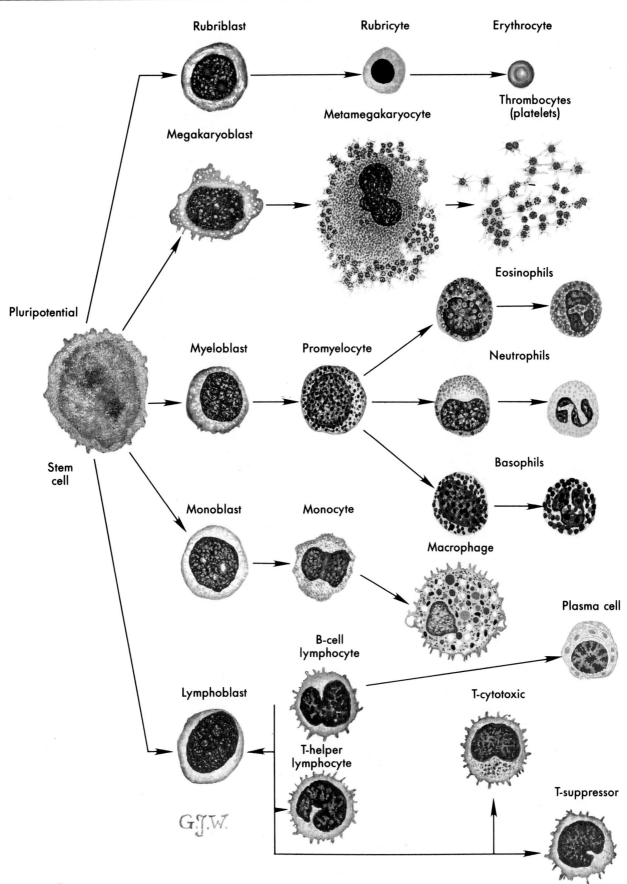

Rubriblast   Rubricyte   Erythrocyte

Thrombocytes (platelets)

Metamegakaryocyte

Megakaryoblast

Eosinophils

Pluripotential

Myeloblast   Promyelocyte   Neutrophils

Basophils

Stem cell

Monoblast   Monocyte

Macrophage

Plasma cell

B-cell lymphocyte

T-cytotoxic

Lymphoblast

T-helper lymphocyte

G.J.W.

T-suppressor

FIGURE 1-5
Components of blood derived from a single stem cell.

red compound called heme, which contains iron and porphyrin. The total amount of iron in the body ranges from 2 to 6 grams, two thirds of which is contained in hemoglobin.

Leukocytes

About 5,000 to 10,000 leukocytes, or white blood cells (WBCs), are present in a cubic millimeter of blood. White blood cells are divided into three major categories: granulocytes, lymphocytes, and monocytes. Granulocytes, which make up 70% of all white blood cells, are produced by the bone marrow and function according to the type of granulocyte:

- Polymorphonuclear leukocytes (PMNs, or neutrophils), whose main function is to fight bacterial infections through a process of phagocytosis
- Eosinophils, which are particularly important in digesting bacteria and appear to play a role in combating allergic reactions
- Basophils, which contain enzymes thought to play a role in combating acute systemic allergic reactions

Lymphocytes, which are mainly produced in the lymph nodes, make up about 25% of the white blood cells and are primarily concerned with producing antibodies and maintaining tissue immunity. Monocytes, which are derived from components of the reticuloendothelial system, are responsible for the phagocytosis of dead red blood cells and white blood cells in the blood. They also play a role in the processing of antigenic information.

Thrombocytes

There are approximately 250,000 to 500,000 thrombocytes per cubic millimeter of blood. Formed in the bone marrow, they maintain capillary integrity, initiate coagulation, and retract clots.

LYMPHATIC SYSTEM

The lymphatic system also has numerous functions, including:

- Transporting lymph
- Producing lymphocytes and antibodies
- Phagocytosis
- Absorption of fats and fat-soluble matter from the intestine

The lymphatic system has three major characteristics: (1) the formation of lymph is regulated by the ex-

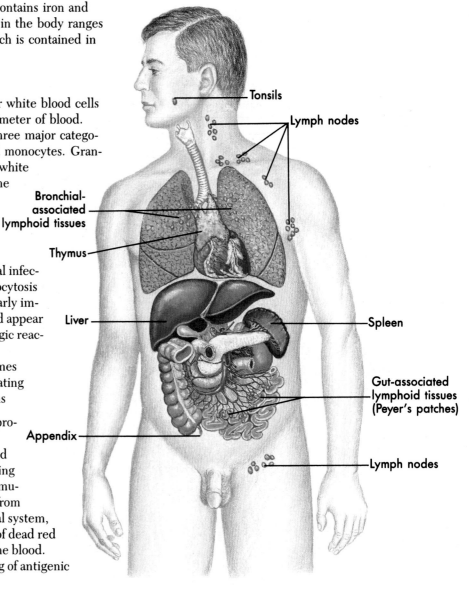

FIGURE 1-6
Components of the lymphatic system. (From Seidel et al.[53])

change of fluid between capillaries and tissue spaces; (2) the muscle pump is responsible for the movement of lymph; and (3) the amount of lymphoid tissue and the distribution of lymph nodes are related to age. The lymphatic system includes peripheral lymphatics, regional nodes, main lymphatic ducts, and the thoracic duct (Figure 1-6). Lymph nodes are present in virtually every area of the body. The most familiar nodes are those palpable in the neck and groin. The nodes serve as filters along the course of lymphatic channels and have a rich blood supply, which is important in transporting lymphocytes (Figure 1-7). The spleen is a mass of lymphoid and reticuloendothelial cells found under the ribs in the upper left quadrant of the abdomen. Its structure allows close inter-action among lymphocytes, macrophages, and materials carried in the blood-stream. The thymus is located in the thorax anterior to the upper part of the heart and great vessels and contains lymphatic follicles and lymphocytes. The bone marrow is considered an important part of the lymphoid system, because millions of lymphocytes are scattered throughout it.

The various lymphatic channels in the body drain fluid from organs and tissues, con-duct it centrally, and introduce it to the blood-stream via a large vein (the vena cava) in the thorax. Many lymphocytes are found in the lymph and are recycled for varying periods of time.

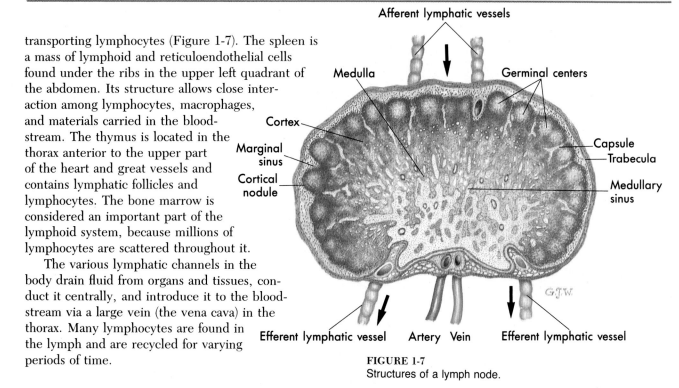

FIGURE 1-7
Structures of a lymph node.

IMMUNE SYSTEM

The functions of the immune system are to recognize and destroy harmful foreign substances, including bac-teria, viruses, and malignant cells. The system's ability to differentiate "self" from "nonself" is an essential characteristic; failure of this self-recognition results in autoimmune disease. The components of the immune system include the bone marrow, thymus, spleen, lymphatic vessels and fluid, lymph nodes, other lym-phoid tissue (tonsils and adenoids, appendix, and Pey-er's patches), and parts of the liver and lungs.

The early lines of defense against foreign sub-stances from the external environment include the skin, which serves as a passive barrier; ciliated epithe-lium in the respiratory tract; the composition and flushing action of urine; saliva; and lysozyme in human tears.

If the foreign substance passes the early lines of defense and if the substance (antigen) is being intro-duced for the first time, the immune system's re-sponse is nonspecific. If the substance (antigen) has been introduced before or is very similar to the initial agent, the immune system's response is specific. The system's memory of an earlier contact enables it to mount an accelerated response.

In addition to the surface defenses and nonspecific resistance factors, there are three other aspects of the immune system: the phagocytic-inflammatory system; the cell-mediated immune system; and humoral immu-nity (Figure 1-8). All are interrelated and interdepen-dent.

When an antigen enters the body, the phagocytic response begins. A chemical is elaborated by the anti-gen or by the tissue it has injured, which stimulates the body's initial efforts to find the antigen and destroy it. Blood flow to the injured area increases, and with vaso-dilation the walls of the blood vessels become more per-meable, allowing the neutrophils to migrate to the site of tissue injury. Once the neutrophils are in contact with the antigen, phagocytosis (engulfment) (Figure 1-9) is followed by lysis, which is accomplished by the release of digestive enzymes from the granules within each neu-trophil. If this initial attack is inadequate, the mononu-clear macrophages provide the second line of defense. The result of this effort is an increase in the total periph-eral white blood cell count, although viral infections or bone marrow suppression will decrease this count.

Complement is a group of at least 11 proteins that normally circulate in the blood in an inactive, nonfunc-

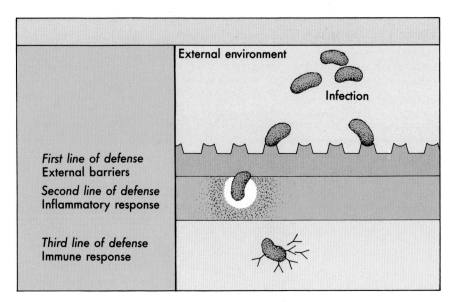

FIGURE 1-8
Lines of defense against infection. (From Grimes.[24])

tional form. However, once activated during the immune response, complement promotes inflammation and phagocytosis. It becomes activated in the complement cascade, a series of reactions in which each component of the series activates the next component.

Phagocytosis has limitations; certain bacteria, almost all viruses, and many fungi can resist digestion by the neutrophil after they have been ingested, then safely multiply and live within and off of their host cells (intracellular parasites). Because the body is in constant contact with potential pathogens, the phagocytic system would soon be overwhelmed if it responded to full capacity each time an antigen appeared. Thus other systems assist to ensure the host's survival. In general, humoral immunity (B cell–dependent immunity) protects against bacterial infections, and cell-mediated immunity (T cell–mediated immunity) guards against intracellular parasites and is a factor in immune surveillance and graft rejection.

Humoral immunity, which occurs in the blood and tissue fluid, involves specific antigen recognition, synthesis of antibody (immunoglobulins) by B lymphocytes, an immediate hypersensitivity reaction (allergy), binding of the immunoglobulin to the antigen, and ingestion by phagocytes.

Each B cell is genetically programmed to recognize and react with only one specific antigen. The humoral immune system can manufacture 1 million to 100 million different types of immunoglobulins in response to the antigens produced by the millions of microbes that exist in nature.

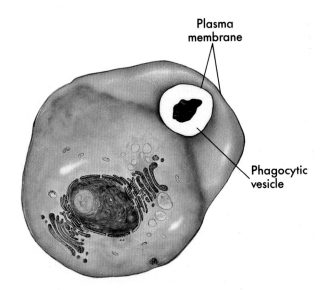

FIGURE 1-9
Phagocytosis. Cell processes (pseudopodia) extend from the cell and surround the particle to be taken into the cell by phagocytosis. Once the pseudopodia have surrounded the particle, they fuse to form a vesicle, which contains the particle. The vesicle is then internalized into the cell. (From Seeley et al.[52])

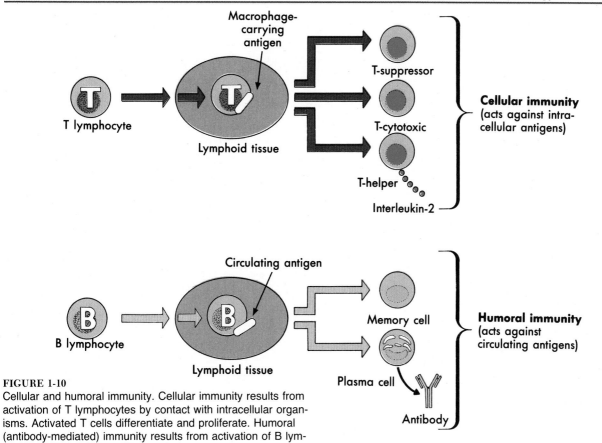

FIGURE 1-10
Cellular and humoral immunity. Cellular immunity results from activation of T lymphocytes by contact with intracellular organisms. Activated T cells differentiate and proliferate. Humoral (antibody-mediated) immunity results from activation of B lymphocytes. (From Grimes.[24])

The antibody initially manifested in a primary humoral response is of the IgM immunoglobulin class; this initial response takes 4 to 10 days and requires help from the cell-mediated immune system. If the same antigen is encountered again at a later time, IgM does not respond with a significant elevation because this primary defense is no longer needed. After the IgM response, IgG immunoglobulin rises at a slower rate and in larger amounts; the IgG carries the memory of exposure. The reappearance of the antigen jogs the B cell's memory, and a massive, rapid response occurs; the host is said to be immune to this antigen (Figure 1-10).

Cell-mediated immunity has as its active component the T lymphocyte. When a T cell meets its antigen, it triggers the release of cytokines (also called lymphokines), producing an inflammatory response and attracting macrophages to the area. These macrophages assist neutrophils in the phagocytosis of antigens and display the antigens on their own surface like a red flag.

The red flag alerts highly specialized lymphocytes, called helper T cells (thymus-derived cells), which bind to the macrophage and begin to multiply. Some helper T cells also rush to the spleen and lymph nodes to stimulate the production of (1) killer T cells, which chemically puncture the viral membranes, spilling the contents, which are then removed by phagocytes, and (2) B cells, which produce antibodies that bind to the surface of the virus. Suppressor T cells then release substances that turn off the B cells and command helper T cells to "cease and desist." Memory T and B cells are left in the blood and lymph system, ready to respond more quickly if the antigen reappears. When this occurs, immunoglobulins (Ig) bind to the specific antigens and neutralize them.

As noted previously, T cells work primarily by secreting lymphokines, which bind to specific receptors on target cells and call into play many other cells and substances, including the elements of the inflammatory response. Lymphokines encourage cell growth, promote cell activation, direct cellular traffic, destroy target cells, and incite macrophages.

Interferon, one of the first cytokines (lymphokines) to be discovered, is a protein that protects the body against viral infection and perhaps some forms of cancer. It does not protect the cell that produces it or act directly against viruses, but it does bind to the surface of other cells, where it stimulates production of antiviral proteins that prevent production of new viral nu-

Table 1-1 _____

PROMINENT BIOLOGIC PROPERTIES OF HUMAN CYTOKINES

Lymphokine	Biologic properties
Interleukin-1 (alpha and beta)	Activates resting T cells; is cofactor for hematopoietic growth factors; induces fever, sleep, release of adrenocorticotropic hormone (ACTH), neutrophilia, and other systemic acute-phase responses; stimulates synthesis of lymphokines, collagen, and collagenases; activates endothelial and macrophagic cells; mediates inflammation, catabolic processes, and nonspecific resistance to infection
Interleukin-2	Growth factor for activated T cells; induces the synthesis of other lymphokines; activates cytotoxic lymphocytes
Interleukin-3	Supports the growth of pluripotent (multilineage) bone marrow stem cells; growth factor for mast cells
Colony-stimulating factor (CSF)	
Granulocyte-macrophage CSF	Promotes neutrophilic, eosinophilic, and macrophagic bone marrow colonies; activates mature granulocytes
Granulocyte CSF	Promotes neutrophilic colonies
Macrophage CSF	Promotes macrophagic colonies
Interleukin-4 (B-cell stimulating factor-1)	Growth factor for activated B cells; induces histocompatibility module expression on B cells; growth factor for resting T cells and mast cells; enhances cytolytic activity of cytotoxic T cells
B-cell stimulating factor-2 (B-cell differentiating factor)	Induces the differentiation of activated B cells into immunoglobulin-secreting plasma cells; identical with beta$_2$-interferon, plasmacytoma growth factor, and hepatocyte-stimulating factor
Gamma-interferon	Induces class I, class II (histocompatibility module), and other surface antigens on a variety of cells; activates macrophages and endothelial cells; augments or inhibits other lymphokine activities; augments natural-killer-cell activity; exerts antiviral activity
Interferon (alpha and beta)	Exerts antiviral activity; induces class I antigen expression; augments natural-killer-cell activity; has fever-inducing and antiproliferative properties
Tumor necrosis factor (alpha and beta)	Direct cytotoxin for some tumor cells; induces fever, sleep, and other systemic acute-phase responses; stimulates the synthesis of lymphokines, collagen, and collagenases; activates endothelial and macrophagic cells; mediates inflammation, catabolic processes, and septic shock

From Dinarello C and Mier J: Current concepts: lymphokines, *N Engl J Med* 317(5):940, 1987.

cleic acid and proteins, thus stopping viral reproduction. Interferon also can stimulate production of defective viruses, which cannot infect other cells, and can prevent release of a virus from the infected cell. It also activates macrophages and natural killer cells that attack tumor cells.

Other cytokines whose basic structure has been identified have been renamed interleukins (IL), messengers between leukocytes (Table 1-1). Interleukin-1 (IL-1) is a product of macrophages that helps activate B cells and T cells. Interleukin-2 (IL-2) is produced by antigen-activated T cells and promotes the rapid growth of mature T cells and B cells. Interleukin-3 (IL-3) is a T cell–derived member of the protein mediators known as colony-stimulating factors (CSF); one of its many functions is to nurture the development of immature precursor cells into a variety of mature blood cells. Interleukin-4 (IL-4) helps B cells grow and differentiate.

IMMUNOSURVEILLANCE

Some T cells are responsible for immunosurveillance. When a cell becomes malignant, it carries a tumor-specific antigen on its membranes that is recognized as nonself and destroyed. If T cell function is suppressed by age, drugs (e.g., corticosteroids), poor nutrition, alcohol, serious infections, or certain disease processes (e.g., neoplastic invasion of bone and lymph tissue), the risk of cancer increases. To suppress T cell rejection of a transplanted organ, steroids and other drugs are administered. The resultant loss of immunosurveillance increases the risk of certain cancers. Other causes of impaired immunosurveillance are thought to be inefficient tumor burden (too small to excite immunologic recognition); production of tumor suppression factors such as prostaglandins, which inhibit stimulation of lymphocytes; and tolerance caused by continued recurrence of tumor cells.

Cell in center with abnormal tripolar spindle

Giant multinucleate tumor cell

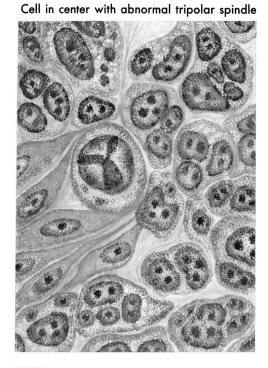
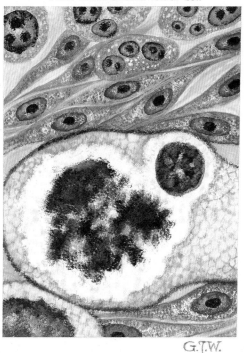

FIGURE 1-11
Multinucleate anaplastic tumor cells (cancer cells).

CARCINOGENESIS

In describing the nature and possible causes of cancer, it is important to understand that cancer cells, unlike normal cells, proliferate without organization and often without differentiation. Certain stimuli are believed to initiate this process, which subsequently overpowers the normal control mechanism. The results are uninhibited growth (autonomy), uncontrolled function (anaplasia), and uncontrolled motility, permitting spread to other parts of the body (metastasis) via blood or the lymphatic system.

ABNORMAL CELL STRUCTURE, DIVISION, AND DIFFERENTIATION

The cellular features of cancer cells are: a local increase in the number of cells; loss of normal cellular arrangement; variation in cell shape and size; increased nuclear size and density of staining (reflects an increase in total DNA); increased mitotic activity; and abnormal mitosis and chromosomes (Figure 1-11).

Two types of disorganization usually are seen. One involves the chaotic nuclear and cytoplasmic changes characteristic of cells undergoing transformation (the process by which a normal cell becomes a cancer cell), with pronounced cellular proliferation and great variation in the size and shape of cells. Cancer cells divide in an uncoordinated fashion, invading and destroying neighboring tissue. The other type of disorganization is the disordered relationship of the component cells to each other. This is caused by differences between the cell surfaces of normal cells and those of cancer cells. The surfaces of normal cells bind to each other better than do the surfaces of cancer cells, which lose an adhesive called fibronectin. This reduction in adhesiveness of malignant cells has been suggested as the physical basis of malignancy.

The nuclei of malignant cells often are enlarged and vary in shape, and mitosis frequently proceeds more quickly. Changes in chromosomes include breaks, deletions, ring forms, and abnormal chromosomal karyotypes. For example, consistent changes are reported in chromosomes 1 and 17 in a number of hematologic cancers. Changes in chromosome 22, where the long arm is translocated to chromosome 9, have made that chromosome well known in chronic granulocytic leukemia as the Philadelphia chromosome (Figure 1-12).

The plasma membranes of cancer cells have altered surface characteristics, fewer glycolipids, decreased amounts of membrane proteins, altered membrane fluidity, and loss of contact inhibition. Changes in internal membrane function include increased glucose transport, which is associated with surface alterations in cancer cells.

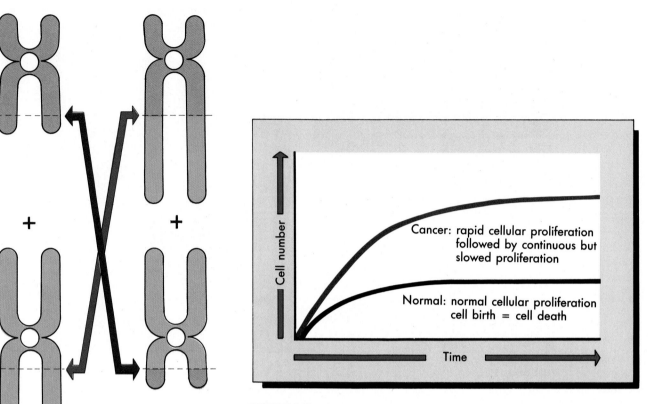

FIGURE 1-13
Doubling time of cancer cells.

FIGURE 1-12
Reciprocal chromosome translocation.

ALTERATIONS IN CELLULAR KINETICS

Tumors develop in progressive steps from normal to malignant growth, with the origin from a single cell or from several cells, depending on the type of tissue affected. The growth rates of tumors also vary and are influenced by vascular supply and the tumor's structural and functional integrity. New growth of blood vessels to vascularize tissues (angiogenesis) is essential to the development of solid tumors. One measure of a tumor's growth rate is the doubling time, which is the mean length of time for division of all the tumor cells present. It has been calculated that approximately 30 doubling times are required for a tumor to reach 1 cm in diameter. The growth process is thought to be enhanced by growth factors, prostaglandin E_1, proteolytic enzymes, and possibly a tumor angiogenesis factor (TAF). It has been suggested that tumor angiogenesis factor is the stimulus for increasing the network of blood vessels in the tumor. Tumor growth may slow because blood vessels become compressed, cells divide more slowly, or cells enter a dormant state.

Dedifferentiation, the process by which cells lose the characteristics of normal cells, may be caused by the abnormal differentiation of committed but immature stem cells or conversion of mature cells to proliferating cells that become increasingly immature because of changes in the way genes are transcribed. Dedifferentiated cells lose their contact inhibition and have altered antigen expression and enhanced cloning efficiency. As cancer cells become more undifferentiated, they also require lower concentrations of growth factors to reproduce; use higher rates of anaerobic glycolysis, making them less dependent on oxygen; produce autogenic (self-stimulating) growth factors; produce greater amounts of prostaglandins, which may assist in the tumor's escape from immune surveillance and in establishment of metastases; and produce more cell-surface enzymes, which aid the cancer cells in invasion and metastasis.

INVASION AND METASTASIS

Tumors spread throughout the body by direct invasion of contiguous organs or local spread; by metastasis to distant organs by lymphatics and blood vessels; and by metastasis by implantation. The spread of a tumor depends on its growth rate and degree of differentiation and the anatomic presence or absence of barriers and other unknown factors. Invasion and local spread are thought to occur because the tumor builds up pressure that forces fingerlike projections along the lines of least mechanical resistance. Pressure from the growing tumor also may block local blood vessels, leading to local tissue death and reduced mechanical resistance. Periosteum, cartilage, muscle, and dense connective tissues are barriers that slow but do not prevent the spread of a tumor. Normal fibrinolytic and proteolytic enzymes may enhance tumor invasion by modifying or destroying surrounding host tissue.

Metastasis is the spread of cancer cells from a primary site of origin to a distant site. This process is the life-threatening characteristic of cancer, because removal of the primary tumor does not affect growth at other sites, and the primary tumor may not be diagnosed before metastasis has occurred. Some tumors can grow in any organ, whereas others have preferred sites of growth. For example, cancers of the prostate, breast, thyroid, and kidney metastasize and grow in bone. Metastases occur frequently in the lungs, bone, brain, and liver (Figure 1-14).

Distant spread of cancer involves invasion and penetration of tumor cells into blood vessels or lymphatics or both. Lymphatics and thin-walled venules offer relatively little mechanical resistance to penetration by tumor cells. Blood vessels within tumors offer malignant cells direct access to the circulation. Clumps of malignant cells that arise close to a serous surface can penetrate that surface, implant, and become distant metastases (Figure 1-15).

Tumor cells can invade and implant themselves in surrounding proximal serous cavities, as evidenced by cancers of the ovary that spread to the peritoneal surface. Once tumors reach serous cavities (e.g., pleural and peritoneal cavities), loose tumor cells are free to implant themselves anywhere in that cavity. These effusions, also known as seeding, occur in the pleural space surrounding the lung and in the peritoneal space surrounding the abdominal cavity. Implantation is also known to occur from the circulating blood because of surgical procedures; therefore unnecessary diagnostic procedures and surgical manipulation should be avoided.

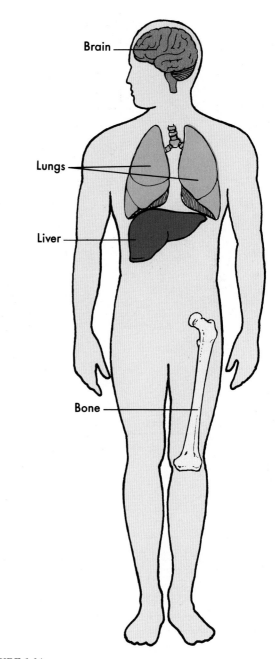

FIGURE 1-14
Common sites for metastasis: brain, liver, lungs, and bone.

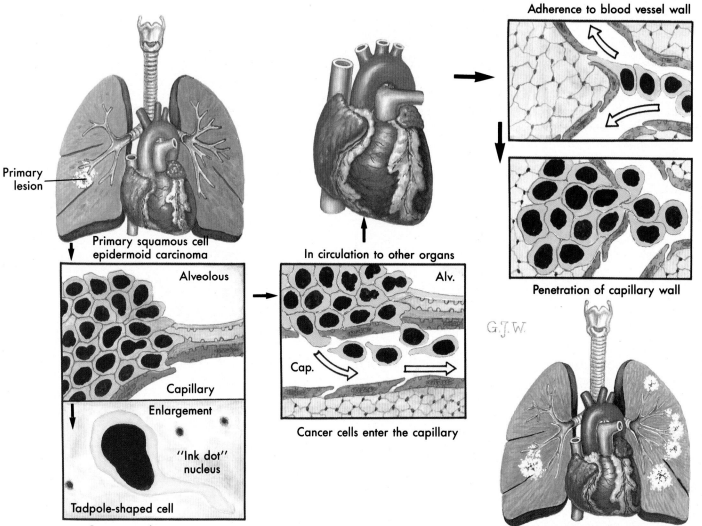

Adherence to blood vessel wall

Penetration of capillary wall

Metastases in other lung

Primary lesion

Primary squamous cell epidermoid carcinoma

Alveolous

Capillary

Enlargement

"Ink dot" nucleus

Tadpole-shaped cell

Common in lung carcinoma

In circulation to other organs

Cancer cells enter the capillary

Alv.

Cap.

FIGURE 1-15
Metastasis of cancer.

DIFFERENCES BETWEEN BENIGN AND MALIGNANT TUMORS

Characteristic	Benign tumor	Malignant tumor
Structure and differentiation	Typical of tissue origin	Atypical of tissue origin
Rate of growth	Usually slow	May be slow, rapid, or very rapid
Progression	Slowly progressive (may remain stationary; may regress); rarely fatal if treated	Usually progressive; almost always fatal if untreated
Mode of growth	Expansion (encapsulated)	Infiltration and/or metastasis
Tissue destruction	No	Common (ulceration and necrosis)
Recurrence	Rare	Common
Prognosis	May be fatal if inaccessible	Fatal if uncontrolled

Modified from Mettlin C and Dodd G: American Cancer Society guidelines for cancer-related check-ups: an update, *CA* 41(5):281, 1991.

TYPES OF CANCER

Malignant tumors can be classified according to the tissue of origin (see box), as determined by examination of specimens under a microscope. Using this system, neoplasms can be described as carcinomas (cancers of epithelial cells), sarcomas (cancers of bone, muscle, or connective tissue), leukemias (cancers of blood-forming organs), or lymphomas (cancers of infection-fighting organs).

CLASSIFICATION OF NEOPLASMS

Tissue of origin	Benign	Malignant
Connective tissues		Sarcoma
Embryonic fibrous tissue	Myxoma	Myxosarcoma
Fibrous tissue	Fibroma	Fibrosarcoma
Adipose tissue	Lipoma	Liposarcoma
Cartilage	Chondroma	Chondrosarcoma
Bone	Osteoma	Osteogenic sarcoma
Epithelium		Carcinoma
Skin and mucous membrane	Papilloma	Squamous cell carcinoma
Glands	Polyp	Basal cell carcinoma
		Transitional cell carcinoma
	Adenoma	Adenocarcinoma
	Cystadenoma	
Pigmented cells (melanoblasts)	Nevus	Malignant melanoma
Endothelium		Endothelioma
Blood vessels	Hemangioma	Hemangioendothelioma
		Hemangiosarcoma
Lymph vessels	Lymphangioma	Lymphangiosarcoma
		Lymphangioendothelioma
Bone marrow		Multiple myeloma
		Ewing's sarcoma
		Leukemia
Lymphoid tissue		Malignant lymphoma
		Lymphosarcoma
		Reticulum cell sarcoma
		Lymphatic leukemia
Muscle tissue		
Smooth muscle	Leiomyoma	Leiomyosarcoma
Striated muscle	Rhabdomyoma	Rhabdomyosarcoma
Nerve tissue		
Nerve fibers and sheaths	Neuroma	Neurogenic sarcoma
	Neurinoma	
	(Neurilemoma)	
	Neurofibroma	(Neurofibrosarcoma)
Ganglion cells	Ganglioneuroma	Neuroblastoma
Glia cells	Glioma	Glioblastoma
		Spongioblastoma
Meninges	Meningioma	Malignant meningioma
Gonads	Dermoid cyst	Embryonal carcinoma
		Embryonal sarcoma
		Teratocarcinoma

From Luckmann J and Sorensen KC.: Medical-surgical nursing: a psychophysiologic approach, ed 3, Philadelphia, 1987, WB Saunders.

CHAPTER 2

Assessment

Cancer nursing assessment involves careful, systematic evaluation of a person's medical, family, social, cultural, psychologic, and occupational history and a systematic physical examination.

The patient and nurse should be relaxed to help ensure a more comprehensive assessment. Technical terms should be avoided, and language should be matched to the person's age, ethnicity, and life experiences. The purposes of the assessment process are to determine the person's current complaint, health status, life-style, and family health history; to discover elements in the person's history that relate to the current problem and the risk of developing cancer; and to allow the nurse to observe the person for clues to the person's health and emotional status. The assessment interview provides an opportunity for the nurse to establish a rapport with the person. By demonstrating interest and concern, the nurse can elicit valuable information that will be useful in the evaluation of risk and symptoms.

Awareness of nonverbal communication during the interview increases the nurse's understanding of the person. Facial expression, body position, and tone of voice can provide important assessment clues. Responses to questions are recorded in the person's own words.

The person's chief complaint is best elicited by asking, "What has brought you here?" or "What is bothering you?" The nurse determines when the person first began having symptoms. The nature of the complaint directs the line of questioning. Complete information should be obtained through specific questions about the following: the location, radiation, quality, and quantity (severity, duration) of the symptom or symptoms; precipitating or aggravating factors; relieving factors; associated findings; and treatments sought.

A person's response to stress and a person's coping methods sometimes are difficult to assess directly in the initial interview, but this information is important. Direct questioning about recent stress and major life changes often can elicit pertinent information about the individual's coping abilities and symptoms. However, the nurse should never assume that a major life change was stressful for a person simply because it *sounds* stressful. Similarly, an event that seems minor may be interpreted as extremely stressful by the individual.

General information

Name, age, gender, ethnicity, date and place of birth, marital status

Presenting complaint

Severity: location, quality, and quantity
Temporality: onset, duration, frequency, precipitators
Alleviating or aggravating factors
What the person thinks may be happening

Concurrent disorders

Cardiac disease, pulmonary disease, diabetes, obesity, renal disease, and so on

Previous state of health

Infancy and childhood
Previous disorders
Injuries
Hospitalizations and surgeries

Allergies

Present state of health and life-style

Prescription and over-the-counter medication pattern
Diet and fluid intake
Oral hygiene and dental status
Sleep patterns
Elimination patterns
Educational level
Occupation, including exposure to carcinogens
Cultural and religious or spiritual values
Economic resources, including health insurance
Life-style, including exercise, consumption of caffeine, alcohol ingestion, use of tobacco products, sexual practices, exposure to sun, self-examination practices

Family medical history

Age and state of health of family members, including grandparents, parents, siblings, children; if one of these is deceased, specify cause of death; if one has been diagnosed as having cancer, specify site and outcome

General review of systems

Weight—present weight, usual weight
Performance status—present level of activity, usual level of activity, fatigue, weakness
Skin and mucous membranes—color, integrity, turgor, color of nail beds; presence of edema, slow-growing lesions, new moles, changes in old moles, scaly patches, clubbing
Head and neck—difficulty chewing, dysphagia, local pain or tenderness, swelling, hoarseness, nasal discharge, asymmetry, adenopathy
Respiratory tract—new or persistent productive or nonproductive cough, hemoptysis, chest wall pain, dyspnea with or without exertion
Cardiovascular function—hypertension, dyspnea, orthopnea, chest pain; pain, redness, swelling in extremities
Gastrointestinal function—anorexia, early satiety, abdominal pain or bloating, nausea, vomiting, hematemesis, change in bowel pattern, melena, tenesmus, date and result of Hemoccult stool test
Urinary tract and bladder—frequency, hesitancy, urgency, dysuria, hematuria, pelvic or flank pain or mass
Gynecologic system—vaginal discharge, abnormal vaginal bleeding, lesions, pelvic pain, abdominal enlargement, date and result of Pap test, pattern of menses
Breasts—lumps, discharge, tenderness, skin changes, axillary swelling, gynecomastia (male), date and result of mammogram
Male genitalia—enlargement of testis, pain, one or more external lesions, date of most recent digital rectal examination of prostate
Musculoskeletal system—swelling, pain, stiffness, redness, limitation of movement
Neurologic function—headache, convulsions, visual disturbances, syncope, vertigo, sensory deficits
Endocrine system—sweating, tachycardia, palpitations, flushing; menstrual irregularities
Hematologic system—fever, sweating, painless lymphadenopathy, pruritus, bruising, anemia, petechia, purpura

PHYSICAL EXAMINATION

The physical examination for a person in whom cancer is suspected should include all body systems, with an emphasis on identifying deviations from normal structure and function. These areas should be further assessed with specific diagnostic procedures. Because cancer may have metastasized by the time the person seeks treatment for a chief complaint, it is important to include common sites of spread in the initial examination.

> Cancer risk assessment may or may not include a physical examination. In many cases the risk assessment is conducted in an occupational setting as an interview, and the person identified as being at risk for one or more cancers is referred to a physician or nurse for further evaluation.

SKIN

Inspection and assessment of color, warmth, moisture, integrity, turgor
Lesions—type, size, location, distribution (Figure 2-1)
   Moles—change in color, size, shape, or sensation; presence of bleeding; inspection of soles of feet, axillae, scalp, interdigital webs, mucous membranes, nail beds; also face, neck, trunk, and extremities
   Purpura—petechia or ecchymosis
   Scaly patches or plaques
   Ulcerative or exophytic areas
   Edema
Nails—color, clubbing (Figure 2-2)

HEAD AND NECK

Inspection
   Face—note asymmetry at rest or with movement
   Eyes—note abnormal protrusion (unilateral or bilateral), scleral jaundice, lumps, or swelling around eyes
   Oral cavity—erythroplasia or leukoplakia (Figure 2-3)
   Trachea—note deviation from midline; rise of larynx, trachea, and thyroid with swallowing (Figure 2-4)
Palpation—tenderness, masses, nodules, enlargement
   Frontal and maxillary sinuses
   Nodes—presence of small, mobile, nontender nodes is common; if node or nodes are enlarged, firm, or fixed, further examination is needed (Figure 2-5)
   Thyroid (Figure 2-6)
Digital examination of oral cavity and tongue

THORAX

Inspection—rate and rhythm of breathing, movement of chest, asymmetry
Palpation—tenderness, masses, cutaneous nodules, enlargements of mediastinum, supraclavicular and infraclavicular nodes
Percussion—note presence and location of abnormal findings such as hyperresonance, dullness
Auscultation—pitch, intensity, duration; if alterations are heard, listen to spoken voice (Figure 2-7)

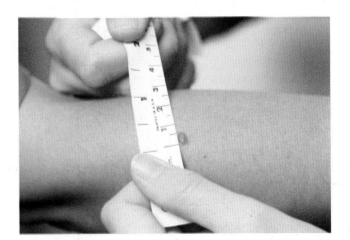

FIGURE 2-1
Measuring a skin lesion with a centimeter ruler.

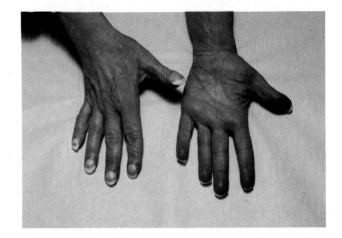

FIGURE 2-2
Severe clubbing. (From Canobbio.[11])

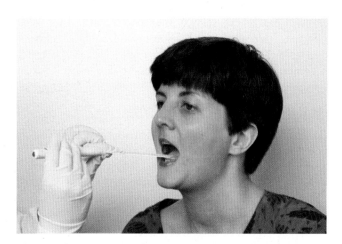

FIGURE 2-3
Examination of the oral cavity.

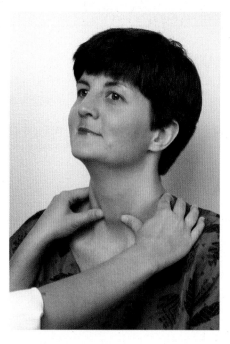

FIGURE 2-4
Evaluation of midline position of trachea.

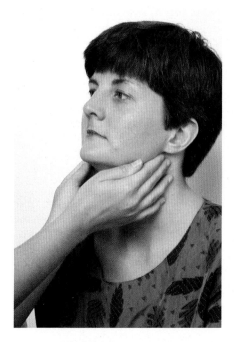

FIGURE 2-5
Palpation of cervical lymph nodes.

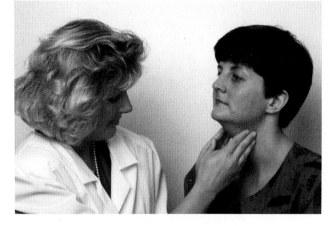

FIGURE 2-6
Palpation of thyroid.

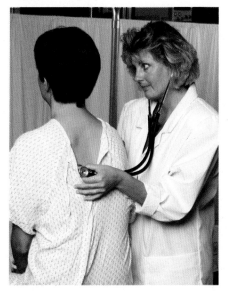

FIGURE 2-7
Auscultation of lungs.

BREASTS AND AXILLAE

Inspection—look for dimpling, peau d'orange, edema; nipple retraction, inversion, asymmetry, bleeding or other discharge; venous prominence

Palpation—thickening or lump in breast; determine size, shape, mobility; check axillary lymph nodes for evidence of swelling (Figure 2-8)

CARDIOVASCULAR

Inspection of anterior chest for thrills and heaves

Auscultation of apical rate and rhythm; note presence of abnormal sounds, murmurs

Arterial palpation—rate, rhythm, intensity; carotid, brachial, femoral, dorsalis pedis

ABDOMEN

Inspection—note dilated veins, asymmetry, organ enlargement, masses, ascitic fluid

Auscultation—presence or absence of bowel sounds, presence of bruits or hepatic or splenic friction rubs

Percussion of liver, spleen—note area of dullness

Palpation—tenderness, masses, borders, contour, size, and consistency of liver, spleen, kidneys, inguinal nodes (Figures 2-9 and 2-10)

BLADDER, KIDNEYS, URETERS, RENAL PELVIS

Inspection—note abdominal or flank asymmetry or masses; presence of lower extremity edema or edema of genitals

Palpation—tenderness, masses, consistency, contour, shape of pelvis and abdomen, flank area

FEMALE GENITALIA AND RECTUM

Inspection—note abnormal hair distribution, masses or asymmetry, lesions

Palpation—tenderness, masses, shape, consistency, fluid over ovaries, uterus, lower abdominal region (Figure 2-11)

Pelvic and rectal exam—mucosal integrity and color, lesions, bleeding or discharge, constriction, masses, nodules, extent of tumor if present; includes external genitalia, vagina, cervix, uterus and ovaries, rectum (masses, constriction, tenderness) (Figure 2-12)

MALE GENITALIA AND RECTUM

Inspection—abnormal hair distribution, masses or asymmetry, lesions, cutaneous nodules

Palpation—tenderness, masses, consistency, contour, shape of scrotum, scrotal contents, inguinal lymph nodes, supraclavicular lymph nodes, breasts (presence of gynecomastia) (Figure 2-13)

Digital rectal examination of prostate (masses, tenderness, firmness, size, contour), rectum (masses, constriction, tenderness) (Figure 2-14)

MUSCULOSKELETAL

Inspection—note skeletal or soft tissue swelling, masses, visible bone enlargement, lower extremity edema, proptosis

Palpation—tenderness, masses

Range of motion (Figure 2-15)

NEUROLOGIC

Note any of these signs or symptoms—headache, convulsions, intermittent dizziness, papilledema, lateralized sensory deficits, paresthesia, ataxia, altered reflexes, sudden sensory or motor loss, or personality changes (Figures 2-16 and 2-17)

HEMATOLOGIC

Inspection—note pallor, petechiae, purpura, cranial nerve dysfunction, gingival enlargement, hepatomegaly, splenomegaly, or lymphadenopathy

Palpation—tenderness, masses, enlargement of sternum, liver and spleen, nodes

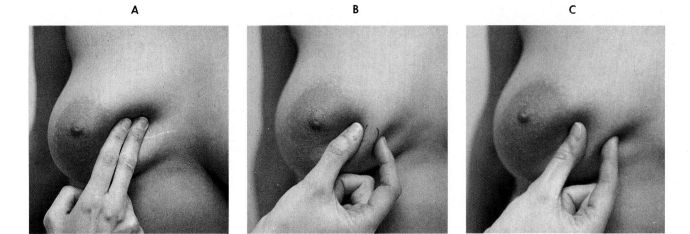

FIGURE 2-8
A, Palpating for consistency of a breast lesion. **B,** Palpating for delineation of borders of breast mass. **C,** Palpating for mobility of breast mass. (From Seidel et al.[53])

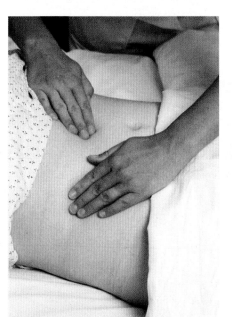

FIGURE 2-9
Palpation of liver.

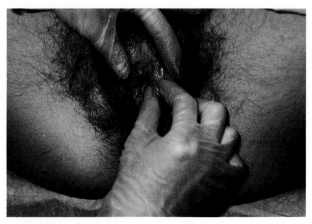

FIGURE 2-10
Palpation of superior superficial inguinal lymph nodes. (From Seidel et al.[53])

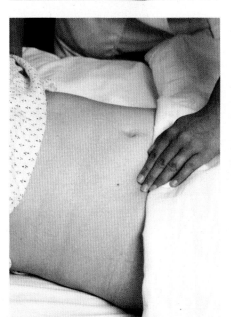

FIGURE 2-11
Palpation of ovaries.

FIGURE 2-12
Palpating the labia as part of pelvic examination. (From Seidel et al.[53])

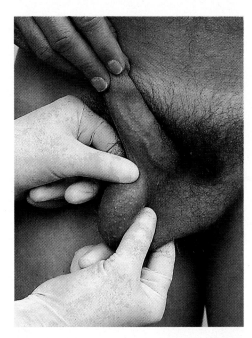

FIGURE 2-13
Palpating contents of the scrotal sac. (From Seidel et al.[53])

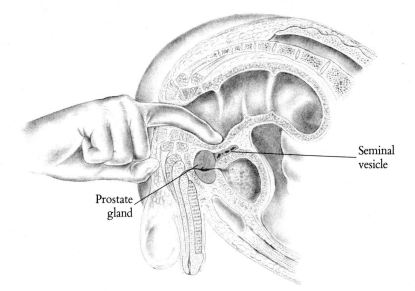

Seminal vesicle

Prostate gland

FIGURE 2-14
Palpation of the anterior surface of the prostate gland. (From Seidel et al.[53])

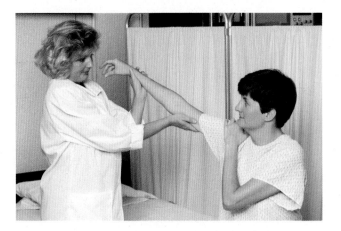

FIGURE 2-15
Examination of range of motion of the upper extremity.

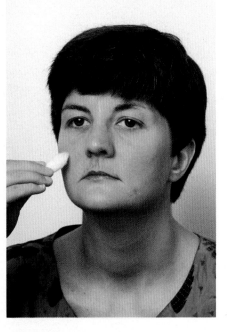

FIGURE 2-16
Examination of sensory function.

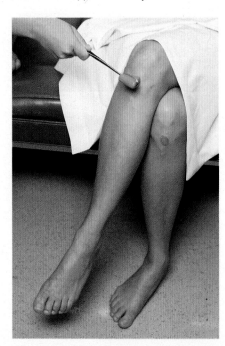

FIGURE 2-17
Examination of patellar reflex.

EARLY DETECTION OF CANCER

The earlier cancer is detected, the more likely it is to be cured. Early detection techniques, which enable health care providers to screen for and diagnose cancer while it is localized and potentially curable, include the Papanicolaou (Pap) test and pelvic examination, endometrial tissue sample, clinical breast examination, mammography, digital rectal examination, and stool blood test and sigmoidoscopy (see Diagnostic Procedures). Techniques that individuals can be taught for early detection include breast, testicular, skin, and vulvar self-examinations (see Patient Teaching Guides).

The American Cancer Society has issued recommendations for early detection of cancer in asymptomatic individuals at average risk (Table 2-1). The nurse should share these guidelines with all clients and patients, with particular focus on individuals whose lifestyle, occupation, medical history, or family history increases their risk of developing cancer.

Table 2-1

SUMMARY OF AMERICAN CANCER SOCIETY RECOMMENDATIONS FOR EARLY DETECTION OF CANCER IN ASYMPTOMATIC PEOPLE AT AVERAGE RISK

Examination	Sex	Age	Periodicity
Sigmoidoscopy	M and F	Age 50 and older	1 examination every 3 to 5 years
Stool blood test	M and F	Age 50 and older	Every year
Digital rectal examination	M and F	Age 40 and older	Every year
Pap test and pelvic examination	F	Women who have been sexually active or have reached age 18 or older	Every year. After 3 or more satisfactory, consecutive, normal annual examinations, the Pap test may be performed less frequently at the discretion of the physician
Endometrial tissue sample	F	At menopause; women at high risk*	At menopause
Breast self-examination*	F	Age 20 and older	Every month
Clinical breast examination	F	20-39	Every 3 years
		Age 40 and older	Every year
Mammography	F	35-39	Baseline
		40-49	Every 1 to 2 years
		50 and over	Every year
Health counseling†	M and F	20-40	Every 3 years
Cancer checkup‡	M and F	Age 40 and older	Every year

From American Cancer Society.[1]
*History of infertility, obesity, failure to ovulate, abnormal uterine bleeding, or estrogen therapy.
†To include counseling about tobacco control, sun exposure, diet and nutrition, risk factors, sexual practices, and environmental and other occupational exposures.
‡To include examination for cancers of the thyroid, testicles, prostate, ovaries, lymph nodes, oral cavity, and skin.

CANCER DETECTION IN THE ELDERLY

Special attention must be given to cancer detection in the elderly, because cancer is increasingly a disease of old age. There are two theories as to why, in general, the incidence of cancer increases as a person ages: first, the elderly may be less resistant to carcinogenesis, particularly with decreased immunologic function; second, the elderly have a greater number of cells that already have been transformed by initiating factors and that are now being exposed to promoting factors.

Several myths held by the public and by some health care providers serve as obstacles to early detection of cancer in the elderly. These myths include the following:

1. Many elderly people are senile or demented and thus cannot give a reliable history.
2. Many elderly people are unhealthy and cannot care for themselves without assistance.
3. Elderly people have undergone an aging process that is inevitable and that results in general physical deterioration.

Actually, most elderly people are not mentally disturbed, are healthy enough to carry on their normal life-styles, and have varying rates of declining organ and system function. However, there are other barriers to early detection of cancer in the elderly, some of which they themselves create. These barriers include:

1. Taking their aches and pains for granted
2. Regarding ill health and disability as inevitable
3. Having fewer relatives and friends to use as a lay referral system
4. Being without accurate health information or access to it
5. Being unable or reluctant to work outside the home, which decreases stimulation, incentives to stay well, and income to support health care expenses
6. Having negative and often fatalistic attitudes about cancer and its treatment

Nurses must help both the elderly and other health care providers avoid the error of assuming that a symptom or change in functional status reflects the aging process rather than a specific disease. Elderly individuals should be taught to do self-assessment, to follow the American Cancer Society's guidelines for screening examinations, and to seek medical evaluation of symptoms, whatever their nature and probable cause.

CHAPTER 3

Diagnostic Procedures

X-RAY EXAMINATION

X-rays (or radiographs or roentgenograms) are a noninvasive tool used to diagnose tumors, metastasis, or abnormal growth in suspected cancer conditions. Radiation is passed through the body, providing images of tissue and bone structure and function (Figure 3-1). X-rays show density changes, irregularities in contour, erosion of surfaces, changes in normal bone or tissue shapes, tumors, and fluid in cavities that should be fluid free.

INDICATIONS

To diagnose:
 Primary and metastatic tumors
 Myxomas
 Soft tissue sarcoma
 Osteogenic sarcoma

CONTRAINDICATIONS

Pregnancy

NURSING CARE

Have the patient remove his clothing when necessary and all metallic objects and jewelry. Provide a gown, if needed, and provide premenopausal women with a metal apron, if there is a chance of pregnancy, to prevent fetal x-ray exposure. A lead shield should protect the reproductive organs in both sexes to prevent radiation-induced abnormalities that may cause congenital deformities in future children. Help the patient into the appropriate position, and instruct him to hold his breath and remain still.

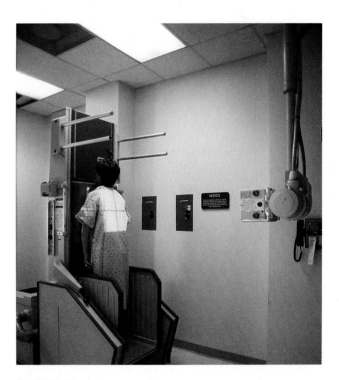

FIGURE 3-1
Patient positioned for chest x-ray. (From Wilson and Thompson.[63])

PATIENT TEACHING

Explain the procedure and its purpose, and stress the need to remain still during the test. Also explain any intake restrictions, and tell the patient how long the test will take. Advise him that this is a relatively painless examination.

MAMMOGRAPHY

Film mammography and xeromammography produce image contrasts with the sensitivity and specificity needed to detect small invasive and even noninvasive breast tumors (Figure 3-2). With both techniques the patient's exposure to radiation has been considerably reduced, and the overall image quality (and thus the screening and diagnostic value) has significantly improved.

INDICATIONS

To diagnose:

Breast cancer	Gross cysts
Suppurative mastitis	Benign tumors
Breast abscess	Intraglandular lymph nodes
Fibrocystic changes	

CONTRAINDICATIONS

Pregnancy

NURSING CARE

Explain the procedure, and tell the patient she may feel some discomfort when her breast is compressed. Reassure her that compression does not harm the breast and that a minimal dose of radiation is used dur-

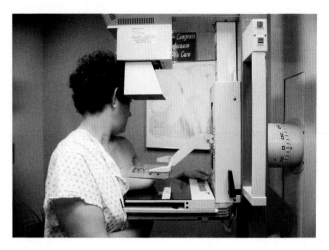

FIGURE 3-2
Clinical setting for mammography.

ing the test. Instruct her to disrobe above the waist and to put on an x-ray gown.

PATIENT TEACHING

In addition to explaining the procedure and the possibility of discomfort, teach the patient how to perform breast self-examination.

LYMPHANGIOGRAPHY

Lymphangiography is an x-ray examination of the lymphatic system that involves injecting a contrast medium into a lymphatic vessel of the hand or foot. An examination of this system is crucial to the monitoring of many cancers, because the disease often spreads by means of the lymphatic system.

INDICATIONS

To diagnose:

Lymphoma	Metastatic lymphatic tumor

To evaluate:

Level of lymphatic metastasis	Staging of lymphoma
Results of chemotherapy or radiation therapy	

CONTRAINDICATIONS

Allergy to iodine dye or shellfish	Cardiac disease
Severe chronic lung disease	Liver disease
Advanced kidney disease	

NURSING CARE

Explain the procedure, and obtain informed consent if required. No fasting or sedation is required. Assess for and inform the radiologist of any allergy to iodinated contrast material. After the procedure, observe the injection and incision sites for cellulitis.

PATIENT TEACHING

Explain that the procedure, performed by a radiologist, takes approximately 3 hours, with additional films sometimes taken 24 to 48 hours later. Apprise the patient that his urine may have a blue tint if blue dye is used. (Excessive use of the dye may give the entire skin surface a temporary blue tint.) Explain that the patient may feel discomfort from the subcutaneous injection and when the hand or foot is locally anesthetized prior to surgical incision of the lymphatic channels for insertion of catheters through which dye is injected. After the procedure, if the patient is returning home, tell him to check the site for redness, pain, and swelling. The sutures should be removed 7 to 10 days after the test.

MAGNETIC RESONANCE IMAGING (MRI)

Magnetic resonance imaging (MRI) provides multiplane, cross-sectional imaging based on the magnetism inherent in certain nuclei in the human body and its interaction with radiowaves (Figure 3-3). A huge electromagnet is used to detect hidden tumors by mapping the vibrations of the various atoms in the body on a computer screen. MRI has some advantages over CT scanning: the patient is not exposed to ionizing radiation; cross-sectional views can be obtained in any plane, not just axially; MRI does not "see bone"; and various types of pathologic tissue can be recognized.

INDICATIONS

To detect primary and metastatic tumors in the following areas:
  Head, face, and surrounding structures
  Spine and surrounding structures
  Neck
  Mediastinum
  Heart and great vessels
  Liver
  Kidneys
  Prostate
  Bone and joints
  Breasts
  Extremities and soft tissue

CONTRAINDICATIONS

Obesity (>300 pounds)
Pregnancy
Confusion, agitation
Claustrophobia
Unstable conditions requiring continuous life support
Implanted metal objects or fragments

NURSING CARE

Explain the procedure, and obtain informed consent if required. Assess the patient for contraindications (see above). Antianxiety agents may help those with mild claustrophobia. Stress the need for patient compliance (i.e., remaining still) during the entire procedure. Ask the patient to remove all metal objects and to empty his bladder before the test.

PATIENT TEACHING

In addition to explaining the procedure, inform the patient that there is no exposure to radiation with MRI; parents may remain with a child in the scanning room during the procedure. Also, a patient can drive without

---

| **TUMOR IMAGING** |

The current roles of tumor imaging are to define the extent of disease (tumor staging) and to assess the patient's progress during and after treatment. Currently imaging techniques are not widely used for screening and early detection because of questions about their sensitivity and specificity, as well as the cost. The one exception to these limitations is mammography for breast cancer screening.

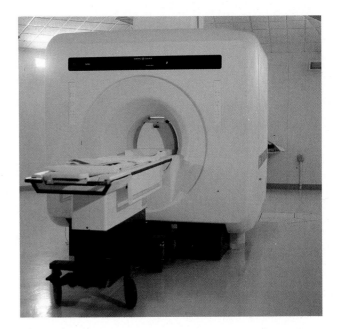

FIGURE 3-3
Magnetic resonance imaging equipment. (From Mourad.[46])

---

assistance after the procedure. The only discomfort he may have may be from lying still on a hard surface or a possible tingling in metal teeth fillings. If possible, use a picture of the scanning machine to encourage the patient to talk about any anxieties he may have. The patient should be apprised that he may hear a thumping sound during the procedure. Tell the patient that the procedure is performed by a radiologic technologist and takes 30 to 90 minutes.

COMPUTED TOMOGRAPHY (CT)

Computed tomography (CT) produces cross-sectional views of soft tissue anatomy by passing several x-ray beams through the body at different angles and then restructuring the information in the shape of a picture, using a computer (Figures 3-4 and 3-5). CT can be done with or without a contrast agent. The technique is highly accurate in distinguishing between benign and malignant lesions. It frequently is used to evaluate the central nervous system, the head and neck, the lungs, and the abdomen. When CT is used with ultrasonography, the radiologist can determine the exact site (e.g., liver, pancreas, or gallbladder) and nature of the obstructing lesion. CT-guided percutaneous skinny-needle techniques (with or without injection of a contrast medium) can be used for aspiration biopsy to define pancreatic, hepatic, or renal tumors.

INDICATIONS

To diagnose:
Kidney tumor
Liver, pancreatic, or splenic tumor
Biliary or gallbladder tumor
Uterine or ovarian tumor
Prostate tumor
Retroperitoneal tumor
Lymphadenopathy
Pulmonary tumor
Granuloma
Esophageal tumor
Mediastinal tumor
Primary or metastatic chest wall tumor
Intracranial tumor
Hematoma
Meningioma
Adenoma
Carcinoma
Pheochromocytoma

CONTRAINDICATIONS

Allergy to iodinated dye or shellfish
Pregnancy
Unstable vital signs
Obesity (>300 pounds)
Claustrophobia

NURSING CARE

Explain the procedure and the importance of patient compliance. Obtain informed consent if required. Assess for allergies to contrast medium (iodinated dye or

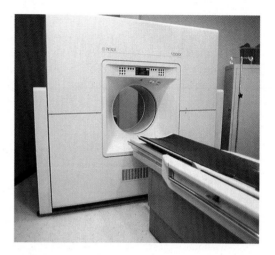

FIGURE 3-4
Clinical setting for computed tomography. (From Wilson and Thompson.[63])

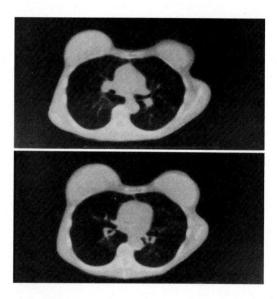

FIGURE 3-5
Transverse CT scan of female patient. Bilateral breast shadows, heart, pulmonary arteries, and main bronchi are visible. (From Thompson et al.[60])

shellfish); inform radiologist if an allergy is suspected. Inform the patient that wigs, hairpins or clips, and partial dental plates must be removed if the scan will include the head.

Keep the patient NPO for at least 4 hours before the oral contrast is administered, except in emergency situations. After the test, encourage the patient to drink fluids to avoid renal complications and to promote excretion of the dye.

PATIENT TEACHING

Use a picture of the CT machine to explain the procedure, and encourage the patient to express her concerns. Many claustrophobic patients can undergo the procedure if given an antianxiety agent beforehand.

Apprise the patient of the discomforts associated with an abdominal or kidney study (e.g., lying still on a hard surface, peripheral venipuncture, mild nausea). Some patients experience a salty taste, flushing, and warmth during injection of the dye. Inform the patient that the test is performed by a radiologist, usually in less than 30 minutes; if a contrast dye is used, the procedure may take about an hour. Patients receiving a CT scan of the brain may hear a clicking noise as the machine moves around the head.

COMPLICATIONS

Allergic reaction to iodinated dye (potentially life threatening)
Acute renal failure

ULTRASONOGRAPHY

Ultrasonography is an inexpensive, noninvasive technique that uses high-frequency sound waves to obtain a cross-sectional image, either through direct-contact scanning or through water bath techniques. It is highly accurate in distinguishing between cystic and solid masses but does not detect small, nonpalpable cancers; nor does it distinguish between benign and malignant solid tumors. Prostatic ultrasonography (using a rectal probe that produces ultrasonic waves to obtain an image of the prostate) is being studied as a screening tool for early detection of occult prostate cancer.

Since radiation is not used with ultrasonography, repeat studies and numerous images can be obtained over a brief period with little risk. In addition, because no radiation exposure is involved, this test can be done in a physician's office or clinic. Ultrasonography is used most often to assess the pelvis, abdomen, heart, and pregnant uterus.

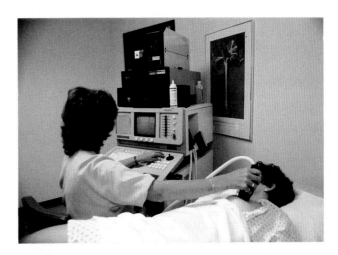

FIGURE 3-6
Ultrasonography of breast.

INDICATIONS

To diagnose or detect:
  Abdominal mass
  Primary and metastatic tumors

CONTRAINDICATIONS

Uncooperative patient

NURSING CARE

Consent forms may be required. The patient undergoing a pelvic sonogram must have a full bladder, whereas the patient undergoing a gallbladder examination must be kept NPO before the procedure. A greasy paste is applied to the skin above the area being examined to enhance sound transmission. No other special nursing measures are needed.

PATIENT TEACHING

Explain the procedure, and reassure the patient that ultrasonography is painless, noninvasive, and does not involve any radiation.

BONE SCANNING

Bone scanning involves several steps. First, a radioactive material is injected into a vein in the arm. The patient then is encouraged to drink water over the next 1 to 3 hours to aid renal clearance of any radioisotope not picked up by the bone. After the patient has voided, a scanning camera reveals the degree of radionuclide uptake in the target area (Figure 3-7). Areas of concentrated nucleotide uptake may represent a tumor or other abnormality. These areas of concentration can be detected days or weeks before an ordinary x-ray can reveal a lesion.

INDICATIONS

To detect metastatic tumor; all malignancies capable of metastasis may reach the bone, especially those of the following:
    Breasts
    Kidneys
    Lungs
    Prostate
    Thyroid
    Urinary bladder

CONTRAINDICATIONS

Pregnancy
Lactation

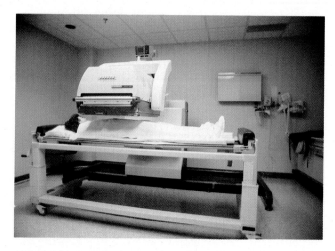

FIGURE 3-7
Patient positioned for bone scan. (From Mourad.[46])

NURSING CARE

Before the test the patient must remove all jewelry and metal objects. After the IV injection of the radioisotope, encourage the patient to drink several glasses of water to aid excretion of circulating radioisotope not picked up by the bone. The patient should void before scanning to clear the pelvic region of the tracer. Check the injection site for redness or swelling; apply warm soaks to relieve any pain.

PATIENT TEACHING

Explain the procedure, and assure the patient that the dose of radiation involved is less than the amount received from regular diagnostic x-rays. The radioactive substance will not affect other people and usually is excreted in the urine within 6 to 24 hours. Explain that the scanning machine itself does not *emit* radiation; rather, it detects radiation from the patient. Thus the scanning process does not cause radiation effects. Apprise the patient that the machine makes a clicking sound during scanning.

After the IV injection, tell the patient the exact time when the scanning will be done, and encourage her to drink water to aid renal clearance.

LUMBAR PUNCTURE/SPINAL TAP

A lumbar puncture and spinal tap allow the spinal fluid to be examined for diagnosis of brain or spinal cord malignancies. A needle is placed in the subarachnoid space of the spinal column to obtain the fluid (Figures 3-8 and 3-9). Pressure within the subarachnoid space can be measured by attaching a sterile manometer to the needle used in lumbar puncture. A pressure above 200 mm H_2O, an increase in the protein content, a decrease in the glucose level, or the presence of shed malignant cells may indicate the presence of a tumor.

INDICATIONS

To diagnose:
Brain or spinal cord tumor
Cerebral hemorrhage
Meningitis
Encephalitis
Degenerative brain disease
Autoimmune disorders of the central nervous system
Acute demyelinating polyneuropathy

CONTRAINDICATIONS

Uncooperative patient
Increased intracranial pressure
Severe degenerative spinal joint disease
Psychosomatic tendencies
Infection near the lumbar puncture site

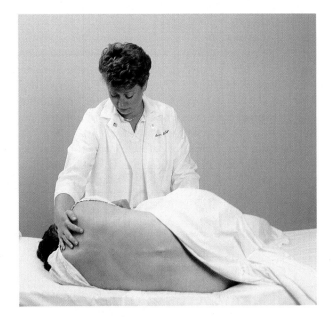

FIGURE 3-8
Patient positioned for lumbar puncture. (From Grimes.[24])

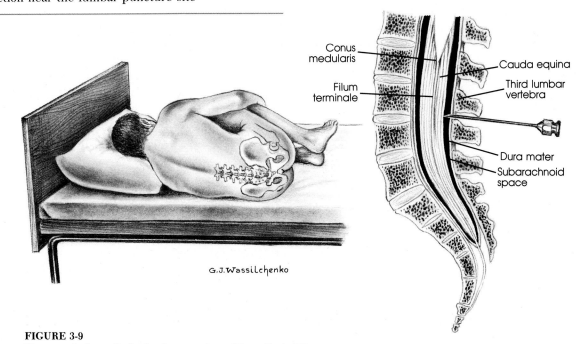

G.J.Wassilchenko

FIGURE 3-9
Placement of needle for lumbar puncture. (From Rudy EB: Advanced neurological and neurosurgical nursing, St Louis, 1984, Mosby–Year Book.)

NURSING CARE

To minimize anxiety and ensure cooperation, explain the procedure to the patient. Obtain written and informed consent. The patient should void both bladder and bowels before the procedure and must be told to lie very still throughout the procedure to avoid traumatic injury.

Help the patient assume the appropriate position (i.e., lying on one side with the head, neck, and knees flexed into the chest). A pillow between the patient's legs may prevent the upper leg from rolling forward. If necessary, help the physician hold the manometer straight. Specimens must be labeled, numbered, and delivered to the laboratory immediately.

After the procedure the patient must remain in bed with her head flat to minimize the risk of spinal fluid leakage, which can cause a severe headache. To keep her head flat, the patient should be encouraged to drink through a straw, although she may turn from side to side. Assess the patient for movement of extremities, pain at the injection site, drainage of blood or fluid at the injection site, and ability to urinate.

PATIENT TEACHING

Relieve the patient's fears by explaining the procedure and its aftermath. Because paralysis is a common fear, the patient should be assured that this procedure does not cause paralysis because the needle is inserted below the spinal cord.

Explain to the patient the importance of lying very still throughout the procedure to prevent traumatic injury. After the procedure, explain the need to keep the patient's head flat because of the risk of spinal headache, most likely caused by the loss of cerebrospinal fluid at the puncture site.

GASTRIC CYTOLOGY

Gastric cytology involves collecting shed tumor cells by aspiration for microscopic examination. The test's value depends on the cytologist's ability to read slides accurately; a negative cytologic report does not rule out malignancy but reinforces the assumption of benignancy. A positive report indicates malignancy.

Specimen cells can be obtained during gastroscopy or by insertion of a nasogastric tube, with instillation of approximately 100 ml of saline solution. The patient is turned 360 degrees several times while the fluid is aspirated, and then it is sent for analysis in a covered container. The fluid is centrifuged, and the precipitate containing the cells is smeared on a microscopic slide for evaluation by the cytologist.

INDICATIONS

To detect:
  Gastric malignancy

CONTRAINDICATIONS

Patients who cannot cooperate fully
Severe UGI bleeding
Esophageal diverticula

NURSING CARE

The patient must be kept NPO after midnight. Obtain written permission if required. Provide emotional support, explaining that discomfort may be felt with activation of the gag reflex.

The patient must remove dentures and eyeglasses before the test, and oral hygiene procedures should be performed both before and after the test. With gastroscopy, have an Ambu bag and physostigmine ready in case of respiratory arrest. Anesthetize the patient's throat with lidocaine; no eating or drinking will be allowed until the gag reflex returns (in about 2 to 4 hours).

After the procedure, administer cool fluids and gargles to relieve possible sore throat. Observe for bleeding, abdominal pain, fever, dyspnea, and dysphagia, and observe safety precautions until sedative effects have worn off.

PATIENT TEACHING

Explain the procedure, and identify the drugs that will be used and their effects. The patient should be told that although the procedure is not painful, discomfort and vomiting may occur when the gag reflex is initiated. Encourage the patient to talk about his fears, and provide appropriate support.

Before the test, explain to the patient that he will not be able to speak when the scope is in the GI tract. Explain that he may be hoarse and have a sore throat for several days after the procedure.

THORACENTESIS AND PLEURAL FLUID ANALYSIS (PLEURAL TAP)

A pleural tap is an invasive procedure that involves inserting a needle into the pleural space to remove fluid or air (Figure 3-10). No fasting or sedation is necessary, and a cough suppressant is given as needed before the procedure. The patient is placed in an upright position with the arms and shoulders raised and supported on a padded overbed table. The procedure is performed under strict sterile technique; the needle is positioned in the pleural space, and the fluid is withdrawn with a syringe and three-way stopcock. A spring or Kelly clamp may be placed on the needle at the chest wall to stabilize needle depth during fluid collection. Fluid may be aspirated through insertion of a short polyethylene catheter. After the procedure the needle is removed and the site bandaged. The patient is then turned onto her unaffected side for 1 hour.

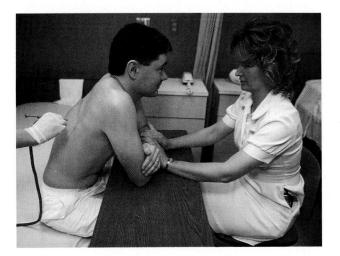

FIGURE 3-10
Patient positioned for thoracentesis. (From Wilson and Thompson.[63])

INDICATIONS

To relieve:
 Pain
 Dyspnea
 Symptoms of pleural pressure
To diagnose:
 Pleural effusion

CONTRAINDICATIONS

Uncooperative patient
Thrombocytopenia
Use of heparin or warfarin

NURSING CARE

Explain the procedure, and caution the patient that she must not move or cough during the test to prevent trauma. Give the patient a cough suppressant before the procedure if necessary. Obtain informed consent.

Make the patient's chest x-ray or ultrasound scan available before thoracentesis. Help position patient appropriately. During the test monitor the patient for reflex bradycardia, diaphoresis, and feeling of faintness. When labeling the specimen, be sure to record the exact location of the thoracentesis, the quantity of fluid obtained, and the gross appearance of the fluid, in addition to the patient's name, the date, the source of the fluid, and the diagnosis.

After the procedure obtain a chest x-ray to check for the complication of pneumothorax. Monitor vital signs as ordered, and observe for coughing or hemoptysis, signs of pneumothorax, tension pneumothorax, subcutaneous emphysema, pyogenic infection, and pulmonary edema or cardiac distress. Listen to the patient's lungs, and compare breath sounds to baseline breath sounds. If no signs of dyspnea appear, normal activity can be resumed 1 hour after the procedure.

PATIENT TEACHING

Explain the purpose of the procedure, and warn the patient that moving or coughing during the test may induce trauma. Apprise the patient of the possibility of diaphoresis and faintness.

PAPANICOLAOU (PAP) SMEAR

The Pap smear is used to detect neoplastic cell secretions taken from the cervix and vagina; the test can detect early cellular changes in premalignant or existing malignant conditions (Figure 3-11). It is 95% accurate in detecting cervical carcinoma and 40% accurate in detecting endometrial carcinoma.

A Pap smear should be part of the routine pelvic examination for women over 18 years of age. The American Cancer Society recommends that a Pap smear be performed annually for two negative examinations, then repeated every 3 years until age 65 in asymptomatic women. More frequent testing may be indicated for more susceptible patients.

INDICATIONS

To diagnose:
Cervical cancer
Endometrial cancer
Cervical intraepithelial neoplasia
Premalignant conditions

CONTRAINDICATIONS

Menses

NURSING CARE

The patient should not douche or take a tub bath for 24 hours before the examination and must empty her bladder just before the procedure.

Help the patient into the lithotomy position. After the physician obtains the specimen, it must be immediately applied to a clean slide and fixed before drying. Label the slide with the patient's name, age, and parity and the date of her last menstrual period. The patient's medication history and the reason for the examination should be written on the laboratory form.

PATIENT TEACHING

Explain the procedure, and instruct the patient not to douche or tub bathe for 24 hours before the test. Some physicians ask that the patient refrain from sexual intercourse for 24 to 48 hours before the smear. Explain that no discomfort is associated with this procedure except for insertion of the speculum.

CYTOLOGY

Exfoliative cytology has been used as both a screening and a diagnostic technique since the development of the Papanicolaou (Pap) smear. The method is based on the exfoliation (desquamation) of cells from the epithelium into the surrounding body fluid. The specimen obtained by aspiration or voiding is smeared onto a slide, stained, and examined under a microscope for histologic classification (see Grading, page 54). Target organs for cancer detection by cytologic technique include the female genital tract (uterine cervix, vagina, endometrium, ovaries, and fallopian tubes), the lower urinary tract (bladder, ureters, and renal pelvis), the respiratory tract (oral cavity, larynx, and bronchi), and the gastrointestinal tract (esophagus, stomach, and colon). The diagnostic advantage of this technique is that it is noninvasive (e.g., sputum or voided urine can be used for samples) or only minimally invasive, so it can be used for sampling at the time of esophagoscopy or gastroscopy or thin-needle aspiration biopsy (see Biopsy, page 43).

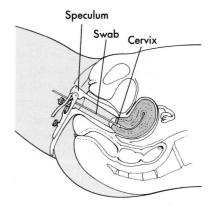

FIGURE 3-11
Obtaining cervical specimen. (From Grimes.[24])

SPUTUM STUDIES

Tumors in the pulmonary system frequently shed cells into the sputum. By examining sputum cultures, it is possible to diagnose a lung tumor. If no malignant cells are seen, either no cancer exists or the tumor is not sloughing cells. Thus, although a positive test result indicates malignancy, a negative result does not rule out cancer.

Sputum is collected as soon as the patient awakens in the morning, before he eats or drinks. Only sputum that has been coughed up from deep in the lungs should be collected. Other methods include endotracheal aspiration, transtracheal aspiration, and fiberoptic bronchoscopy.

INDICATIONS

To diagnose:
    Lung tumor

CONTRAINDICATIONS

None

NURSING CARE

Explain the procedure, stressing that sputum must be coughed up from the lungs (saliva is not sputum). List any drugs being taken on the laboratory slip; withhold antibiotics until after sputum has been obtained. The patient should be given the sterile container the night before so that the morning specimen can be obtained immediately. The patient should rinse his mouth with water before collection but should avoid oral hygiene products until after the specimen has been obtained. It may be wise to wrap the sputum container in paper so that the contents cannot be seen, for aesthetic reasons. Finally, the sample should be delivered to the laboratory as soon as possible after collection.

PATIENT TEACHING

While explaining the procedure, emphasize that the sputum must be coughed up from the lungs and that saliva is not sputum. Instruct the patient to rinse his mouth with water on arising but not to use toothpaste or mouthwash, since these may interfere with the viability of the microorganisms in the specimen. If an aerosol will be needed to stimulate coughing and expectoration, explain the purpose and procedure to the patient.

Instruct the patient to use the sterile container provided and to contact the nurse as soon as the specimen has been collected.

BRONCHOSCOPY

Bronchoscopy has a multitude of uses in diagnosing and treating disorders of the tracheobronchial tree. It allows direct inspection of the larynx, trachea, and bronchi to localize bleeding or tumors. Biopsies can be obtained, and secretions can be collected for cytologic or bacteriologic examination for culturing fungi, acid-fast bacilli, *Pneumocystis carinii*, and *Legionella pneumophila*. Bronchoscopy can also be used to remove foreign bodies and mucus plugs and to implant radioactive gold seeds for treating tumors.

The flexible fiberoptic bronchoscope is the instrument of choice in most cases because it is small and permits visualization of the segmental and subsegmental bronchi. Figure 3-12 illustrates both the instrument's structure and its application. The flexible fiberoptic bronchoscope has an external diameter between 3 and 6 mm and contains four channels: two light channels, one vision channel, and one open channel that accommodates biopsy forceps, cytology brush for obtaining samples, suction tube, lavage tube, anesthetic, or oxygen. With the aid of a fluoroscope, forceps and brushes can be advanced beyond the bronchoscope field of vision to obtain specimens. When alveolar tissue is obtained, this is termed a transbronchial biopsy.

The rigid bronchoscope is necessary to remove foreign bodies, excise endobronchial lesions, evaluate tracheal lesions, and control massive hemoptysis. The rigid bronchoscope is a hollow metallic tube with a light at its end.

General anesthesia is sometimes used. However, in most cases the patient is sedated and a local anesthetic is sprayed or swabbed over the mouth, tongue, and throat. An oxygen tube is inserted into one nostril and left in place throughout the procedure. Lidocaine jelly is generally used to both lubricate the bronchoscope and suppress the gag and cough reflexes. The bronchoscope is introduced through the nose or mouth, through the trachea, and into the mainstem bronchi.

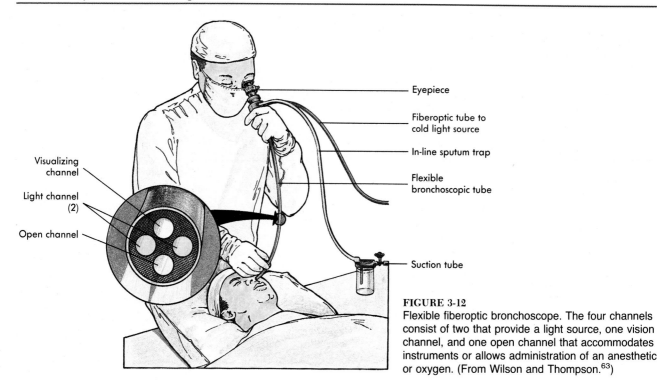

Eyepiece

Fiberoptic tube to
cold light source

In-line sputum trap

Flexible
bronchoscopic tube

Visualizing
channel

Light channel
(2)

Open channel

Suction tube

FIGURE 3-12
Flexible fiberoptic bronchoscope. The four channels
consist of two that provide a light source, one vision
channel, and one open channel that accommodates
instruments or allows administration of an anesthetic
or oxygen. (From Wilson and Thompson.[63])

Evaluation of distal lesions or transbronchial biopsy requires fluoroscopic guidance.

Just before the procedure the patient is given atropine to dry respiratory secretions. A narcotic for sedation and a sedative or tranquilizer (such as Valium) for muscle relaxation are also given.

Complications of bronchoscopy include bleeding, infection, and pneumothorax.

INDICATIONS

Severe or chronic lung infection	Foreign body
	Mucus plug
Lung tumor	Implant radioactive seeds
Hemoptysis	

CONTRAINDICATIONS

None

NURSING CARE

The patient should be kept NPO for 6 to 8 hours before the procedure. Remove any dental prosthesis and warn the physician about any loose teeth. Administer sedative as ordered.

After the procedure, the patient should be kept in a semi-Fowler's position, although he may be turned from side to side. Talking should be discouraged; in fact, temporary loss of voice is common. Provide the patient with pencil and paper to communicate. Oxygen may be ordered.

Fluids may be given after the gag and swallow reflexes return, usually about 2 hours after the procedure. Throat discomfort is to be expected. Warm drinks, warm saline gargles, and throat lozenges will help to ease the soreness. If swallowing is painful, a soft diet can be offered.

Assess breath sounds and respiratory rhythm and be alert for signs of pneumothorax. Subcutaneous emphysema, which presents as crepitus around the patient's neck and face, indicates a leak in the pleura. Laryngeal stridor and dyspnea suggest laryngeal edema or laryngospasm. Pink-tinged secretions after bronchoscopy are normal, but hemoptysis suggests hemorrhage. Vigorous coughing after a biopsy must be discouraged because it could dislodge a clot.

PATIENT TEACHING

Before bronchoscopy is performed, explain the purpose of the procedure. Assure the patient that he will be sedated to minimize the discomfort. Explain that he must breathe through the tube, which initially may produce a feeling of suffocation, but that he should try to relax and not fight against it. He will not be able to talk while the tube is in place. Bronchoscopy takes about 45 to 60 minutes. Results of most tests usually are available the following day, although the acid-fast bacilli test may take up to 6 weeks. Patients who are undergoing bronchoscopy to determine whether a malignancy is operable may need extra support.

PERITONEOSCOPY

The development and refinement of fiberoptic endoscopes have made it possible to inspect many internal organs and structures directly and to photograph, biopsy, and either excise lesions or assess their operability. One of endoscopy's primary uses is in a person known to have, suspected of having, or at risk for cancer.

Peritoneoscopy (insertion of one or two telescopes through the abdominal wall) can be used to evaluate patients with intraabdominal tumors who in the past required laparotomy (Figure 3-13). The specific uses for the procedure cited most often are detecting liver metastases, staging of lymphoma, and staging and follow-up of ovarian cancer.

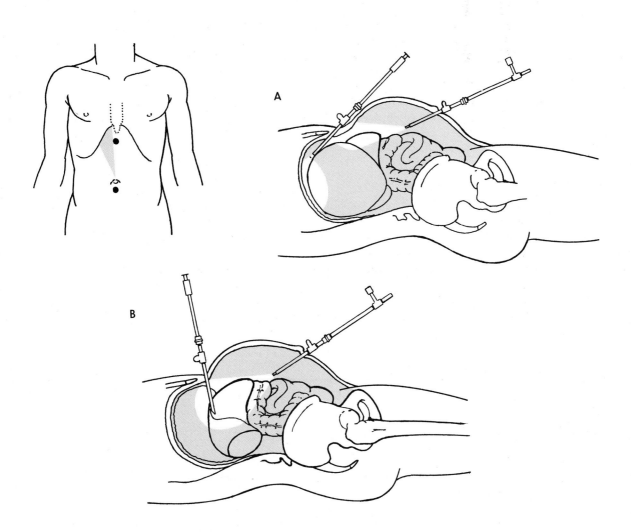

FIGURE 3-13

In double-puncture peritoneoscopy, an end-viewing telescope inserted below the umbilicus transilluminates the abdominal wall and monitors insertion of an oblique-viewing telescope. After both scopes have been used to search for metastases on the liver's superior surface **(A)**, the oblique scope is used to elevate the organ and the other is used to inspect its inferior surface **(B)**.

COLONOSCOPY

The colonoscope can be used not only to diagnose colon cancer and differentiate it from other colonic diseases but also for biopsies of cancers, polyps, and inflammatory bowel diseases and to remove polyps. Colonoscopy replaces the laparotomy and its surgical risks.

INDICATIONS

To diagnose:

Inflammatory bowel disease	Colon cancer
AV malformations	Colon polyps
Ischemic or postinflammatory strictures	Diverticulosis

CONTRAINDICATIONS

Uncooperative patient	Profuse rectal bleeding
Unstable medical condition	Suspected colon perforation

NURSING CARE

Explain the procedure and its associated risks (such as bleeding or perforation) before obtaining informed consent. Instruct the patient on bowel preparation to be done before the examination day, using either 2 days' administration of clear liquids and a strong cathartic or a 1-day preparation of ingestion of Colyte or other intestinal irritant, such as Dulcolax tablets.

On the examination day the patient is given an enema if Colyte was not taken or was ineffective. Avoid using oral bowel preparations in patients with UGI obstructions, suspected acute diverticulitis, or recent bowel resection. Administer preendoscopic sedation and atropine, if prescribed, to minimize secretions.

Establish IV access, and help the patient into the lateral decubitus position for the physician's examination. After the test examine the abdomen for evidence of colon perforation (abdominal distention and tenderness). Assess vital signs, particularly for signs of hemorrhage (decreased blood pressure and increased pulse), and inspect stools for gross blood. Notify the physician of increased pain or significant GI bleeding. If there is no evidence of bowel perforation, allow the patient to eat when she is fully alert and to drink plenty of fluids to prevent or recover from dehydration.

PATIENT TEACHING

Explain the procedure and its risks. Instruct the patient in bowel preparation to be implemented during the 1 to 2 days leading up to the procedure (see above). Assure the patient that she will be appropriately draped during the procedure and that minimal discomfort is associated with the test.

After the test explain to the patient that because air has been introduced into the bowel, she may have flatulence or gas pains. Instruct her to notify the nurse if the pain increases rather than decreases as she recovers from the procedure.

SIGMOIDOSCOPY

Sigmoidoscopy is endoscopy of the lower GI tract (anus, rectum, and sigmoid colon), allowing visualization and removal of biopsy specimens. Because radiographic visualization of the lower GI tract is difficult, direct visualization through sigmoidoscopy is invaluable in diagnosing many lower bowel disorders.

After digital examination and dilation of the anal sphincter, the sigmoidoscope is passed into the rectum and into the sigmoid colon to a distance of about 25 cm. Air insufflation distends the bowel for better visualization. Small amounts of mucus and stool may be removed.

INDICATIONS

To diagnose:
  Tumor
  Polyps
  Ulcerations

CONTRAINDICATIONS

Uncooperative patient
Painful anorectal conditions
Severe rectal bleeding

NURSING CARE

Explain the procedure and associated discomfort; obtain the patient's written consent. Allow him to eat a light breakfast on the morning of the examination, and help with enemas ordered before the test. Drape the patient with sensitivity to potential exposure or embarrassment. After the study, observe for fever, abdominal distention, bleeding, and unusual complaints of pain. Slight rectal bleeding may follow specimen biopsy.

PATIENT TEACHING

Explain the procedure, apprising the patient of the discomfort and the urge to defecate as the sigmoidoscope is passed. Encourage the patient to talk about his fears, and provide emotional support. Assure the patient that he will be properly draped to avoid unnecessary exposure during the procedure. Explain that because of the insufflation of air into the bowel during the procedure, he may have abdominal discomfort.

UPPER GASTROINTESTINAL ENDOSCOPY

Upper GI endoscopy allows direct visualization of the upper GI tract (esophagus, stomach, duodenum) with a flexible fiberoptic scope. The endoscope also can be used to remove polyps and coagulate sources of active GI bleeding and for follow-up after gastric surgery for other conditions. Areas of narrowing can be dilated, and photography equipment can be attached to the viewing lens to record existing conditions. By using a longer scope, the upper small intestine can also be evaluated. Endoscopic retrograde cholangiopancreatography (ERCP) is particularly useful in diagnosing the patient with jaundice.

INDICATIONS

To investigate:
Unexplained dysphagia and weight loss (especially with moderate to heavy use of tobacco and alcohol)
To diagnose:
Tumors
Varices
Inflammations
Hernias
Polyps
Ulcers
Obstructions
Jaundice
To treat:
Gastric polyp (excision)
For follow-up of gastric cancer surgery

CONTRAINDICATIONS

Uncooperative patient
Severe UGI bleeding
Esophageal diverticula

NURSING CARE

Explain the procedure, and obtain written consent. The patient must be kept NPO after midnight to provide optimum visualization of the GI tract and to prevent regurgitation during initiation of the test. The patient must remove his dentures and eyeglasses before the test. Oral hygiene procedures should be done before and after the test. Provide an Ambu bag and physostigmine in case of respiratory emergencies. Once the throat has been anesthetized, do not permit the patient to eat or drink anything until the gag reflex returns.

Place any specimens obtained in an appropriate container, and label them. Observe the patient for bleeding, dysphagia, dyspnea, fever, and abdominal pain. Monitor vital signs as needed. Observe general safety precautions associated with the use of sedatives.

PATIENT TEACHING

Explain the procedure, and encourage the patient to talk about his fears. Assure the patient that the test is not painful but that it may cause discomfort and vomiting when the gag reflex is initiated. Explain, too, that he will not be able to speak when the scope is in position.

Inform the patient that he may have a sore throat for several days after the anesthetic wears off.

LAPAROSCOPY

Inserting a fiberoptic scope through the abdominal wall and into the peritoneum allows visualization of the female abdominal organs. In addition to obvious diagnostic processes, surgery can easily be performed with this procedure.

INDICATIONS

To diagnose:
- Pelvic adhesions
- Ovarian tumors and cysts
- Tubal and uterine causes of infertility
- Endometriosis
- Ectopic pregnancy
- Ruptured ovarian cyst
- Salpingitis
- Stage of carcinoma

Therapeutic uses:
- Adhesion lysis
- IUD removal
- Tubal ligation
- Removal of biopsy specimen
- Cholecystectomy
- Appendectomy

CONTRAINDICATIONS

Local peritonitis
History of multiple surgeries
Suspected intraabdominal hemorrhage

NURSING CARE

After explaining the procedure, obtain informed consent. Help the patient with enemas, if they are ordered, and record the results. Follow the routine general anesthesia precautions associated with the procedure. Shave and prepare the patient's abdomen as ordered. Keep patient NPO after midnight before the test. Give fluids intravenously as needed. Instruct the patient to void before the test. Help the patient into a modified lithotomy or Trendelenburg position for the procedure. A needle is inserted through a small incision into the peritoneal cavity, which is filled with 3 to 4 L of carbon dioxide to enhance visualization. The laparoscope is then inserted for the examination.

After the procedure, do not let the patient walk or stand immediately, since orthostasis may cause dizziness or fainting. Assess the patient frequently for signs of bleeding, perforated viscus, and acidosis. If minor shoulder or subcostal discomfort occurs as a result of pneumoperitoneum, assure the patient that this usually resolves within 24 hours. Administer minor analgesics to relieve discomfort.

PATIENT TEACHING

Explain the procedure, noting that it usually is performed by a surgeon in approximately 20 to 40 minutes. If general anesthesia will be used, inform the patient that she will feel no discomfort, although she may have mild incisional pain and shoulder or subcostal discomfort later; this usually subsides in about 24 hours. She may take minor analgesics for relief.

Explain that the patient should not walk or stand immediately after her legs are removed from the stirrups because of the risk of dizziness.

BIOPSY

In general, the purpose of a biopsy is to obtain a sample of tissue for pathologic examination. The three types of biopsy are incisional, excisional, and needle/aspiration (Figure 3-14). **Incisional biopsy** is the removal of a portion of tissue for examination (e.g., the bite biopy performed during endoscopy). **Excisional biopsy** is the removal of the complete lesion, with little or no margin of surrounding normal tissue removed (e.g., polypectomy).

Another example of excisional biopsy is the dissection of peripheral lymph nodes (e.g., those of the axilla for staging of breast cancer or those of the peritoneal region for staging of various abdominal cancers). **Needle/aspiration biopsy** is the aspiration of fluid or tissue by means of a needle (e.g., breast biopsy is performed with an aspiration needle). The specimen is examined by the pathologist for an immediate decision on surgical intervention (frozen section) as well as for more detailed staging and grading as the basis for determining further treatment and prognosis.

Transcutaneous **aspiration biopsy** has eliminated most of the exploratory laparotomies for diagnosing metastatic cancer of the liver or for primary inoperable pancreatic cancer. Other benefits of this procedure are low cost, speed in reaching an accurate diagnosis, and acceptance by most patients. Organs accessible to thin-needle biopsy under guidance of palpation include breasts, skin, thyroid, prostate, palpable lymph nodes, and salivary glands. The technique is used for imaging guidance of such organs as the lungs and mediastinum, liver, pancreas, spleen, kidneys, brain, retroperitoneum, deep lymph nodes, eyes and orbits, and skeleton.

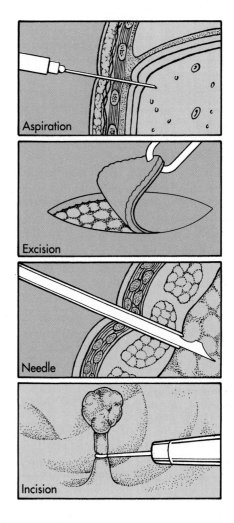

FIGURE 3-14
Types of biopsy.

BONE MARROW BIOPSY

Hematopoiesis can be fully evaluated by examining a bone marrow specimen. The examination will reveal the number, size, and shape of the RBCs, WBCs, and megakaryocytes (platelet precursors). The hematologist may obtain samples either by aspiration or by surgical removal. Microscopic examination involves estimating cellularity, assessing for fibrotic tissue or primary and metastatic neoplasms, and estimating iron storage.

The preferred site for *bone marrow aspiration* is the posterior iliac crest. After the overlying skin and soft tissue, as well as the periosteum, are infiltrated with lidocaine, a large-bore needle with a stylus is slowly advanced through the soft tissue and into the outer table of the bone. Once inside the marrow, the stylus is removed and a syringe is attached. About 0.5 to 2 ml of marrow is aspirated, smeared on slides, and dried. The slides are sprayed with a preservative and sent to the laboratory.

With a *bone marrow biopsy*, the skin and soft tissues are incised, a core biopsy instrument is screwed into the bone, and a biopsy specimen is obtained and sent to the laboratory for analysis.

INDICATIONS

To diagnose:
Leukemias (myeloid, lymphocytic)
Metastatic neoplasia
Neoplastic marrow infiltrative disease
Lymphoma
Multiple myeloma
Hodgkin's disease
Metastatic tumors (breasts, kidneys, lungs)

CONTRAINDICATIONS

Acute coagulation disorders
Patients who cannot remain still
Uncooperative patients

NURSING CARE

Explain the procedure, and obtain written informed consent. Assess coagulation studies, reporting any evidence of coagulopathy. Obtain an order for sedatives if the patient appears extremely anxious; remind the patient to remain very still throughout the procedure.

Help the patient into the preferred position (prone or on his side), exposing the posterior iliac crest. (Other sites less frequently used are the sternum, iliac crest, anterior iliac spine, and proximal tibia.) Prepare and drape area in a sterile manner. The overlying skin and soft tissue, as well as the periosteum, are infiltrated with lidocaine. After an *aspiration* procedure, spray the slides with a preservative and send the slides or specimen to the pathology laboratory.

Apply pressure to the puncture site, and apply a bandage; observe for bleeding, using ice packs when appropriate. Monitor the patient for signs of infection at the site (tenderness and erythema), shock (increased pulse rate, decreased blood pressure), and pain, and report these to the physician. The patient should stay in bed for 30 to 60 minutes after the test. Administering mild analgesics for the first few days after the test may relieve tenderness at the puncture site.

PATIENT TEACHING

When explaining the procedure, encourage the patient to talk about his fears and provide emotional support. Explain whether the procedure is an *aspiration* or *biopsy*, noting that aspiration is performed by either a specially trained nurse or physician and that a biopsy usually is performed by a physician. Each procedure usually takes about 20 minutes. Remind the patient that it is important to remain very still throughout the procedure.

Inform the patient that he probably will feel pain during the lidocaine infiltration and pressure when the syringe plunger is withdrawn for aspiration. He may also feel some anxiety when pressure is applied to puncture the outer table of the bone during either procedure.

LIVER BIOPSY

Liver biopsy is a method of diagnosing liver cancer. It involves inserting a special needle through the skin and abdominal wall into the liver, and then removing a liver tissue specimen for microscopic examination.

After a coagulation profile and blood cross-matching, the patient is kept NPO after midnight on the scheduled examination day. Meperidine and atropine are administered 30 to 60 minutes before the study, and the patient is placed in the supine or left lateral position. After aseptic cleansing and anesthetizing of the skin, a small incision is made in the skin. The patient is instructed to exhale and hold the exhalation to raise the diaphragm and reduce the possibility of pneumothorax. During sustained exhalation, the physician rapidly introduces the needle, obtains the biopsy specimen, and rapidly withdraws the needle. The needle used may be a long aspiration-type needle (with syringe) or an excision needle. Excision needles provide more tissue but are associated with a slightly higher risk of complication.

INDICATIONS

To diagnose:
Unexplained hepatomegaly
Persistently elevated liver enzyme levels
Suspected primary or metastatic tumor
Unexplained jaundice
Suspected hepatitis
Suspected infiltrative diseases

CONTRAINDICATIONS

Uncooperative patient
Impaired hemostasis
Profound anemia
Infection of right pleural space
Septic cholangitis
Obstructive jaundice

COMPLICATIONS

Hemorrhage caused by puncture of blood vessel within or surrounding the liver
Peritonitis caused by inadvertent laceration of bile duct and subsequent leakage
Pneumothorax caused by improper placement of biopsy needle

NURSING CARE

After explaining the procedure, obtain written informed consent. Check the results of hemostasis studies to rule out coagulation disorders. Inform the physician of any abnormal findings. Keep the patient NPO after midnight.

In explaining the procedure, stress the importance of lying very still and sustaining exhalation to avoid laceration of the liver or diaphragm. Administer sedatives if ordered. Assist as needed during the procedure; place tissue sample in the appropriate specimen container and send it to the pathology laboratory.

After the test, place the patient on his right side for 1 to 2 hours to compress the liver capsule against the chest wall and tamponade hemorrhage or bile leakage. The patient must remain in bed for 12 to 24 hours. Assess vital signs as directed (usually four times in the first hour, then q 1 h for 4 hours, then q 4 h) for evidence of hemorrhage and peritonitis. Evaluate for pain; some pain in the right upper quadrant of the abdomen and right shouldertop is common. Report any severe pain immediately.

PATIENT TEACHING

Explain the procedure, encouraging the patient to talk about his fears. Emphasize that it is vital that he lie very still and hold his breath during exhalation to avoid laceration of the liver or diaphragm.

After the procedure, explain the need for the patient to remain on his right side for 1 to 2 hours (to tamponade any hemorrhage or bile leakage).

LUNG BIOPSY

Specimens of pulmonary tissue for detecting lung carcinomas and other disorders must be obtained through invasive lung biopsy, using either an open technique (through limited thoracotomy) or a closed technique (by means of a transbronchial lung biopsy, transbronchial needle aspiration biopsy, or transcatheter bronchial brushing). The patient is kept NPO after midnight on the day of the biopsy and sedated 30 to 60 minutes before the procedure. The positioning of the patient depends on the method used.

The different methods of lung biopsy include the following:

Transbronchial lung biopsy is performed through a flexible fiberoptic bronchoscope using cutting forceps. Before the procedure the patient usually is given meperidine or morphine for sedation and atropine to reduce secretions. Fluoroscopy is used to ensure proper opening, positioning, and visualization of the "tug" of the lung on specimen removal.

Transbronchial needle aspiration biopsy involves a fiberoptic bronchoscope and a needle. As with the transbronchial procedure, the patient usually is given atropine beforehand to reduce secretions. After the bronchoscope has been inserted and the target site has been identified by fluoroscopy, the needle is inserted into the tumor for aspiration with the attached syringe and catheter. The needle is retracted within its sheath, and the entire catheter is withdrawn from the fiberoptic bronchoscope, which is removed last.

Transcatheter bronchial brushing also uses the fiberoptic bronchoscope; a small brush is moved back and forth over the target area to remove cells for microscopic slides. The bronchoscope is then removed.

Percutaneous needle biopsy is done after x-ray films have been used to determine the target site. The specimen is obtained either by using a cutting needle or by aspiration with a spinal-type needle. This procedure carries a risk of damage to major blood vessels.

Open-lung biopsy requires general anesthesia and an operating room. The patient is placed in the supine position, and a small thoracic incision is made in the chest wall so that a piece of lung tissue can be removed. The lung is then closed, and chest tube drainage is used for about 24 hours after the procedure.

INDICATIONS

To diagnose:
Carcinoma
Granuloma
Sarcoidosis
Cause of parenchymal pulmonary disease or pulmonary lesion
Environmental risks, infections, or familial disease

CONTRAINDICATIONS

The following contraindications are relative; the risk must be weighed against the importance of securing a diagnosis by lung biopsy.
Bullae or cysts
Suspected vascular anomalies
Bleeding abnormalities
Pulmonary hypertension
Severe respiratory insufficiency
Uncooperative patient

NURSING CARE

After explaining the procedure, obtain informed and written consent. Ensure that the patient fasts as ordered; the patient usually is kept NPO after midnight on the test day. Administer the prescribed medications 30 to 60 minutes before the test.

Before the lung biopsy, instruct the patient to remain still and avoid coughing; during the procedure observe for signs of respiratory distress and report these immediately. Place specimens in the appropriate containers.

After the lung biopsy procedure is initiated, assess the patient's vital signs frequently and as directed for signs of bleeding, shortness of breath, and signs of pneumothorax (dyspnea, tachypnea, decrease in breath sounds, anxiety, and restlessness). Immediately report any decrease of breath sounds on the biopsy site. A chest x-ray usually is ordered after this procedure to assess for complications.

PATIENT TEACHING

Explain the procedure and specific method, stressing the importance of remaining still. Tell the patient that any movement or coughing could cause the biopsy needle to perforate the lung.

PLEURAL BIOPSY

Pleural biopsy for histologic examination is sometimes necessary when the pleural fluid specimen (see the section on thoracentesis and pleural fluid analysis) contains exudative fluid suggesting a neoplasm or tuberculosis. This test distinguishes between these two diseases.

The test usually is performed by means of needle biopsy of the pleura, by pleuroscopy (insertion of a fiberoptic bronchoscope for biopsy), or by open pleural biopsy (limited thoracotomy requiring general anesthesia). The advantage of this method is that a larger specimen can be obtained for examination.

The procedure usually is performed with the patient in a sitting position, with the shoulders and arms elevated and supported by a padded overbed table. After anesthetizing and subsequent piercing of the skin over the biopsy site, a Cope instrument is inserted. This instrument is made up of a needle with an 11-gauge outer cannula with a sharp cutting edge and a 13-gauge blunt-tipped, hooked biopsy trocar. The hub of the trocar is attached to a metal pointer to indicate the direction of the hook. After the outer cannula has been inserted, the 13-gauge needle is inserted within the cannula until fluid is removed. The inner needle is then removed, and the blunt-tipped trocar is substituted. The patient exhales all air and performs the Valsalva maneuver to prevent air from entering the pleural space. The cannula and trocar are then withdrawn, while the hook catches the parietal wall and takes a specimen with its cutting edge.

Usually three specimens are taken from different sites at the same session. The specimens are placed in a fixative solution and sent to the laboratory immediately. Additional parietal fluid can be removed after the specimens. The procedure usually takes about 30 minutes.

INDICATIONS

To diagnose:
  Tuberculosis
  Neoplasm

CONTRAINDICATIONS

Prolonged bleeding or clotting time

NURSING CARE

Explain the procedure, and obtain signed and informed consent. Position the patient, and instruct him to remain still during the entire procedure. Place the biopsy specimen in an appropriate fixative solution, and send it immediately to the laboratory to ensure accurate interpretation of the test result.

After the test, check the patient's vital signs frequently, observing for signs of respiratory distress (shortness of breath, diminished breath sounds on the side of the biopsy site). Ensure that the chest x-ray is repeated if ordered for a pneumothorax check.

PATIENT TEACHING

Explain the procedure, and encourage the patient to talk about his fears. Offer appropriate reassurance. Instruct the patient in the Valsalva maneuver, and emphasize the importance of remaining still during the entire procedure, explaining that any movement can cause inadvertent needle damage. Inform the patient that the entire test usually takes about 30 minutes, and that biopsy specimens probably will be obtained from three different sites.

ENDOMETRIAL BIOPSY

In addition to determining the occurrence of and the effect of ovulation estrogen, as well as investigating for tuberculosis, polyps, or inflammatory conditions, endometrial biopsy is used to diagnose endometrial cancer. After a bimanual pelvic examination and a cleaning of the cervix, a tenaculum is placed on the cervix for stabilization, and a metal probe is used to determine the size of the uterus. Specimens are obtained from the anterior, posterior, and lateral walls with a suction tube curette or endometrial biopsy curette. The specimens are sent to the pathologist in a 10% formalin solution.

INDICATIONS

For analysis of:
   Occurrence of ovulation
   Effects of estrogen
To diagnose:
   Endometrial cancer   Polyps
   Tuberculosis   Inflammatory conditions

CONTRAINDICATIONS

Patients in whom the cervix fails to visualize
Infection
Uncooperative patients

NURSING CARE

Explain the procedure, offering emotional support. Help the patient into the lithotomy position. After the procedure, assess the patient's vital signs for 48 hours. Report temperature elevations.

Bed rest for 24 hours is recommended after this procedure; heavy lifting should be avoided, and douching and intercourse are not permitted for 72 hours after the biopsy. Excessive bleeding should be reported to the physician.

PATIENT TEACHING

While explaining the procedure, it is important to encourage the patient to talk about her fears and to provide appropriate emotional support. Inform the patient that this procedure usually causes only momentary discomfort, and analgesics should not be necessary.

Encourage the patient to adhere to the recommended 24 hours of bed rest, as well as the 72-hour abstinence from douching and intercourse. Tell her that she will need to wear a pad, because some vaginal bleeding will occur. Remind her to report excessive bleeding (more than one pad per hour) to the physician. Explain how she may obtain her test results from your facility; a report usually is available within 72 hours.

TUMOR MARKERS

Tumor markers are substances produced and secreted by tumor cells that are found in the serum of individuals with cancer. Elevated levels of these substances, along with other data, are used to establish a diagnosis, evaluate the prognosis, and monitor the response to therapy or recurrence of certain cancers. The level of tumor marker seems to correlate with the extent of the disease; for example, in patients with colorectal cancer, elevated levels of carcinoembryonic antigen (CEA) usually relate to the extent of metastasis and the response to treatment. Tumor marker levels also are useful in determining the patient's prognosis; for example, a patient with circulating levels of human chorionic gonadotropin (HCG) above 8,000 ng/ml usually has a poor prognosis unless intensive therapy is administered. Changes in the levels of tumor markers are useful in monitoring the response to therapy; for example, a rise in HCG or alpha-fetoprotein (AFP) levels after a decline during treatment suggests recurrence of testicular cancer and the need to resume chemotherapy (Table 3-1).

ESTROGEN AND PROGESTIN RECEPTOR ASSAYS

Analyses of estrogen (ER) and progestin (PR) receptors provide information that is useful in treating breast cancer. There is a relationship between the quantity of these receptor proteins in a tumor biopsy and the disease-free survival of patients. The presence of the specific steroid receptor appears to be a prerequisite for hormonal responsiveness of the target tissues. Specific binding capacity is expressed in femtomol per milli-

Table 3-1 _____

CLINICALLY USEFUL TUMOR MARKERS

Tumor marker	Normal value	Cancers in which marker may be found
Carcinoembryonic antigen (CEA)	0-2.5 ng/ml*	Colorectal cancer; metastatic breast cancer; lung cancer
Alpha-fetoprotein (AFP)	10 ng/ml	Testicular cancer (nonseminomatous); liver cancer
Human chorionic gonadotropin (HCG)	0-1 ng/ml	Choriocarcinoma; testicular cancer (nonseminomatous/seminomatous†)
Prostatic acid phosphatase (PAP)	1399-9833 ng/ml	Metastastic prostate cancer
Prostate-specific antigen (PSA)	<4 ng/ml	Primary and metastatic prostate cancer
Cancer antigen (CA) 125	34 U/ml	Ovarian cancer
Immunoglobulins	IgM, 80-170 mg/dl; IgG, 750-1750 mg/dl; IgA, 170-280 mg/dl; IgD, 2-4 mg/dl; IgE, 0.1-1 mg/dl	Multiple myeloma
Calcitonin	Male, 0-14 pg/ml; female, 0-28 pg/ml	Medullary cancer of the thyroid

*A nanogram (ng) is a millionth of a milligram.
†Seminomatous testicular cancer may cause a small elevation in HCG but not an elevation in AFP.

Table 3-2 _____

USING ENZYMES IN CANCER DIAGNOSIS

Enzyme	Normal range	Cancers in which elevation may occur
Amylase	Adult: 15-200 mg/dl	Some lung and ovarian tumors
Amylase isoenzymes		Some bronchogenic or serous ovarian tumors
Lactate dehydrogenase (LDH) and LDH isoenzymes	Pyruvate to lactate 210-420 U/L; lactate to pyruvate 45-90 U/L	Extensive dehydrogenase carcinomatosis and malignant processes; acute leukemia
Leucine aminopeptidase (LAP)	Males: 80-200 U/ml; females: 75-185 U/ml	Pancreatic cancer with liver metastases
Lysozyme	4-13 mg/L	Acute monocytic or myelomonocytic leukemia and chronic myeloid leukemia
Serum gamma glutamyl transpeptidase (SGGT)	Males: 6-37 U/ml; females: 4-24 U/ml	Some cases of renal cell cancer and liver metastases
Serum glutamic oxaloacetic transaminase (SGOT)	Adult: 5-40 U/ml	Liver metastases or infiltration
Serum glutamic pyruvic transaminase (SGPT)	Adult: 5-35 U/ml	Some liver cancers

gram of cytosol protein (fmol per mcp). For breast cancer it is generally accepted that finding fewer than 3 fmol/mcp represents a receptor-negative tumor, which correlates with lack of response to hormonal therapy. A level of 10 fmol/mcp or more represents a receptor-positive tumor and correlates with response to hormonal manipulation. When estrogen is present in a tumor, a higher progestin concentration frequently is seen; if estrogen is absent, a lower level of progestin is seen. Estrogen receptors are more often present in tumors of postmenopausal women than in those of premenopausal women. Estrogen and progestin are not only useful as a predictive index of the patient's response to hormonal therapy, they also can serve as a prognostic index of the course of the disease (e.g., patients with primary breast cancer containing estrogen receptors live disease free longer).

OTHER HORMONES

Some tumors inappropriately produce hormones such as adrenocorticotropic hormone (ACTH), insulin, parathyroid hormones, human chorionic gonadotropin (HCG), and erythropoietin. The term "ectopic hormone production" is used to describe hormone production by tumors of nonendocrine origin. Certain tumors can be detected by measuring the serum levels of hormones and substrates produced by the hormone (e.g., cortisol).

ENZYMES

The abnormalities of enzyme expression in cancer include expression of an immature or fetal form of an enzyme and ectopic production of enzymes. Isoenzymes are variable forms of an enzyme, such as amylase and lactate dehydrogenase. The enzymes or isoenzymes produced by the tumor are not new or unique; they normally are produced by the noncancerous tissue from which the cancer develops. The changes occur primarily within the tumor itself and are detected in the circulation only when the tumor is very large or when widespread metastasis has occurred (Table 3-2).

MONOCLONAL ANTIBODIES

Monoclonal antibody reagents have a promising future in the diagnosis of cancer. The high specificity of monoclonal antibodies for antigen can reduce the number of false results. When combined with the appropriate assay system, monoclonal antibodies may provide methods for detecting cancer earlier. For example, highly purified monoclonal antibodies could be used to detect circulating tumor antigens, providing a method for periodic screening of individuals at high risk for a specific type of cancer. When bound to a radionuclide, monoclonal antibodies could be used for radiologic imaging. Also, monoclonal antibodies could be developed that are specific for tumor antigens; these would mediate tumor rejection without affecting normal tissues. Thus monoclonal antibodies have potential value in screening and early detection of cancer, as well as monitoring in tumor response to therapy.

CHROMOSOMAL ANALYSES

Chromosome abnormalities have been found in several types of cancer (e.g., leukemias and lymphomas) and may be prognostic indicators of response to therapy. Cytogenetic studies are routinely included in the diagnostic evaluation of individuals suspected of having any of a variety of cancers. Most chromosomal changes involve translocations of genetic material from one autosome to another and may be the reason for neoplastic changes that occur in normal cells.

The presence of these malignancies can be confirmed by analyzing the chromosome set, or karyotype, for morphologic abnormalities. For example, in Burkitt's lymphoma, material from chromosomes 8 and 14 is rearranged, written as t(8;14)(q24;q32). The letter *t* indicates a translocation between the two chromosomes at the respective regions, or bands (q24 of chromosome 8 and q32 of chromosome 14), which are symbolized by the letters in these examples.

TUMOR ANTIGENS

Tumor-associated antigens (TAA) may be categorized as tumor-specific transplantation antigens (TSTA), which are unique for each tumor, and cross-reactive tumor-associated transplantation antigens (TATA), which are shared by different tumors. The TSTA cause the stronger immune response; the best recognized example is the immunoglobulin idiotype antigens expressed by B cell lymphomas.

The viral antigens are products expressed by virally transformed cells that are encoded by viral genes and are common to all tumors induced by the same virus. For example, Burkitt's lymphoma and nasopharyngeal cancer are caused by the Epstein-Barr virus. Individuals with Burkitt's lymphoma have higher antibody titers to Epstein-Barr virus antigens than do unaffected people of the same age, gender, and geographic location. The tumor cells have copies of the virus incorporated into their genome, and the titers against the virus in people with nasopharyngeal cancer correlate with the stage of disease, suggesting that viral antigens are continually expressed by tumor cells.

Oncofetal antigens are molecules expressed by cells during certain stages of embryonic development but absent or expressed at very low concentrations by normal adult cells. The two best examples of antigens in this group are alpha-fetoprotein and carcinoembryonic antigen (see the section on tumor markers).

BLOOD CHEMISTRIES

Although the individual blood chemistry tests differ as to fasting requirements and whether anticoagulants are used, they usually are done as a unit on the fasting person. Either serum or plasma may be used for most of the blood chemistry tests. Individuals suspected of having cancer, as well as those who have been diagnosed and are undergoing treatment, may require evaluation of a variety of electrolytes, enzymes, hormones, and amino acids. For example, calcium is known to be elevated with certain tumors, particularly those involving the bone (e.g., multiple myeloma). Creatinine and urea nitrogen values should be obtained before initiating chemotherapy, which requires adequate renal function. Likewise, bilirubin and lactate dehydrogenase values, which indicate liver function, would predict the liver's ability to metabolize various chemotherapeutic agents.

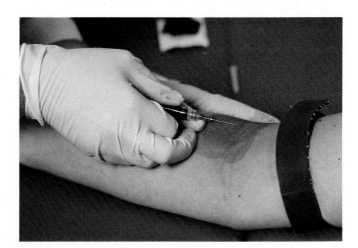

FIGURE 3-15
Performing venipuncture. (From Grimes.[24])

HEMATOLOGY

A complete blood count (CBC) consists of a white blood count (WBC) and differential, red blood count (RBC) and hematocrit, hemoglobin, erythrocyte indices, platelet count, and inspection of the peripheral blood smear. When these values are determined accurately, most hematologic diagnoses can be made and a significant amount of information can be gathered for several purposes, such as evaluating the stage of a particular disease (e.g., leukemia), diagnosing diseases not directly related to the hematopoietic system (e.g., gastrointestinal cancer), or monitoring the impact of therapy (e.g., the effect of radiation therapy on the white blood cell, red blood cell, and platelet counts).

ROUTINE URINALYSIS

Routine urinalysis involves noting the color and odor of the specimen; determining its pH, specific gravity, and levels of protein or albumin, glucose, and ketone bodies; and microscopic examination of the urinary sediment. The test results are used to determine the presence and severity of renal disease, which may indicate cancer or a disorder that will affect treatment decisions.

DNA FLOW CYTOMETRY

DNA flow cytometry is used to measure the characteristics and amount of DNA in individual cells obtained by biopsy. The cytometer produces a histogram of the cells' DNA content, which is reported in terms of the S-phase index (SPI) and ploidy. The SPI is a measure of the tumor cells' proliferative capacity. Normal tissue value is 3% to 5%; a high value (>5% to 8%) indicates a rapidly proliferating tumor. Ploidy is a measure of the amount of DNA in tumor cells when compared to normal cells; those with a normal amount of DNA are diploid; those with an abnormal amount are aneuploid.

The SPI and ploidy, when considered with the tumor's size, steroid hormone receptors, histopathology, and nuclear grade, are thought to have predictive validity in the treatment of node-negative breast cancer.

STAGING OF CANCER

The purpose of staging is to describe the extent of a malignant tumor in order to aid the physician in planning treatment, determining the prognosis, evaluating the results of treatment, and standardizing communication among health care providers for consultation, referral, and research. Staging should be done during the pretreatment phase of the disease and, when applicable, after surgical resection. Staging also will be necessary if the disease recurs after a disease-free interval. Clinical staging includes a physical examination, with careful inspection, palpation, auscultation, and percussion as applicable. The pathologic assessment is based on evaluation of incisional, excisional, or aspiration biopsy specimens and may include dissection of regional lymph nodes.

TNM STAGING SYSTEM

A general staging system developed by the International Union Against Cancer (UICC) and revised by the American Joint Committee on Cancer (AJCC) is based on measurement of the primary tumor, lymph node involvement, and metastic spread (TNM classification). Using the TNM staging system, the disease is categorized as follows:

T Extent of the primary tumor; based on size, depth of penetration, and invasion of adjacent structures

N Presence, extent, and location of regional lymph node involvement

M Presence or absence of distant metastases and the degree of dissemination (Table 3-3)

Table 3-3

TNM STAGING SYSTEM

Tumor		
T0	No evidence of primary tumor	
Tis	Carcinoma in situ	
T1, T2, T3, T4	Progressive increase in tumor size and involvement	
Tx	Tumor cannot be assessed	
Nodes		
N0	Regional lymph nodes not demonstrably abnormal	
N1, N2, N3	Increasing degrees of demonstrable abnormality of regional lymph nodes. (For many primary sites an "a" may be added [e.g., $N1_a$] to indicate that metastasis to the node is not suspected; a "b" may be used [e.g., N_{1b}] to indicate that metastasis to the node is suspected or proved)	
Nx	Regional lymph nodes cannot be assessed clinically	
Metastasis		
M0	No evidence of distant metastasis	
M1, M2, M3	Ascending degrees of distant metastasis, including metastasis to distant lymph nodes	

From the American Joint Committee for Cancer Staging and End Results Reporting Clinical Staging System for Carcinoma of the Esophagus. *Cancer* March-April 1975, pp 25-51.

GRADING

Grading is the histologic classification of a tumor, which may be useful in determining the prognosis. The pathologist evaluates tissue within the primary site for any prognostically important tumor characteristics, reviews surgical specimens to determine if lines of resection are free of tumor, and evaluates regional lymph nodes for histologic confirmation of cancer. Cancers usually are classified as grades 1 to 4, based on increasing anaplasia (see box).

The more poorly differentiated a tumor is, the less it resembles normal cells and the poorer the prognosis. Grading systems vary according to the site of the disease.

METASTATIC WORKUP

The most common sites of metastatic disease are the lungs, liver, bones, bone marrow, adrenal glands, and brain. The physician selects the studies needed to determine the anatomic extent of the disease and those whose results would affect the course of treatment. A variety of techniques, including radiographic, ultrasonographic, and radioisotopic scanning; magnetic resonance imaging; aspiration and biopsy; and tumor marker tests, may be used, based on the nature of the primary tumor and its usual pattern of spread.

GRADING OF TUMORS

G_X Grade cannot be assessed
G1   Well differentiated
G2   Moderately well differentiated
G3 and G4   Poorly to very poorly differentiated

CHAPTER 4

Lung Cancer

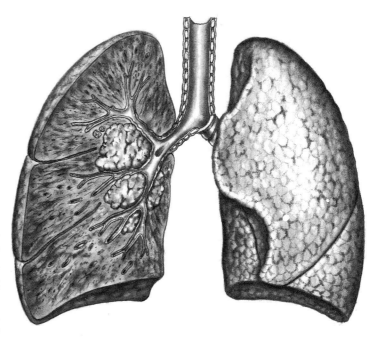

Carcinoma of the lung, the leading cause of death from cancer in both men and women, has reached almost epidemic proportions in the United States. Lung cancer causes 21% of cancer deaths in women and 34% of cancer deaths in men. In women, the death rate from lung cancer now exceeds that of breast cancer.

The overall 5-year survival rate for all persons with lung cancer is 13%. A major reason for this poor prognosis is that only 21% of these individuals have localized disease when diagnosed. Fifty percent of those diagnosed are considered inoperable.

EPIDEMIOLOGY

Approximately 80% of lung tumors are linked to cigarette smoking. The risk of developing lung cancer is 10 times greater in men who smoke and five times greater in women who smoke. The people at highest risk began smoking in their teens, inhale deeply, and smoke at least half a pack a day. The length of each cigarette and its tar content are other factors affecting the incidence of lung cancer. When an individual quits smoking, the risk gradually declines, eventually reaching levels similar to those of nonsmokers. "Passive smoking" (breathing in side-stream smoke) brings as many, if not more, carcinogens into the body as inhaled smoke.

Another etiologic factor in the development of lung cancer is occupational exposure to such substances as asbestos, polycyclic aromatic hydrocarbons, radon, nickel, and chromium. Smoking tobacco has a synergistic effect on individuals exposed to these substances, because it increases their risk of developing lung cancer beyond that of coworkers who do not smoke. Air pollutants have not yet been proved a risk factor for cancer, but the incidence of the disease is higher in urban populations.

Vitamin A deficiency may increase a person's risk of lung cancer. Siblings and children of individuals with lung cancer are at slightly greater risk. Lung cancer occurs with greater frequency among African-American men than among white men. The incidence is also higher in lower-income and less-educated groups, whatever their ethnicity. The average age of onset is 60 years.

PATHOPHYSIOLOGY

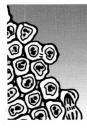

The period between a person's initial exposure to a carcinogen and the onset of lung cancer can range from 10 to 30 years. A lesion detected by sputum cytology and found by fiberoptic bronchoscopy can easily be resected and is potentially curable. This generally is not true of a lesion first found on a chest x-ray; the smallest detectable tumor on an x-ray is 1 centimeter in diameter.

The major histologic types of lung cancer are divided into two categories, non–small cell lung cancer (NSCLC) and small cell lung cancer (SCLC).

Non–small cell lung cancers (NSCLC) usually are not as aggressive as small cell lung cancers but have limited potential for response to treatment, except for surgery. This category includes three subtypes:

Squamous cell (epidermoid) cancer is the most common type of lung tumor, accounting for 35% of NSCLC. Ninety percent of these tumors occur in men. The tumors tend to be centrally located and often cause bronchial obstruction.

Adenocarcinoma accounts for 35% of all lung tumors, and is often located peripherally. A common scar carcinoma that arises in an area of fibrosis at the site of previous pulmonary damage, this cancer has less association with smoking than the other types. Adenocarcinomas frequently spread through the submucosal lymphatics to regional lymph nodes and often metastasize to the brain and other distant organs by vascular invasion.

Large cell undifferentiated cancer constitutes 15% of lung tumors and may appear in any area of the lung. This type tends to disseminate early in its course and is associated with a poor prognosis. Giant cell and clear cell carcinomas are subtypes.

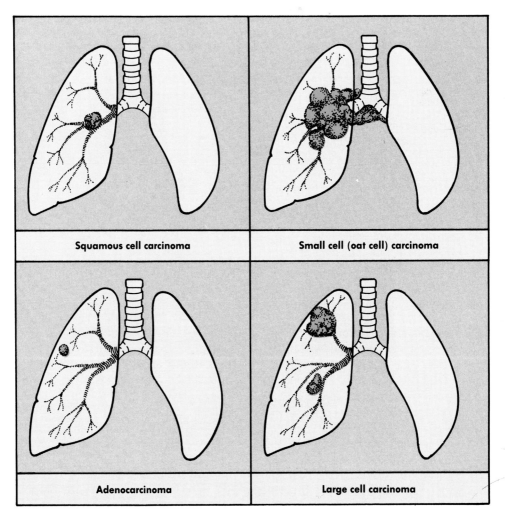

FIGURE 4-1
Predominant sites of types of lung cancer. (From McCance and Huether.[43])

Small cell lung cancer (SCLC), or oat cell cancer, accounts for 10% of lung tumors and usually is centrally located. It is the most aggressive cancer, with lymphatic and distant metastases usually present at the time of diagnosis. Paraneoplastic syndromes are more common with this type. It tends to be highly sensitive to both chemotherapy and radiation therapy.

All types of lung cancer show lymphatic metastasis early in the course of the disease, beginning in the bronchial and mediastinal nodes and extending upward to the supraclavicular nodes and downward to the nodes below the diaphragm and to the liver and adrenal glands. Distant metastasis via the bloodstream to the brain, bones, and contralateral lung may occur.

SIGNS AND SYMPTOMS

A chronic cough, a change in the volume or odor of sputum, dyspnea, dull chest pain, and frequent upper respiratory infections are the most common early symptoms of lung cancer. Other symptoms are fatigue, chest tightness, and aching joints. Late but clinically significant signs include hemoptysis, clubbing of the fingers, weight loss, and pleural effusion. Invasion of the superior vena cava causes edema of the neck and face. Phrenic nerve involvement causes paralysis of the diaphragm. Hoarseness indicates recurrent involvement of the laryngeal nerve. A superior sulcus tumor involving the brachial plexus may be manifested as shoulder and arm pain and paresthesia.

The chest lesion may be relatively asymptomatic, with the chief complaint caused by metastatic disease. Metastasis to the brain may result in headache, unsteady gait, and other neurologic signs. Weight loss, jaundice, or anorexia may occur with liver involvement. Localized bony pain or pathologic fractures may accompany skeletal involvement. Asymptomatic patients usually are diagnosed by routine chest x-ray.

Paraneoplastic syndromes (see box) may be associated with lung cancer. For example, some patients with small cell cancer develop inappropriate antidiuretic hormone production or Cushing's syndrome, caused by secretion of ectopic adrenocorticotropic hormones. Other syndromes include hypercalcemia (caused by production of an ectopic parahormone-like substance), carcinomatous neuropathy and myopathy, dermatomyositis, and hypertrophic pulmonary osteoarthropathy.

PARANEOPLASTIC SYNDROMES ASSOCIATED WITH LUNG CANCER

Endocrine system

Antidiuretic hormone excess
Cushing's syndrome
Hypercalcemia
Carcinoid syndrome
Ectopic gonadotropin

Neuromuscular system

Myasthenia-like syndrome
Subacute cerebellar degeneration
Peripheral neuropathy
Myopathy

Dermatologic type

Acanthosis nigricans
Dermatomyositis

Skeletal system

Hypertrophic pulmonary osteoarthropathy
Clubbing

Hematologic type

Anemia
Intravascular coagulopathy
Leukocytosis
Red cell aplasia

Vascular system

Thrombophlebitis
Nonbacterial endocarditis

From Holleb, Fink, and Murphy.[33]

COMPLICATIONS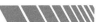

Superior vena cava syndrome
Paraneoplastic syndromes

```
┌─────────────────────────────────────┐
│   PROGNOSTIC FACTORS FOR             │
│        LUNG CANCERS                  │
└─────────────────────────────────────┘
```

Cell type
    Best with well-differentiated squamous cell cancer
    Worst with small cell lung cancer
Extent of disease
    Stage I: 5-year survival 40%-60%
    Stage II: 5-year survival 12%
    Overall: 5-year survival <10%
Performance status (e.g., Karnofsky Performance Scale, page 214)
Other factors
    Age (physiologic more so than chronologic)
    Gender (women survive longer than men)
    Nutritional status (weight loss of more than 10 pounds in 6 months is a
      bad sign)
    Immune status

DIAGNOSTIC STUDIES AND FINDINGS

Diagnostic Test	Findings
Sputum cytology	Positive for malignant cells
Chest x-ray	Tumor; invasion of chest wall or mediastinum
Computed tomography (CT) scan of the chest	Precise delineation of nodule, its density, and presence of calcium; invasion or compression of vascular structures; abnormal mediastinal lymph nodes
CT scan of the upper abdomen	Metastatic disease in liver or adrenal glands
Magnetic resonance imaging (MRI) study	Invasion or compression of vascular structures by tumor
Fluoroscopy	Paralysis and phrenic nerve involvement
Barium esophagram	Extension of tumor into central mediastinum
Bronchoscopy with bronchial brushing and biopsy	Malignant cells
Mediastinoscopy and mediastinotomy	Malignant cells in mediastinal lymph nodes
Transthoracic or transbronchial needle aspiration	Malignant cells
Thoracentesis	Malignant cells
Scalene or supraclavicular node biopsy	Malignant cells in palpable lymph nodes
Bone marrow biopsy	Malignant cells in centrally located small-cell tumor
Pulmonary function tests	50% reduction in predicted forced vital capacity (FEV_1), maximum voluntary ventilation (MVV), or vital capacity (VC)
Arterial blood gas analysis	Partial pressure of arterial oxygen (Pao_2) under 65 mm Hg
	Partial pressure of arterial carbon dioxide ($Paco_2$) over 45 mm Hg
Ventilation and perfusion radionuclide scanning	Little or no function in lung tissue to be resected
Abdominal CT or ultrasound scan	Metastatic disease to liver
CT or MRI study of the brain	Metastatic disease to brain
Bone scan	Metastatic disease to bone

MEDICAL MANAGEMENT

SURGERY

Thoracotomy: Surgical incision of the chest wall (exploratory); collection of biopsy specimen (ribs are spread and pleura is opened).

Limited pulmonary resection (segmental, wedge).

Lobectomy: Removal of a lobe of the lung and regional node dissection.

Pneumonectomy: Surgical removal of an entire lung.

Extended resection: En bloc removal of portions of the chest wall, vertebral body, left atrium, and/or diaphragm.

Other: Resection of the subcarinal, lobar, and mediastinal nodes. Surgical excision of solitary metastatic disease to brain.

RADIATION THERAPY

External beam; interstitial/endobronchial bradytherapy with iridium-192 (^{192}Ir).

CHEMOTHERAPY

For advanced non−small cell lung cancer: VdP (vindesine, cisplatin); VbP (vinblastine, cisplatin); CAMP (cyclophosphamide, doxorubicin, methotrexate, procarbazine); MVbP (mitomycin, vinblastine, cisplatin); PtVP-16 (etoposide/VP-16, cisplatin); CAP (cyclophosphamide, doxorubicin, cisplatin); CBP (cyclophosphamide, bleomycin, cisplatin); FOMi (5FU, vincristine, mitomycin-C).

For small cell lung cancer: CAV (cyclophosphamide, doxorubicin, vincristine); CEA (cyclophosphamide, etoposide, doxorubicin); CEV (cyclophosphamide, etoposide [VP-16], vincristine); EVAC (etoposide [VP-16], vincristine, doxorubicin, cyclophosphamide); Hansen's (cyclophosphamide, lomustine, vincristine, methotrexate); Hansen's VP (cyclophosphamide, lomustine, vincristine, etoposide); VP-16+P (etoposide, cisplatin).

Biologic response modifiers: Monoclonal antibody KC4 for NSCLC.

Endobronchial laser therapy

Photodynamic therapy (PDT)

Sclerosis: To treat malignant pleural effusion

SURGERY

Surgery may be as simple as a pulmonary resection for a limited primary or second primary tumor or as complex as an extended resection for widespread disease. Lobectomy is the standard procedure for all stage I and stage II lung cancers (Table 4-1) with no or limited lymph node involvement (e.g., intrapulmonary or hilar nodes or both). Pneumonectomy is used for large centrally located tumors, involvement of a main-stem bronchus, or invasion of the main pulmonary artery.

COMPLICATIONS OF SURGERY

Respiratory insufficiency
Tension pneumothorax
Cardiac failure or myocardial infarction
Thrombosis or pulmonary embolism
Atelectasis
Bronchopleural fistula
Pulmonary edema
Subcutaneous emphysema
Infection

Table 4-1 _____

STAGE GROUPING FOR LUNG CANCER*

Occult carcinoma	T_X	N_0	M_0
Stage 0	T_{is}	N_0	M_0
Stage I	T_1	N_0	M_0
	T_2	N_0	M_0
Stage II	T_1	N_1	M_0
	T_2	N_1	M_0
Stage IIIA	T_1	N_2	M_0
	T_2	N_2	M_0
	T_3	N_0, N_1, N_2	M_0
Stage IIIB	Any T	N_3	M_0
	T_4	Any N	M_0
Stage IV	Any T	Any N	M_1

From Beahrs OH and others, editors: Manual for staging of cancer, ed 3, Philadelphia, 1988, JB Lippincott.
*T, tumor; N, nodes; M, metastasis. See p. 53 for an explanation of the TNM system.

Preoperative Care

It is essential to determine the patient's preoperative status based on the current respiratory status (amount and extent of dyspnea, cough, hemoptysis, tachypnea), baseline pulmonary function studies, arterial blood gas analysis, electrocardiogram (ECG), blood counts and chemistry, general nutrition, and hydration.

The patient should be encouraged to stop smoking in preparation for the surgery. He should be instructed in deep-breathing and coughing techniques; range-of-motion and leg and arm exercises; the need for early ambulation; and the need for and technique of suctioning and closed chest drainage after surgery.

Postoperative Care

Patients who undergo a thoracotomy, resection, or lobectomy have closed chest drainage after surgery. The nurse should note fluctuation in the water-seal chamber and the drainage tubing near the patient; observe and record the amount and character of drainage; and check the status of the dressing at the entry site of the chest tube. Stripping of the tube or tubes is used to remove clots and maintain the flow of drainage into the chamber (see box for specific aspects of care of the patient with closed chest drainage).

Patients who undergo a pneumonectomy do not usually have closed chest drainage. It is preferred that the thoracic cavity on the affected side fill with serous exudate, which eventually consolidates. The surgeon may sever the phrenic nerve on the affected side, allowing the diaphragm to assume an elevated position, which also helps fill the empty thoracic space.

CARE OF THE PATIENT WITH CLOSED CHEST DRAINAGE

- If the chest tube (or tubes) is in place for the treatment of pleural effusion, bubbling in the water-seal chamber could indicate a leak in the system. Clamp the drainage tube near the patient with a booted hemostat. If the bubbling stops, the leak probably is at the insertion site or inside the pleural cavity. If the bubbling does not stop, there is a leak in the system; most likely it is in the link between the chest tube and the drainage system. The link should be secured with adhesive tape at all times.
- Other than in the situation described above, it is rarely necessary to clamp a chest tube. Even when a tube is disconnected, it is easier to reconnect it than to clamp the tube, reconnect it to the drainage system, and then unclamp the tube. In addition, not clamping the tube helps prevent tension pneumothorax.
- Stripping and milking of tubes are also dangerous because the suction created affects the patency of the pleural space. Milking, the gentler of the two procedures, may be used to clear the tube of obstructing blood clots or other materials.
- Although it is better not to raise the closed drainage system above the level of the patient's chest, this can be done if there is no fluid in the drainage tube. The only harm to the patient would be the return of fluid to the pleural space.

The patient should be assessed frequently for signs of airway obstruction, atelectasis, aspiration, or impaired gas exchange. Pain management, fluid replacement, exercise (including movement of the shoulder on the affected side) and rest, skin care, and pulmonary toileting are important aspects of nursing care.

RADIATION THERAPY

Radiation therapy (RT) may cure stage I or stage II non–small cell lung cancer in patients with poor preexisting lung function, but it is used most often in stage II disease.

In small cell lung cancer, it is advocated that external beam therapy be administered concurrently with the start of chemotherapy, after chemotherapy has been completed, or as a split course between cycles of chemotherapy. Radiation therapy is also used postoperatively with N_1 or N_2 disease or neoadjuvant with cisplatin or 5FU as radiation sensitizers. Endobronchial bradytherapy involves the use of remote afterloading units of iridium-192 for recurrent cancer and in patients who have received previous external radiation therapy. Radiation therapy is also used for the management of metastases to the brain and bone, for relief of superior vena cava syndrome, and for relief of nerve paresthesia and pain in the shoulder and arm caused by a superior sulcus tumor.

Radiation therapy is given in daily doses for 5 to 6 weeks, for a total of 5,000 to 6,000 rad. The patient may be placed on a split schedule of two courses with 2 to 3 weeks of rest before the next course to allow normal tissues to recover and the tumor to shrink. Patients receiving palliative radiation therapy undergo 1 to 2 weeks of therapy, for a total of 2,000 to 4,000 rad. Radiation therapy is used more frequently as palliation for lung cancer than for any other cancer.

Preprocedural Care

The patient needs instruction in the preparations for radiation therapy, which include CT for treatment planning; creation of individually designed blocks for defining the treatment field; and care of the skin during and after the period of treatment. The patient also should learn how to maintain or improve his nutritional status and avoid fatigue.

Postprocedural Care

The patient's respiratory status should be monitored throughout the course of treatment. The nurse should also assess the status of the skin and nutrition and the patient's ability to perform activities of daily living (ADL). Problems identified in any of these areas require prompt intervention.

With regard to acute radiation pneumonitis, the patient may complain of a hacking cough or mild chest pain (first signs); other symptoms include dyspnea and hypoxia, fever, and night sweats. If the reaction is severe, the patient may require hospitalization for oxygen therapy, steroids, antibiotics, sedatives, and cough suppressants. Antibiotics may be prescribed empirically. Steroids are the cornerstone of therapy (at least 60 mg of prednisone per day with gradual tapering).

SIDE EFFECTS OF RADIATION THERAPY

Early effects

Skin reactions
Nausea and vomiting, esophagitis, anorexia
Fatigue

Late effects

Pneumonitis
Pericarditis
Pleural effusion

CHEMOTHERAPY

Non–small cell lung cancer (NSCLC) is quite resistant to chemotherapy. In addition, previous surgery or radiation therapy (or both) often have compromised the tumor's blood supply, so that direct drug delivery is impaired. Chemotherapy may be useful for palliation in patients with few symptoms. Rapid physiologic deterioration of patients caused by the common complications of non–small cell lung cancer limits the clinician's ability to evaluate the effectiveness of chemotherapy. It generally is believed that the high risk of toxicity outweighs the minimum improvement in the patient's quality of life or survival.

Patients who have not received previous chemotherapy, who can still move about, and who are maintaining their weight seem to respond better to chemotherapy and to survive longer. The highest response rate has been observed in regimens containing cisplatin.

Other criteria used to determine the patient's eligibility for chemotherapy include no medical contraindications, evidence of disease progression, the presence of measurable disease, a life expectancy of longer than 2 months, and a clear understanding of the risks and benefits associated with treatment.

For patients with small cell lung cancer (SCLC) chemotherapy is the treatment of choice. Three drug regimens have been found to be the most effective. Cyclophosphamide is the cornerstone of SCLC chemotherapy. Clinical trials currently under way include (1) intensification strategies, in which high drug doses are administered at specified intervals during treatment; (2) cross-over regimens, in which specific non-cross-resistant drugs are alternated; and (3) the use of high drug doses with autologous bone marrow transplant.

Endobronchial Laser Therapy

Palliation of symptoms caused by obstructive primary or secondary cancers can be achieved with laser therapy, preferably with the YAG laser. Debulking the tumor can relieve hemoptysis, distal pneumonitis, and atelectasis and death by strangulation. A rigid bronchoscope is used to remove the tumor.

Photodynamic Therapy

Photodynamic therapy (PDT) is used for treatment of both small, early cancers and bulky, obstructing lesions. Usually a photosensitizer called hematoporphyrin derivative (Hpd) is administered, which localizes in the tumor. It is then activated by visible light, usually the argon pump dye laser. The treatment is useful only for patients with small, early cancer who are deemed inoperable for medical reasons or those with small, multiple cancers.

Sclerosis

Patients who develop malignant pleural effusion may experience some relief of symptoms with the use of tetracycline to sclerose the lung. The effect of the sclerosis is to prevent fluid accumulation, which impairs the patient's breathing and can also be quite painful. Sclerosis is accomplished by instilling the medication through a thoracostomy tube, with the patient having been premedicated with 5 to 10 mg of morphine sulfate. After the tetracycline has been instilled, the tube is clamped for 2 hours, during which time the patient is turned from side to side, onto the stomach, and into the Trendelenburg and reverse Trendelenburg positions every 15 minutes to ensure equal distribution of the medication. The tube then is unclamped and left to drain for 12 to 24 hours, after which time it is removed if drainage is minimal. Sclerosing can be repeated again in 24 hours if necessary.

1 Assess

ASSESSMENT	OBSERVATIONS
Respiratory	Chronic cough, nonproductive or productive; change in sputum volume or odor; dyspnea; orthopnea; tachypnea; wheezing; dull chest pain; fatigue; chest tightness; frequent upper respiratory infections (URIs); hemoptysis; hoarseness; fever; clubbed fingers; enlarged neck with venous distention; shoulder and arm pain with paresthesia
Nutritional	Fatigue, weight loss, anorexia
Psychosocial	Fear

2 Diagnose

NURSING DIAGNOSIS	SUBJECTIVE FINDINGS	OBJECTIVE FINDINGS
Ineffective airway clearance related to bronchial obstruction secondary to tumor invasion	Complains of difficulty breathing	Wheezing, tachypnea, productive or nonproductive cough, dyspnea, labored or irregular breathing
Altered nutrition: less than body requirements related to fatigue and dyspnea	Reports decreased appetite and fatigue	Weight loss; decreased intake of food and fluid; dyspnea

NURSING DIAGNOSIS	SUBJECTIVE FINDINGS	OBJECTIVE FINDINGS
Activity intolerance related to generalized weakness	Complains of fatigue, dyspnea	Dyspneic during activity; decreased activity level
Fear related to cancer, its treatment and prognosis	Expresses fear of disease, treatment, and possibility of death	Appears sad, withdrawn, angry, and depressed

 PLAN

Patient goals

1. The patient will have a patent airway.
2. The patient's nutritional status will improve.
3. The patient will be able to perform usual activities without fatigue or dyspnea.
4. The patient will be less fearful about the diagnosis, treatment, and prognosis.

4 IMPLEMENT*

NURSING DIAGNOSIS	NURSING INTERVENTIONS	RATIONALE
Ineffective airway clearance related to bronchial obstruction secondary to tumor invasion	Auscultate lungs for rhonchi, crackles, or wheezing.	To determine adequacy of gas exchange and extent of airway obstruction from secretions.
	Assess symmetry of chest expansion, depth and rate of inspiration, and use of accessory muscles.	To assess ease of gas exchange.
	Assess characteristics of secretions: quantity, color, consistency, odor; note hemoptysis.	To detect presence of infection or bleeding; infection is indicated by increased, thick and/or yellow secretions that may have a foul odor.
	Assess patient's hydration status: skin turgor, mucous membranes, tongue, intake and output over 24 h, Hct.	To determine need for fluids; fluids are needed if skin turgor is poor, mucous membranes and tongue are dry, intake >output, and/or hematocrit is elevated.
	Monitor arterial blood gases.	To determine acid-base balance and need for oxygen.
	Monitor chest x-rays.	To determine extent and location of lung involvement.
	Monitor results of sputum cytology.	To determine presence of cancer cells.
	Assist patient with coughing as needed.	Coughing removes secretions.

*Pages 63-67 modified from Wilson and Thompson.[63]

NURSING DIAGNOSIS	NURSING INTERVENTIONS	RATIONALE
	Position patient in proper body alignment for optimum breathing pattern (head of bed up 45 degrees; if tolerated, up to 90 degrees).	Secretions move by gravity as position changes; elevating head of bed moves abdominal content away from diaphragm to enhance diaphragmatic contraction.
	Administer humidified oxygen as ordered.	To supply supplemental oxygen and reduce the work of breathing.
	Assist patient with ambulation and position changes (turning side to side).	Secretions move by gravity as position changes.
	Increase room humidification.	To humidify secretions and facilitate their elimination.
	Help patient use blow bottles and incentive spirometry.	Requires deep breathing, which prevents atelectasis by filling alveoli with air.
	Encourage increased fluid intake to 1.5 to 2 L/day unless contraindicated.	To liquify and thin secretions so they can be expectorated more easily.
	Help patient with oral hygiene as needed.	To remove taste of secretions.
Altered nutrition: less than body requirements related to fatigue and dyspnea	Assess dietary habits and needs.	To help individualize the diet.
	Weigh patient weekly.	As nutrition improves, the patient's weight will increase.
	Auscultate bowel sounds.	To document gastrointestinal peristalsis.
	Assess psychologic factors (e.g., depression, anger).	To identify effect of psychologic factors that may decrease food and fluid intake.
	Monitor albumin and lymphocytes.	To assess adequate visceral protein needed for the immune system.
	Measure midarm circumference and triceps skinfold.	To assess protein and fat stores, which indicate malnutrition.
	Provide oxygen while eating as ordered.	To reduce dyspnea by reducing the work of breathing.
	Encourage oral care before meals.	To remove taste of sputum that may curb appetite.
	Provide frequent, small meals.	To lessen fatigue.
	Administer antiemetics before meals.	To reduce nausea that may be interfering with eating.
	Provide foods in appropriate consistency for eating.	To require less energy to eat foods, thereby reducing oxygen requirement.

NURSING DIAGNOSIS	NURSING INTERVENTIONS	RATIONALE
	Provide high-protein diet.	To support immune system.
	Administer vitamins as ordered.	To supplement diet.
Activity intolerance related to generalized weakness	Observe response to activity.	To determine extent of tolerance.
	Identify factors contributing to intolerance (e.g., stress, side effects of drugs).	When causative factors for weakness can be identified, interventions can be planned to counteract their effect.
	Assess patient's sleep patterns.	May document a causative factor of weakness.
	Plan rest periods between activities.	To reduce fatigue by providing additional rest.
	Perform activities for patient until he can perform them.	To meet patient's need without causing fatigue.
	Provide progressive increase in activity as tolerated.	To slowly increase the number and endurance of activities as tolerance allows and promote as much independence as possible.
	Provide oxygen as needed.	To decrease work of breathing during activity.
	Instruct patient or family member in use of equipment.	To ensure proper use and decrease frustration of users.
	Keep frequently used objects within reach.	To provide convenient use for patient; decreases oxygen demand.
	Problem solve with patient to determine methods of conserving energy while performing tasks (e.g., sit on stool while shaving; dry skin after bath by wrapping in terry cloth robe instead of drying skin with a towel).	To identify ways to conserve energy, thereby using less oxygen and producing less carbon dioxide.
Fear related to cancer, its treatment and prognosis	Assess appetite, weight loss, sleep patterns, mobility, and constipation.	Depression may be indicated by decreased appetite, weight loss, inability to sleep or sleeping more than usual, decreased activity, and/or constipation.
	Assess presence and quality of support system.	To determine if people are available to patient and if they are supportive, ambivalent, or disruptive.
	Monitor changes in communication patterns with others.	Changes to withdrawal or silence may indicate depression.

NURSING DIAGNOSIS	NURSING INTERVENTIONS	RATIONALE
	Monitor expressions such as worthlessness, anxiety, powerlessness, abandonment, or exhaustion.	To assess patient's state of mind and guide the nurse's communication with patient.
	Monitor ongoing coping such as withdrawal, denial, rationalization, compliance, dependency.	To assess patient's current coping strategies.
	Encourage eating a balanced diet, regular sleeping habits, active or passive exercise, and comfort measures.	To ensure that physiologic needs are met while patient is unable to do so independently.
	Accept patient's behavior at current level.	To develop trust as the basis for all other interventions.
	Listen and accept expressions of anger without personalizing reaction.	To foster constructive expression of anger and negative feelings.
	Help patient use physical expression geared to his physical capabilities (e.g., walking, punching a pillow).	Physical activity can be used as a means to express anger.
	Encourage patient to keep a "gripe list"; discuss list with patient if patient agrees.	To allow patient to write about and express anger.
	Encourage patient to identify, redefine situation, obtain needed information, generate alternatives, and focus on solutions.	To support coping, problem solving, and decision making.
	Respect patient's need for privacy.	To allow patient and others to grieve together.
	Use humor with patient as appropriate.	To improve mood and self-view.
	Administer antidepressants as ordered.	To improve depressive mood.
Knowledge deficit	See Patient Teaching.	

5 EVALUATE

PATIENT OUTCOME	DATA INDICATING THAT OUTCOME IS REACHED
Airway is patent.	Airways are clear and breathing occurs without secretions; breath sounds and chest x-ray are clear; cough has subsided.
Nutritional status has improved.	Patient has gained weight and is eating a balanced diet. Albumin = 3.2-4.5 g/dl Lymphocytes = 2,100 or 35%-40% per ml^3 blood Triceps skinfold = 12 mm (men), 23 mm (women) Midarm circumference = 32.7 cm (men), 29.2 cm (women)

PATIENT OUTCOME	DATA INDICATING THAT OUTCOME IS REACHED
Patient performs usual activities without fatigue or dyspnea.	Patient performs self-care activities.
Progress is demonstrated in lessening fear.	Patient talks about diagnosis and treatment options.

PATIENT TEACHING

1. Encourage patient to stop smoking, and encourage family members to stop also.
2. Teach importance of exercising to tolerance each day.
3. Teach name, action, dosage, frequency of administration, and side effects of medications.
4. Encourage eating a diet high in protein and calories.
5. Identify resources in the community, such as the American Cancer Society and the American Lung Association, that can help the patient and family with information, support groups, and equipment needs.
6. Instruct the patient and family to notify the physician if the patient experiences any side effects from medications or signs of recurrence such as shoulder or arm pain, difficulty in memory, fatigue, weight loss, increased coughing, or hemoptysis.

CHAPTER 5

Breast Cancer

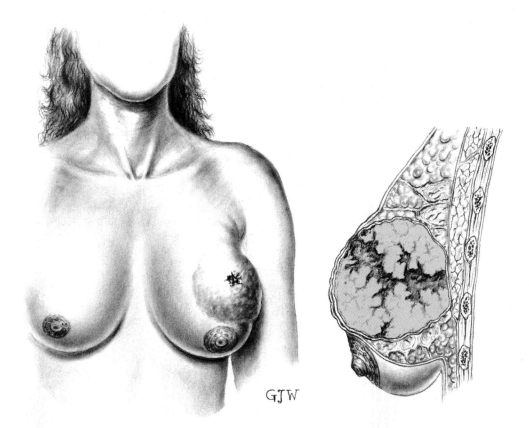

GJW

Breast cancer is the most common malignancy among American women. The American Cancer Society predicted that 150,000 women would be diagnosed with breast cancer in 1991, and that 44,300 would die. In contrast, breast cancer accounts for less than 1% of male cancers. Although breast cancer in men usually is diagnosed at an older age and in a more advanced stage, the pathology, pattern of metastasis, and prognosis are similar to those for women. Breast cancer is believed to be a systemic disease, with the possibility of occult distant metastases occurring early in the disease with or without lymph node involvement.

One of nine women will be diagnosed with breast cancer during her lifetime. Women consider this disease their most serious health problem and frequently equate a diagnosis of breast cancer with loss of a breast and, in many instances, death.

Elderly women (those over 65 years of age) have twice the incidence of breast cancer that women age 45 to 64 do. In the 55 or older age group, 50% more patients have metastatic disease at presentation than do younger women.

EPIDEMIOLOGY

Breast cancer is a multifactorial problem. The major risk factors are shown in the box at right. Other etiologic factors are obesity, a diet high in fat, and use of high doses of exogenous estrogens. It is important to remember, however, that only 25% of cases of breast cancer are associated with known risk factors.

Although the highest incidence of breast cancer occurs in women between 50 to 59 years of age, there is a first-peak occurrence in premenopausal or menopausal women 45 to 49 years of age.

The 5-year survival rate for localized breast cancer is 85% for white women and 79% for black women. Once the disease spreads beyond the breast, the survival rates drop dramatically. Only 48% of whites and 32% of blacks are diagnosed while the cancer is in a localized stage. The differences in survival rate and stage of disease at diagnosis are believed to be the result of differing socioeconomic factors. Breast cancer is the leading cause of cancer deaths among women 15 to 54 years of age.

The most important prognostic factor is the stage of the disease. Of patients with stage I disease, 60% to 75% are cured with local treatment. Women with a higher risk of recurrence in this group have negative estrogen receptor assay, high nuclear grade, and blood vessel and lymphatic invasion.

Among patients with stage II disease, the prognosis depends on the degree of nodal involvement (see box).

PATHOPHYSIOLOGY

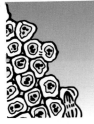

Most breast malignancies occur in the upper outer quadrant (Figure 5-1). More than 75% of breast cancers are invasive ductal carcinomas, usually manifesting as a single, unilateral, solid, irregular, poorly delineated, nonmobile, painless mass. This type grows as a fibrotic, stellate mass with long, tentacled extensions that radiate from a central dense core, invading and distorting surrounding breast structures.

The mean diameter of a lesion detected by a woman on self-examination is 3 to 3.5 centimeters, a size associated with a greater than 50% incidence of occult axillary lymph node metastases.

SIGNS AND SYMPTOMS

A painless mass or thickening in the breast is the most common presenting symptom. Nipple discharge, although more commonly associated with benign breast conditions or hormonal imbalance, can be a sign of malignancy if described as spontaneous, unilateral, from a single duct, watery and clear, serosanguineous, or bloody in color.

MAJOR RISK FACTORS FOR BREAST CANCER

- A mother, sister, grandmother, or aunt who has or has had breast cancer (the risk is increased if the relative developed the disease before menopause and/or has bilateral disease)
- Menarche before 12 years of age
- Menopause after 55 years of age
- No children, or first child after 30 years of age
- Excessive exposure to ionizing radiation, especially before 35 years of age
- Fibrocystic change (atypical epithelial hyperplasia)
- Personal history of breast cancer
- Personal history of other cancers, especially endometrial, ovarian, colon, or thyroid types

PROGNOSIS AND NODAL INVOLVEMENT

Number of nodes	Metastatic recurrence
1-3	50%-60%
4-10	75%-85%
> 10	Even worse prognosis

Signs of advanced disease are skin or nipple dimpling; puckering or retraction; changes in breast size, shape, or contour; skin edema; discoloration; dilated superficial blood vessels; frank skin ulcerations, and a hard, fixed mass in the axilla (Figure 5-2).

Paget's carcinoma manifests crusting, oozing, and bleeding on the nipple surface. Inflammatory breast cancer shows skin erythema and edema with underlying induration. Medullary, colloid, papillary, and intracystic cancer may manifest a well-delineated mass of medium consistency that may feel slightly mobile.

COMPLICATIONS

Metastases, most commonly to lung, liver, bone
Hypercalcemia
Spinal cord compression
Brachial plexopathy
Pleural effusion
Pathologic fracture

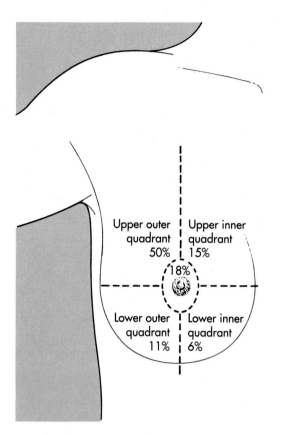

FIGURE 5-1
Right breast. Location of breast cancers. About half of all breast cancers develop in the upper outer quadrant of the breast.

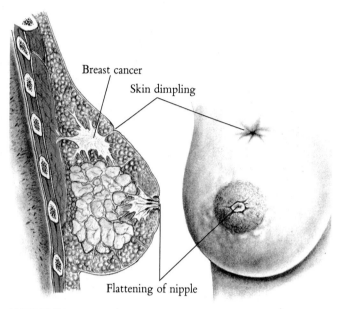

FIGURE 5-2
Clinical signs of breast cancer: nipple retraction and dimpling of skin. (From Seidel et al.[53])

DIAGNOSTIC STUDIES AND FINDINGS

Diagnostic Test	Findings
Clinical examination	Palpation of one or more lesions, usually a painless mass or thickening; restricted mobility of lesion; changes in skin texture (i.e., dimpling, orange peel); skin edema; discoloration of skin; dilated superficial blood vessels; change in breast size, shape, contour; nipple discharge; nipple retraction;
Mammogram	Solid nodule with ill-defined borders; clustered microcalcifications
Biopsy	
Lesion	Evidence of malignant cells
Axillary lymph nodes	Evidence of malignant cells
Estrogen receptors and progestin receptors	<3 fmol/mcp receptor negative tumor >10 fmol/mcp receptor positive tumor
Carcinoembryonic antigen (CEA)	Elevated in metastatic liver disease
S-phase index	>5%-8%
Ploidy	Aneuploid DNA

MEDICAL MANAGEMENT

SURGERY

Lumpectomy: Wide excision and removal of tumor and margin of healthy tissue.

Partial mastectomy: Simple excision of tumor and wider margin of healthy tissue.

Quadrantectomy: Removal of one quarter of breast.

Mastectomy

Subcutaneous: Removal of all breast tissue while preserving overlying skin and nipple-areolar complex.

Total (simple): Complete removal of breast tissue and tail of Spence.

Modified radical: Removal of breast and axillary lymph nodes.

Radical: Removal of breast, underlying pectoral muscles, and axillary nodes.

Superradical: Removal of internal mammary lymphatic chain with breast, pectoral muscles, and axillary lymph nodes.

Breast reconstruction

RADIATION THERAPY

Bradytherapy: Implantation of radioactive sources.

Teletherapy: Use of external beam (photon or electron).

Other: Regional node irradiation.

ADJUVANT THERAPY

Combination chemotherapy: CMF (cyclophosphamide, methotrexate, 5-fluorouracil); CMFVP (CMF with vincristine and prednisone); CA (cyclophosphamide and doxorubicin); CAF (cyclophosphamide, doxorubicin, 5-fluorouracil).

Antiestrogen therapy (ablative): Tamoxifen citrate.

Estrogens (additive): Diethylstilbestrol (DES); ethinyl estradiol.

Androgens (additive): Fluoxymesterone; testosterone; methyltestosterone.

Progestins (additive): Megestrol acetate; medroxyprogesterone.

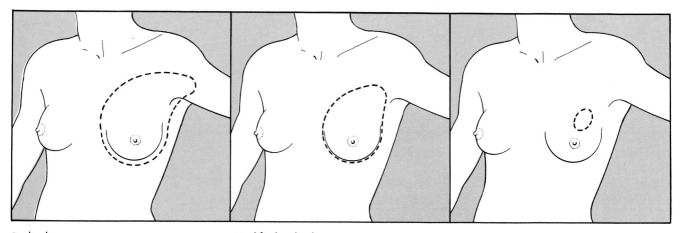

Radical mastectomy   Modified radical mastectomy   Lumpectomy

FIGURE 5-3
The surgical treatment for breast cancer is determined by the size of the tumor, whether it has spread, the woman's age and physical condition, and her preference. Shown above are the radical mastectomy, modified radical, and lumpectomy. A simple mastectomy (not shown) includes removal of the breast and some nodes.

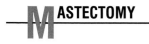ASTECTOMY

Mastectomy, which is still the most common surgical intervention, may be as simple as the removal of all breast tissue while preserving the overlying skin and nipple-areolar complex to radical removal of the internal mammary lymphatic chain with the breast, pectoral muscles, and axillary lymph nodes (Figures 5-3 and 5-4).

COMPLICATIONS

(uncommon in all but radical procedures, which are done less frequently)

Infection in the incision line   Seroma
Lymphedema   Nerve injury
Impaired shoulder mobility

Preprocedural Care

The nurse bases patient preparation on plans for intervention during the initial surgery (one-step procedure) or a scheduled follow-up surgery (two-step procedure). The patient needs to know the types of dressings and equipment that will be used postoperatively, as well as plans for exercises, hand and arm care, and drainage tube management.

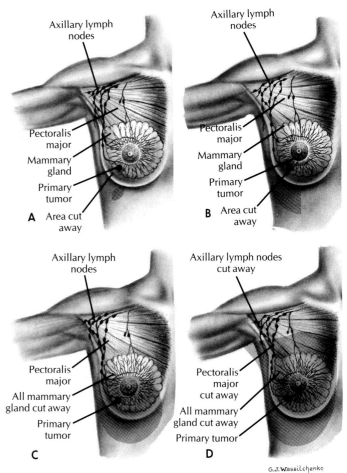

FIGURE 5-4
Surgical treatments for breast cancer highlighting anatomic structures involved. **A,** Lumpectomy (tylectomy). **B,** Quadrectomy (segmental resection). **C,** Total (simple) mastectomy. **D,** Radical mastectomy. (From Bobak et al.[7])

HAND AND ARM CARE INSTRUCTIONS

While the patient is in bed, position the affected arm on one small and one large pillow so that the wrist is slightly higher than the elbow, and the elbow is slightly higher than the shoulder.

The patient should get out of bed on the unaffected side.

Encourage the patient to perform ball-squeezing and range-of-motion exercises as instructed by the physical therapist.

Have the patient avoid using deodorants or antiperspirants until the stitches have been removed from the axilla and the wound has healed.

Encourage the patient to perform activities of daily living (ADL) as tolerated with the following precautions:

1. Wear canvas gloves when gardening.
2. Wear a long, padded glove on the affected arm when reaching into an oven.
3. Wear a thimble when sewing.
4. Wear rubber gloves when using harsh detergents or steel wool.
5. Apply hand lotion to prevent dry skin.
6. Use an electric razor for underarm shaving to avoid nicking the skin.
7. Do not allow injections, intravenous lines, blood to be drawn, or blood pressure to be taken on the affected arm.
8. Use insect repellent to avoid insect bites.
9. Avoid using constricting jewelry or clothing on the affected arm.
10. Use a sunscreen (SPF of 15 or greater), and avoid overexposure to the sun.
11. Use cuticle cream and a nail file to trim fingernails.
12. If the affected arm is burned, apply ice and leave it exposed to the air until the blister breaks. Then wash with soap and water, apply antiseptic solution (e.g., iodine), and cover the area with a bandage. Notify the health care provider if the area does not heal.
13. If the affected arm is cut, wash the area with soap and water, apply an antiseptic (e.g., iodine), and cover the area with a bandage. Notify the health care provider if the area does not heal.
14. Call the health care provider if redness, pain, or increased swelling develops.

From Brown M, Kiss M, Outlaw E, and Viamontes C.[9]

Postprocedural Care

Patients who undergo modified radical or partial mastectomy with axillary node dissection usually have drains placed at the time of surgery. These drains help prevent the collection of serous fluid (seroma), which can precipitate postoperative pain and infection and impair wound healing. Because patients are being discharged earlier, they may go home with one or more drains still in place.

The patient should be taught to change the dressing, assess the appearance of the drain site, empty the drainage container, and record the amount of drainage. The patient should also know to report to her health care provider any redness or drainage around the drain, fever, blood in the drain, and inability to keep the container flat.

Hand and arm care instruction is essential to prevent infection after axillary node dissection (see box). The patient will learn appropriate exercises as well. The use of pain medication to regain the preoperative activity level is also important.

The incidence of phantom breast experience varies from 8% to 64%, with time of onset immediately after surgery to up to 4 years later. The areas involved usually have been the total breast or nipple. The incidence is greater in younger women. Twinges and itching are the sensations most frequently reported. The nurse should reassure the patient that these sensations are real and probably will become less noticeable as time passes. If the sensations cause intense discomfort, the physician should be consulted about medical or surgical interventions.

BREAST RECONSTRUCTION

In patients who have undergone a mastectomy for local recurrence, a transverse rectus abdominis musculocutaneous (TRAM) flap from the abdomen can provide sufficient tissue for breast reconstruction. Patients who have had irradiation to the internal mammary lymph nodes can more safely have a pedicle based on the contralateral internal thoracic and superior epigastric vessels (Figure 5-5).

The tissue expander is a silicone breast implant with an attached valve. During the postoperative period, it is gradually filled with saline by percutaneous injection, thus stretching local breast tissues. The surgeon can later insert a larger, permanent silicone breast implant. The controversy surrounding the safety of silicone implants should be discussed with the surgeon prior to selection of this procedure.

Nipple-areolar reconstruction usually is performed as a separate procedure after breast reconstruction and when satisfactory breast symmetry has been achieved.

COMPLICATIONS

Infection in incision line or prosthesis pocket
Hematomas under skin flaps
Skin necrosis
Deflation of expander
Paresthesia of ipsilateral arm

Preprocedural Care

The nurse may use preoperative and postoperative photographs of breast reconstruction, as well as a visit from someone who has had the surgery, to reassure a patient who has voiced questions and concerns about the procedure. Preoperative teaching should include instruction about postoperative coughing, deep breathing, and pain management strategies. Information about tissue expanders, the inflation process, and possible complications can be initiated.

Postprocedural Care

The nurse should assess the skin for redness, swelling, drainage, odor, and tenderness, and the incision and flap for heat, blanching, and duskiness. Pressure on the flap or suture lines should be avoided. The patient should be kept warm and may receive nasal oxygen to increase circulation and oxygenation to the flap. Further explanation about the inflation procedure will be helpful to the patient.

REACH TO RECOVERY PROGRAM

Sponsored by the American Cancer Society (ACS), the Reach to Recovery program sends qualified, trained volunteers who have experienced breast cancer to visit the patient in the hospital by appointment after the physician authorizes the visit. If the patient wishes to be visited before or after the surgery at home, she may call the local unit of the ACS.

The volunteer visitor provides literature and other useful materials such as a temporary prosthesis. In addition to relating her own positive experience, offering support, and serving as a role model, she can provide information about breast conservation and reconstruction surgeries, radiation therapy, and chemotherapy.

The program is designed for one face-to-face visit with a follow-up telephone call. Support groups are available.

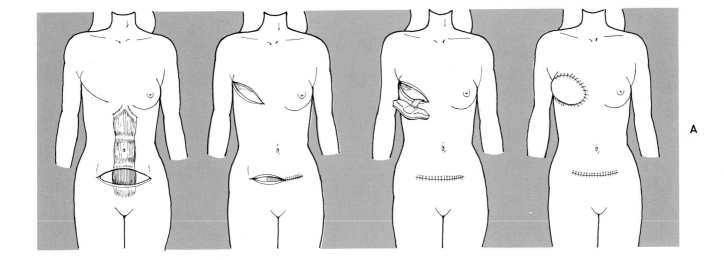

FIGURE 5-5

Breast reconstruction. **A,** The myocutaneous flap has made reconstruction possible for most patients who have undergone mastectomy—even when the pectoralis muscles have been removed or when nerve damage has resulted in muscle atrophy. The flap receives its blood supply from muscle but it can include an overlying layer of skin. At the same time that this procedure is done, a silicone breast implant may be inserted or, if enough pedicle tissue is available, no implant is needed. In rectus abdominis reconstruction, an abdominoplasty is performed, bringing the rectus muscle up on a superior pedicle. **B,** An alternative procedure brings the latissimus dorsi muscle from the posterior aspect of the chest.

RADIATION THERAPY

In the treatment of breast cancer, radiation therapy may be used as primary or adjuvant therapy. It may be delivered by means of an external beam (high-energy photons from a linear accelerator) or by using interstitial iridium implants (^{192}Ir) to surround the malignant tissue (bradytherapy). A "boost dose" may be directed to the excisional site with the implantation of radioactive sources or use of the electron beam. Radiation may be used palliatively in stage IV disease to relieve pain caused by bony metastases.

SIDE EFFECTS

Fatigue
Skin reactions

Preprocedural Care

(See p. 205 for use of external beam therapy.)

The patient receiving iridium should understand that it is implanted surgically by inserting hollow plastic catheters in parallel rows into the involved breast; the number and location depend on the size of the breast, the location and size of the original tumor, and the dosage of radiation to be delivered (see Figure 5-6). The catheters are placed in the operating room. When the patient awakens in the recovery room, she is taken to the simulation room in the radiation oncology department, where x-rays are taken to calculate the length and strength of radiation material needed in each catheter. Localization x-rays are used to check the position of the catheters before afterloading (placement of iridium in the catheters) is done.

The radioactive strands are placed in the catheters in the patient's private room and secured by a button at the end of each catheter. A dressing is placed over the site, and a thin, rubberized lead shield is placed over the dressing. The patient should understand that the private room and limited contact with nurses and visitors are to protect them from exposure to the radiation.

Postprocedural Care

The patient may have a feeling of pressure or heaviness at the site of the catheters, which should be treated with a prescribed analgesic. The radioactive material is left in place about 24 hours, and both it and the catheters are removed in the patient's room, after which a dry gauze dressing is applied and the patient is discharged.

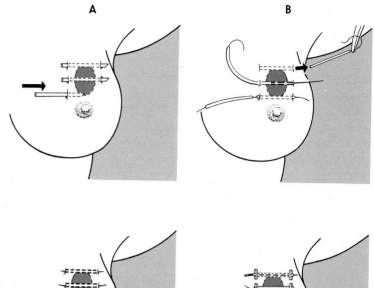
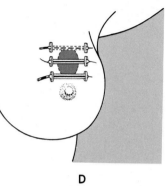
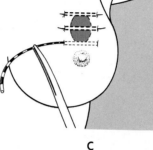

FIGURE 5-6
Radiation implants. **A,** Placement of hollow needles. **B,** Replacement of hollow needles by plastic catheters. **C,** Loading of iridium sources. **D,** Interstitial implant in place with buttons to secure catheters.

The response of breast tissue to radiation depends on the dosage and on tissue sensitivity. Acute, localized inflammatory reactions such as erythema can cause skin ulceration weeks after treatment (see page 249 for care of skin reactions). Residual shrinkage of the breast and changes in skin color may last several months. In the axilla, fibrotic tissue may partially obstruct the lymphatics, causing lymphedema. Patients must also be observed for the development of pneumonitis and fibrosis.

The nurse should urge the patient to avoid irritating garments and topical preparations that contain fragrance (e.g., deodorant). Exercise should be performed to maintain muscle tone and prevent lymphedema. A padded bra can be worn to compensate for breast shrinkage.

CHEMOTHERAPY

In breast cancer, adjuvant chemotherapy may be recommended for disease beyond stage I and for stage I cancer in selected cases. The best results occur in premenopausal women with hormone-dependent (estrogen receptor positive [ER+]) tumors. Single-agent therapy is rarely used, but it may be used with elderly individuals who may not tolerate more aggressive therapy.

The mainstay of therapy for premenopausal women with 1 to 3 positive lymph nodes has been CMF (cyclophosphamide, methotrexate, and 5-fluorouracil). Other frequently used combinations are CAF (cyclophosphamide, doxorubicin, and 5-fluorouracil), CMFVP (CMF with vincristine and prednisone), and CA (cyclophosphamide and doxorubicin). Therapy usually lasts 6 months, and the chemotherapy may be combined with hormones. For example, antiestrogens frequently are prescribed for postmenopausal patients with ER+ tumors and stage II disease.

Hormonal therapy is based on the premise that the development of breast cancer may depend on female hormones. Thus hormonal manipulation, which may inhibit cancer growth, may be (1) additive, increasing the level of circulating hormones such as estrogens, progestins, androgens, or glucocorticoids; or (2) ablative, which includes surgical removal or irradiation of the ovaries and adrenal or pituitary glands or administration of medications that inhibit the production or effect of specific hormones. Because only one third of women with breast cancer respond to hormonal therapy, it is important to predict which patients are most likely to benefit with resultant increased survival time. Postmenopausal women have more favorable responses.

Almost all aspects of breast cancer management are enmeshed in controversy. What is the treatment of choice for newly diagnosed stage I breast cancer? What factors should be considered when making such a decision (i.e., recent survival data, treatment side effects, or cosmetic results)? How are patients selected for different types of surgery, for radiation therapy, hormonal therapy, and for adjuvant chemotherapy? The physician's criteria for recommending treatment options are the size and extent of the tumor, the margins of resection, and the tumor's histologic pattern.

Legislation in some states mandates that the physician discuss all breast cancer treatment options with the woman, so that she has an active role in the decision-making process. Whatever the treatment decision, the best prognostic indicators are tumor size and nodal status.

1 ASSESS

ASSESSMENT	OBSERVATIONS
Skin	Redness, warmth; open wound; tenderness; drainage (serous, serosanguineous); flaking, peeling; swelling, as in the arm on the affected side
Vital signs	Tachycardia; hypertension; altered respiratory rate
Psychosocial	Fear; anxiety; withdrawal; avoidance of physical intimacy; restlessness; fight or flight behavior; increased alertness

→ › ›

2 DIAGNOSE

NURSING DIAGNOSIS	SUBJECTIVE FINDINGS	OBJECTIVE FINDINGS
Potential impaired skin integrity related to surgery, node dissection, or radiation therapy	Complaints of itching, pain, drainage at site of surgery and/or radiation; pain or heaviness in arm at site of node dissection	Redness, warmth; tenderness to touch; drainage; flaking; lymphedema
Pain related to surgery, node dissection, or pressure of tumor	Description of sensation, location, aggravating and relieving factors	Guarding behavior; facial mask of pain; altered muscle tone; diaphoresis; tachycardia, hypertension; altered respiratory rate; pupillary dilation
Body image disturbance related to alteration in breast caused by presence of tumor	Feelings of shame and disfigurement; feelings of powerlessness; altered sense of femininity and sexual attractiveness	Social withdrawal; isolation; avoidance of sexual interaction and physical intimacy
Decisional conflict related to treatment options	Expresses anxiety and fear about need to choose among treatment options; delayed decision making	Irritability; withdrawal; restlessness; increased muscle tension
Fear related to nature of cancer	Increased tension; apprehension; impulsiveness	Tachycardia, hypertension; increased alertness; wide-eyed; fight or flight behavior

3 PLAN

Patient goals

1. The patient's skin will be intact and free of infection in the area of disruption.
2. The patient will obtain relief from pain.
3. The patient will accept the change in her body and incorporate it into her self-concept.
4. The patient will select and implement a course of treatment that is informed, consistent with personal values, and congruent with behavior.
5. The patient's fear will be eased.

4 IMPLEMENT

NURSING DIAGNOSIS	NURSING INTERVENTIONS	RATIONALE
Potential impaired skin integrity related to surgery, node dissection, or radiation therapy	Cleanse skin frequently; apply warm, moist compresses.	To prevent infection and promote circulation and drainage.
	Apply antibiotic ointment and sterile dressing; expose draining area to air (depends on patient's immunocompetence); elevate arm.	To prevent infection and promote healing and to enhance venous return.

NURSING DIAGNOSIS	NURSING INTERVENTIONS	RATIONALE
	Observe for increased drainage or change in its character, skin changes (color, dimpling), swelling, or skin lesions.	To detect infection or further breakdown.
Pain related to surgery, node dissection, or pressure of tumor	Administer analgesic as prescribed; monitor character, intensity, and frequency of pain.	To relieve pain and to evaluate the effectiveness of the analgesic (and determine the need for a change in amount, route, or frequency).
	Teach patient to use relaxation, guided imagery, and diversional activities.	To enhance analgesic effect or to decrease the need for analgesic.
	Use massage, heat, and cold, as appropriate.	To increase comfort.
Body image disturbance related to alteration in breast caused by presence of tumor	Help patient identify personal meaning of loss of breast.	To clarify fears, concerns, and needs brought on by loss of breast.
	Encourage patient to discuss change in her body with husband or significant other.	To use social support.
	Refer patient to appropriate resources (e.g., health care providers, support group).	To provide external support.
Decisional conflict related to treatment options	Explain treatment options in a nonjudgmental way; use objective, factual materials (such as reports) and encourage the patient to discuss the options with her family or significant others; provide sufficient time for making a decision.	To enable the patient to select an option consistent with her values and expectations.
Fear related to nature of cancer	Encourage patient to talk about specific fears and feelings about each fear.	To help patient clarify what fears are.
	Help patient identify previously helpful coping skills, and teach patient newer coping skills.	To use present skills and add to choices.
	Deal with distorted perceptions and misinformation.	To dispel misconceptions.
	Encourage use of such comfort measures as music, religious practices, and presence of family and friends.	To distract self from focus on fears.

→ › ›

5 EVALUATE

PATIENT OUTCOME	DATA INDICATING THAT OUTCOME IS REACHED
Skin will be intact and free of infection in the area of disruption.	The patient's skin is clean, dry, and warm and has normal color and turgor.
The patient has obtained relief from pain.	The patient's facial expression is calm and relaxed, and she reports that she is comfortable; vital signs are within normal limits.
The patient has accepted the change in her body image.	The patient expresses acceptance of altered body image and altered self-concept.
A treatment option has been selected and implemented.	The patient has chosen a course of treatment that is assessed as being informed and consistent with her personal values.
The patient's fears have been resolved.	The patient acknowledges her fears of suffering and dying and is able to focus on the need for further treatment and follow-up.

PATIENT TEACHING

1. Teach the patient the importance of caring for the skin at the site of the surgery, as well as the arm on the affected side.
2. Teach the patient the importance of continuing breast self-examination and mammography on the unaffected breast. (See Patient Teaching Guide on Breast Self-Examination.)
3. Teach the patient to use nonpharmacologic interventions such as relaxation exercises, guided imagery, and diversional activities to cope with pain and fear.
4. Encourage the patient to use her social support network, as well as such resources as the Reach to Recovery program, to cope with her altered body image.

CHAPTER 6

Colorectal and Other Gastrointestinal Cancers

Colorectal Cancers

Each year approximately 155,000 new cases of **colorectal cancer** are diagnosed in the United States. These tumors occur almost equally in men and women, usually after the age of 40; 93% occur after the age of 50.

The incidence of colorectal cancer is second only to that of lung cancer. Although colorectal cancer is a disease of aging, the prognosis in the young (under age 40) is very poor. Based on a recent review of malpractice claims and lawsuits for failure to diagnose colon cancer, physicians are being urged to be more alert to the possibility of colorectal cancer in younger patients. The specific recommendations include (1) asking about a family history of colon cancer and (2) performing a baseline colonoscopy at age 30 on those who have such a history. The colonoscopy should be repeated every 4 years if one family member is affected or every 3 years if two first-degree relatives are affected. If the individual has rectal bleeding or polyps, endoscopy, sigmoidoscopy, and a barium enema should be performed.

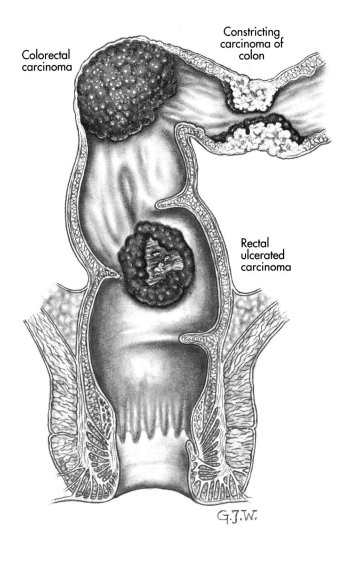

COLORECTAL CARCINOMA

EPIDEMIOLOGY

No definite external etiologic factors have been identified in colorectal cancer, although eating habits such as a diet heavy in refined carbohydrates are suspected. The dietary fiber found in fruits, vegetables, and bran may have a protective effect. Some researchers think that high-fiber diets shorten food's transit time and thus cut down on the amount of time that carcinogens are in contact with the colon.

Some conditions increase the risk of colorectal cancer, such as familial polyposis of the colon or rectum, chronic ulcerative colitis, diverticulosis, and villous adenomas of the colon. Exposure to asbestos has also been identified as a possible cause of these tumors. Families with a tendency to develop uterine, breast, or bladder cancer seem to be at high risk for developing colon cancer. Colorectal cancer also is more common among higher socioeconomic groups and urban populations. Although the incidence of the disease shows no gender or racial differences, African-Americans have a higher mortality rate and a less favorable 5-year survival rate.

PATHOPHYSIOLOGY

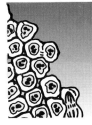

Ninety-five percent of colorectal tumors originate with the development of a benign, adenomatous polyp in the large bowel or rectum; this may degenerate into a malignant tumor over a period of 5 years or longer. Villous adenomas have a 40% to 50% chance of becoming malignant.

Most colorectal tumors are adenocarcinomas; others are carcinoid tumors, leiomyosarcomas, and lymphomas. Regional lymph nodes are involved in at least half of the patients at the time of diagnosis. Most colon tumors spread to periaortic nodes, whereas anal carcinomas spread into perineal nodes. Distant metastasis is most often to the liver and lungs.

The 5-year survival rate for patients with localized disease is 87% for colon tumors and 79% for rectal tumors. These rates are reduced by half with regional or distant involvement. Even with a large tumor and invasion of adjacent structures, the prognosis is favorable if appropriate treatment is provided. Only distant metastases preclude the possibility of a cure.

SIGNS AND SYMPTOMS

The most common symptom of colorectal cancer is rectal bleeding, followed by changes in bowel pattern (constipation or diarrhea), excessive flatus, distention, cramps, obstruction, and unexplained anemia. The type

---

RISK FACTORS FOR COLORECTAL CANCER

Average risk

Age 50 years or older (risk doubles after age 50 with each successive decade)

High risk

Inflammatory bowel disease
    Chronic ulcerative colitis
    Chronic granulomatous colitis
Familial polyposis syndrome
    Inherited adenomatosis
    Gardner's syndrome
    Turcot syndrome
    Oldfield's syndrome
    Juvenile polyposis
Familial cancer syndrome
Family history
    Colorectal cancer or sporadic colorectal adenomas
Past history
    Sporadic colorectal adenomas
    Colorectal cancer
    Breast, endometrial, or bladder cancer

---

of symptoms depends on the tumor's location. Left-sided colonic lesions produce altered bowel habits, decreased stool caliber (pencil-like), urgency to defecate, vague abdominal pain, and hemorrhoids. Right-sided colonic lesions may cause unexplained iron deficiency anemia and gastrointestinal tract bleeding. Tumors of the sigmoid colon are characterized by obstruction from napkin-ring growth. Rectal tumors are evidenced by gross rectal blood and tenesmus with a feeling of incomplete evacuation.

Cancer symptoms in the elderly may take the form of such generalized problems as confusion, weakness, weight loss, or "failure to thrive." For example, a change in bowel habits may be a symptom of colorectal cancer, or it may be due to other factors such as diet, fluid intake, lack of exercise, or medication.

FECAL OCCULT BLOOD SCREENING

- The test is simple and inexpensive.
- The test's predictive value increases with the individual's age. With a positive test result at the initial screening, the risk of colorectal cancer is 50% to 60% in the older age group.
- The survival rate for individuals with colorectal cancer could be increased from 55% to 85% with early detection.
- Reasons given for not participating in screening include lack of knowledge about the test and the perceived unpleasant nature of feces; other factors affecting participation include the person's age, ethnicity, education, income, eyesight, and literacy.

DIAGNOSTIC STUDIES AND FINDINGS

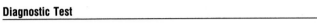

Diagnostic Test	Findings
Hematocrit	Below normal because of blood loss
Occult fecal blood test	Positive for blood
Digital rectal examination	Palpable lesion
Colonic visualization (barium enema, colonoscopy)	Suspicious lesion
Biopsy	Malignant cells
Carcinoembryonic antigen (CEA)	Elevated

MEDICAL MANAGEMENT

SURGERY

Local excision of well-differentiated rectal tumors
Resection of primary colon lesion with all mesentery that contains lymph nodes to which tumor is likely to spread, end-to-end anastomosis (only curative treatment)
En bloc resection of colon, small bowel, bladder, uterus, and/or ovaries
Surgical bypass for inoperable obstructing tumors, with creation of fecal stoma

RADIATION THERAPY

Intraoperative radiation therapy
Radiation seeds
External beam therapy for inoperable obstructing rectal tumors
Transanal irradiation
Postoperative adjuvant therapy with radiation sensitizers for tumors dissecting the bowel wall or with positive lymph nodes
Palliation

CHEMOTHERAPY

Adjuvant regimen of fluorouracil (5FU) with levamisole
Radiation sensitization with 5FU and metronidazole

ENDOSCOPIC LASER

For inoperable obstructing rectal tumors

SURGERY

Colon resection with disease-free margins is the goal of surgery. The tumor and its blood vessels are resected en bloc with proximal vascular and lymphatic structures. Biopsy of the liver and regional lymph nodes is done during the surgical procedure to determine the extent of disease. The tumor's size and location and evidence of metastasis determine the type and extent of surgery (Figure 6-1). Each patient is also evaluated on the basis of age, nutritional status, and presence of perforation or obstruction. In general, surgical treatment of colorectal cancer is as follows:

Tumor in upper rectum (12 cm from anal verge): anterior colectomy
Tumor in middle rectum (7 to 11 cm from anal verge): pull-through procedure
Tumor in lower rectum (7 cm or less from anal verge): abdominal perineal resection and colostomy
Tumor in right colon: right colectomy or colostomy
Tumor in left colon: colectomy or colostomy
Tumor in sigmoid colon: sigmoid resection

Surgery may also be done to relieve pain, odor, or bleeding. More extensive surgery, such as pelvic exenteration (removal of the bladder and rectum and creation of an ileal conduit and sigmoid colostomy), may be required in cases of extensive metastatic disease.

COMPLICATIONS

Infection
Paralytic ileus
Anastomotic leak with possible fistula formation
Stoma retraction or prolapse

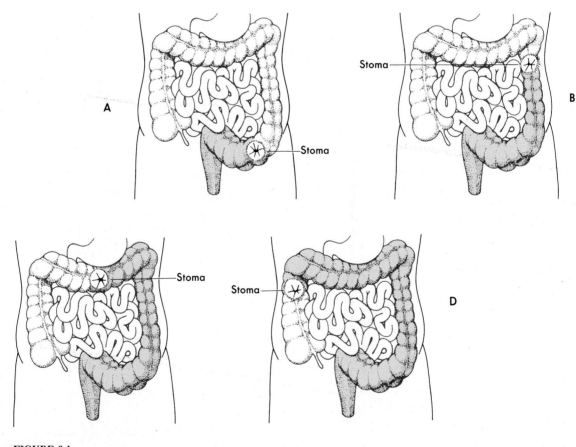

FIGURE 6-1
A, Sigmoid colostomy. **B,** Descending colostomy. **C,** Transverse colostomy. **D,** Ascending colostomy.
(From Beare and Myers.[5])

Preoperative Care

The patient will have some type of bowel preparation, which usually includes 2 or 3 days of liquid diets, a combination of laxatives or enemas, and oral antibiotics to sterilize the bowel. The antibiotic of choice may be neomycin, kanamycin, bacitracin, or erythromycin, each of which suppresses both anaerobic and aerobic organisms in the colon. This regimen is not used for the patient with an obstruction.

Other aspects of preoperative care include instruction in turning, coughing, and deep breathing; wound splinting; and leg exercises. The patient should know that after surgery he will have intravenous lines, a Foley catheter, a nasogastric tube, and abdominal dressings.

If a stoma is to be created, the enterostomal therapist should be notified so that the stoma site can be marked before surgery. The stoma should be away from the waistline, folds, scars, and the abdominal incision. The site usually is below the umbilicus and at the infraumbilical bulge, where the patient can see and reach the pouch easily (Figure 6-2).

Postoperative Care

The patient should be assessed for stable vital signs and return of bowel sounds. The dressing should be checked for drainage or bleeding and changed as needed. The nasogastric tube and Foley catheter should be checked for patency and amount and color of drainage. Accurate intake and output records must be kept to maintain the fluid and electrolyte balance. The stoma site should be observed for size, color (should be pink), and moisture. Drainage should be scant and serosanguineous.

Postoperative coughing, deep breathing, early ambulation, adequate nutrition, pain control, meticulous wound and stoma care, and patency of the nasogastric tube and Foley catheter are important aspects of nursing care for these patients.

Paralytic ileus, a common complication after abdominal surgery, produces the classic signs of increased abdominal girth, distention, nausea, and vomiting. Interventions include decompression of the bowel with a nasogastric tube, NPO status, and increased patient activity.

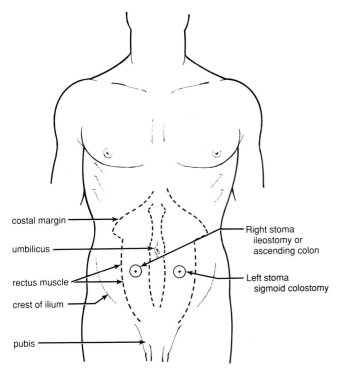

FIGURE 6-2
Best sites for stomas. (From Otto.[48])

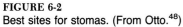

OSTOMY CARE

Includes pouch application, emptying of the pouch, and skin products

- Pouch selection is based on the site of the stoma, the patient's manual dexterity, the cost of the appliance, and the patient's preference. The pouch chosen should protect the skin and should be well fitted and odor free. Additional products are available to help control odor and protect the skin. Certain foods that cause odor should be avoided or eaten in moderation (see Patient Teaching Guide).

- Colostomy irrigations generally are discouraged; patients are taught to use food and fluids to maintain adequate bowel elimination.

- Special dietary needs, as well as restrictions (e.g., no seeds, nuts, excessive bulk, or foods in the cabbage family), focus not only on avoiding odor and gas but also on preventing obstruction. Certain medications may not be absorbed in the intestine but instead may be expelled through the colostomy.

- The patient should be given skin care products, including skin barriers, and taught how to use them.

- Changes in the patient's perception of body image and sexuality need to be addressed before and after surgery. An ostomy visitor may be most helpful to the patient in discussing such fears as rejection, disfigurement, and others' reactions to the ostomy. Sexual counseling may include discussing changes in sexual position, concealing underwear and nightwear, and impotence.

RADIATION THERAPY

Adjuvant radiation therapy, combined with surgical resection of all known disease, has reduced the incidence of local recurrence in patients with colorectal cancer. The primary advantage of preoperative radiation is to decrease the number of cancer cells that may spread locally or to distant sites during surgery. The advantage of waiting until after surgery is that therapy can be determined on the basis of surgical staging.

When given postoperatively, radiation therapy is initiated 3 to 6 weeks after surgery. The total dosage of 4,500 to 5,500 rad, fractionated over 5 to 6 weeks, is delivered by linear accelerator or a cobalt machine. The field of radiotherapy includes the tumor bed and the interior iliac and presacral nodes.

SIDE EFFECTS

Diarrhea or bloating	Skin reactions
Nausea	Vaginal dryness
Fatigue	Temporary sterility

Preprocedural Care

The patient should understand the importance of adequate nutritional status, caring for the skin, balancing activity with rest, and dealing with alterations in sexuality.

Postprocedural Care

The nurse should monitor the patient's weight, nutritional intake, and incidences of nausea and diarrhea. Interventions should focus on maintaining an adequate food and fluid intake while using medications and other measures to treat specific side effects (see box on Managing Diarrhea and Rectal Irritation).

The patient's skin should be assessed at each treatment and the guidelines for skin care reviewed. It is also important to discuss the patient's pattern of activity and rest to avoid severe fatigue.

Temporary sterility occurs in individuals receiving radiation therapy for rectal cancer because of the scattering effect of the radiation. If the patient or partner is of childbearing age, birth control measures should be used while the patient is undergoing radiation therapy. A woman over age 40 may have permanent arrest of menses. Intercourse may be uncomfortable because of dryness of the vaginal mucosa. In such cases a water-based lubricant should be used during intercourse. Douching is discouraged. Men undergoing radiation therapy may develop impotence at any time after radiation; those who experience it usually do not recover from it.

MANAGING DIARRHEA AND RECTAL IRRITATION

Eighty-five percent of patients receiving radiation to the bowel develop diarrhea. The severity of the diarrhea depends on the total radiation dose, preexisting lactose intolerance, and the patient's prior bowel habits. The diarrhea usually occurs within 2 weeks after treatment ends.

Nursing care

- Encourage the patient to avoid milk, alcohol, coffee, spices, fresh fruits and vegetables, high-fiber foods, and fried foods. Advise her to eat less irritating foods such as rice, bananas, applesauce, mashed potatoes, and dry toast.
- Advise the patient to increase her fluid intake, emphasizing less irritating fluids such as apple juice, nectars, weak tea, broth, and gelatin.
- Suggest to the patient that she drink three or four glasses of liquid 30 minutes before radiation therapy. This results in a full bladder, which pushes some of the bowel out of the radiation field.
- Discourage the patient from rubbing, scratching, or applying a commercial product to the rectal area. The patient should also be instructed not to use enemas, suppositories, or rectal thermometers while undergoing therapy or for 1 month afterward unless her physician directs her to do so.
- Encourage the patient to soak in a bathtub or small tub of warm water three times a day. The physician may prescribe a medication to add to the bath treatments.

CHEMOTHERAPY

Therapy for colorectal cancer may involve a single agent or multidrug protocols, as well as combinations of chemotherapy, radiation, and biotherapy.

SIDE EFFECTS

Usually dosage, drug, and patient specific
Nausea and vomiting
Diarrhea
Bone marrow suppression

Diarrhea is a particular concern in the patient with an ostomy, because of skin irritation. A protective barrier and additional paste or powder may be needed. It is important to keep a record of the number and consistency of stools and to suggest ways the patient can control the problem (see the box on page 86). If the patient receives vincristine, constipation may be the problem. Fluids, stool softeners, laxatives, and irrigation of the stoma may be needed.

Stomatitis may occur around the peristomal skin and the stoma itself. Protective skin barriers, careful pouch changes, and thorough skin cleansing are needed.

Fungal infections near the site of the stoma may result from the chemotherapy-induced bone marrow suppression. Antifungal powders may be helpful. The pouch must be removed carefully to prevent bleeding near the stoma because of the low platelet count.

1 ASSESS

ASSESSMENT	OBSERVATIONS
Gastrointestinal	Blood in stool, gross rectal bleeding, tenesmus, feeling of incomplete evacuation, pencil-like stool, urgency to defecate, abdominal distention, excessive flatus, abdominal cramping, constipation or diarrhea
Psychosocial	Fear

2 DIAGNOSE

NURSING DIAGNOSIS	SUBJECTIVE FINDINGS	OBJECTIVE FINDINGS
Constipation related to colorectal obstruction by tumor	Complains of cramping, distention, incomplete evacuation	Absence of bowel movement; hard or pencil-like stool; absence of bowel sounds; blood in stool
Diarrhea related to colorectal obstruction by tumor	Complains of cramping, burning in rectal area, weakness, urgency	Frequent loose or liquid stools; blood in stool
Fluid volume deficit related to blood loss through rectum	Complains of weakness, palpitations, restlessness, dyspnea, and dizziness	Blood in stool; gross rectal bleeding; pallor; tachypnea; tachycardia; hypotension; anemia
Fear related to diagnosis, treatment, and prognosis	Expresses fear of disease, treatment, disfigurement, and death	Appears sad and withdrawn, angry, and depressed

→ → →

3 PLAN

Patient goals

1. The patient will have normal bowel elimination.
2. The patient will have no bleeding.
3. The patient will be less fearful about the diagnosis, treatment, possibility of disfigurement, and prognosis.

4 IMPLEMENT

NURSING DIAGNOSIS	NURSING INTERVENTIONS	RATIONALE
Constipation* related to colorectal obstruction by tumor	Ambulate patient frequently, and encourage physical exercise.	To enhance GI motility and relieve pressure on abdomen.
	Place patient comfortably in sitting position.	To relieve abdominal pressure.
	Change patient's position frequently; increase movement if tolerated.	To relieve distention.
	Encourage increased intake of high-bulk foods and fluids; give fresh fruits, prune juice, hot coffee, and warm and iced liquids.	To increase GI motility.
	Give small, frequent feedings.	To prevent further distention.
	Restrict liquids at mealtime; give warm liquids after meals.	To relax abdomen.
	Give bland foods.	To relieve GI irritation.
	Encourage decreased intake of fatty foods.	To decrease formation of flatus.
	Refrain from giving iced liquids and carbonated beverages.	May increase cramping.
	Avoid use of straws and swallowing of air.	Causes gas formation in GI tract.
	Discourage smoking.	Smoking may increase distention.
	Increase fluid intake to 2,000 ml/day.	To maintain soft stool.
	Give stool softeners and laxatives.	To enhance elimination.
	Administer enemas.	To cleanse bowel.
	Measure intake and output.	To monitor hydration and quantity of feces.
	Give nonprescription drugs, such as simethicone.	To relieve flatus.
	Inspect abdomen for distention; auscultate abdomen for abnormal bowel sounds.	To determine need for further intervention.
	Remove restrictive clothing.	To relieve pressure on abdomen.

*Constipation alternates with diarrhea depending on location of tumor and extent of disease.

NURSING DIAGNOSIS	NURSING INTERVENTIONS	RATIONALE
	Apply heat to abdomen.	To relax abdomen and relieve cramping.
	Apply warm, moist compresses to rectal area, or provide sitz bath.	To relax anal sphincter.
	Evaluate pain for duration, intensity, and quality; evaluate effectiveness of pain relief measures.	To determine interventions needed.
Diarrhea* related to colorectal obstruction by tumor	Provide fluids so that intake equals output.	To prevent dehydration.
	Give clear-liquid or full-liquid diet.	To maintain hydration.
	Administer antidiarrhea drugs as ordered.	To control diarrhea.
	Discourage oral stimulants and intake of high-bulk foods.	They increase GI motility.
	Refrain from giving hot or iced liquids, enemas, or laxatives.	They irritate bowel.
	Cover patient with warm blankets.	To prevent loss of body heat.
	Encourage adequate rest.	To decrease energy expenditure.
	Do not insert rectal tube or take rectal temperatures.	To avoid irritating bowel.
	Check for impaction; use caution with pancytopenic patients.	To prevent bleeding.
	Auscultate abdomen for abnormal bowel sounds.	To assess GI status.
	Measure body weight and intake and output.	To monitor hydration and nutrition.
	Monitor blood studies for acid-base and electrolyte abnormalities resulting from loss of electrolytes and acid.	Loss is caused by dehydration.
	Be alert for complaints of pain caused by abdominal cramping or anal irritation.	May be precursors to diarrhea.
Fluid volume deficit related to blood loss through rectum	Apply ice bag to rectal area.	To enhance vasoconstriction.
	Change patient's position slowly.	To avoid vascular trauma.
	Cover patient with warm blankets.	To maintain warmth and comfort.
	Maintain complete bed rest if bleeding is severe.	To avoid excessive blood flow.

*Diarrhea alternates with constipation depending on location of tumor and extent of disease.

→ › ›

NURSING DIAGNOSIS	NURSING INTERVENTIONS	RATIONALE
	Elevate foot of bed.	To maintain blood flow to vital organs.
	Do not give enemas or laxatives, insert rectal tube, or take rectal temperatures.	To avoid tissue trauma and bleeding.
	Estimate blood volume loss.	To determine replacement needed.
	Monitor blood pressure and blood studies.	To determine blood volume.
Fear related to diagnosis, treatment, and prognosis	Assess appetite, weight loss, sleep patterns, and activity level.	Depression may be manifested by changes in these areas.
	Assess presence and quality of support system.	To determine whether friends and family are available and helpful to patient.
	Monitor changes in communication with others.	Withdrawal or silence may indicate anger or depression.
	Listen to and accept verbalized fears and anger.	To foster constructive expression of negative feelings and fears.
	Encourage patient to use physical means of expression geared to capabilities.	Physical activity can be used as means to express fear and anger.
	Use visitors (e.g., ostomy visitor) to help patient deal openly with fears of disfigurement and rejection.	Talking with someone who has had the same experience can validate fears and stimulate problem solving.
Knowledge deficit	See Patient Teaching.	

5 EVALUATE

PATIENT OUTCOME	DATA INDICATING THAT OUTCOME IS REACHED
Bowel elimination is normal.	Stools are soft and formed; abdomen is soft and not distended; patient reports regular bowel movements.
There is no evidence of rectal bleeding.	Vital signs are within normal limits; results of stool occult blood test are negative; blood counts are within normal limits; patient reports usual energy and activity levels.
Progress has been made in easing patient's fears.	Patient discusses plans for treatment, interacts with ostomy visitor and others who have had similar experiences, and plans realistically for ostomy and its consequences.

PATIENT TEACHING

1. Inform the patient of the need to monitor gastrointestinal function and to maintain regularity.
2. Explain bowel changes that should be reported to the physician (e.g., rectal bleeding).
3. Instruct the patient in care of the ostomy if one is created.
4. Help the patient contact available resources and support groups such as the United Ostomy Association.

Esophageal Cancer

Esophageal cancer usually occurs in individuals 50 years of age or older; it predominates in men. It also is more common among African-Americans. The current 5-year survival rate is 20% overall. The only prognostic variable is the stage of disease (which indicates the importance of early diagnosis).

EPIDEMIOLOGY

Some evidence indicates that esophageal cancer is related to tobacco and alcohol use, nutritional deficiencies, and environmental carcinogens. These tumors occur most often in the Caspian Sea area, in Transkei in southern Africa, and in northern China.

Some of the environmental or nutritional factors implicated in the development of esophageal cancer are nitrosamines or fungi contamination in pickled vegetables or in grains; chronic addiction to morphine, particularly in areas where opium is eaten; tobacco residue; silica fragments associated with millet bran (northern China); and abuse of alcohol. Of these suggested carcinogens, alcoholism is the one with a clear relationship with epidermoid carcinoma of the esophagus. Chronic inflammation of the esophagus is also associated with a higher incidence of cancer. Cancer of the esophagus has been linked to squamous cell carcinoma of the oropharynx or larynx, which is probably a result of exposure of the oral cavity, respiratory tract, and esophagus to the same carcinogenic factors. People with achalasia also have a higher incidence of esophageal cancer.

PATHOPHYSIOLOGY

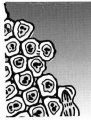

Approximately half of esophageal tumors develop at the esophagogastric junction. These tumors generally are adenocarcinomas that arise from the stomach. Twenty-five percent of esophageal tumors are found in the upper thoracic esophagus, 17% in the lower esophagus, and 8% in the cervical esophagus. Two thirds of these carcinomas are the squamous cell type. Adenocarcinomas are the second most common.

The squamous cell carcinoma begins as a small mucosal patch that eventually grows, ulcerates, and protrudes into the lumen of the esophagus. Local extension to the recurrent laryngeal nerve or tracheobronchial tree is common. Unfortunately, local extension often is present at the time of diagnosis. Metastasis to local lymph nodes includes those around the hilum of the lung and in the neck. Metastasis to the abdominal

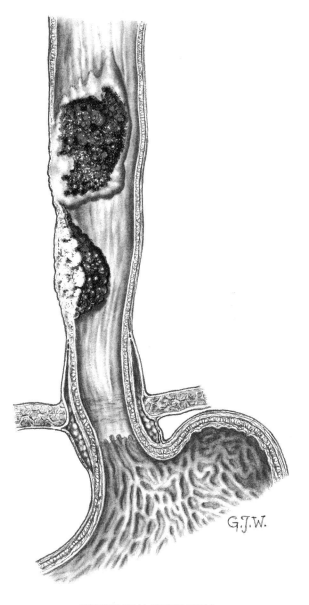

ESOPHAGEAL CARCINOMA

lymph nodes of the celiac axis also occurs. Satellite lesions develop several inches away from the primary lesion.

Carcinomas of the bronchus or stomach often metastasize to the esophagus. Mediastinal lymph node metastasis from other organ carcinomas may lead to esophageal involvement and symptoms of obstruction. Breast carcinomas may metastasize to the esophagus. Primary adenocarcinoma of the esophagus is rare and should be considered the result of Barrett's esophagus or of spread from an adenocarcinoma of the stomach cardia.

SIGNS AND SYMPTOMS

Dysphagia (difficulty swallowing) is the most common complaint of people with esophageal cancer. It usually is first noticed when bulky foods are eaten; later it occurs with soft foods, and finally with liquids. Weight loss, regurgitation, and aspiration pneumonitis may also be noted. The most prevalent symptoms in people without dysphagia are odynophagia (pain on swallowing) and symptoms of gastroesophageal reflux.

Signs and symptoms of advanced disease include cervical adenopathy, a chronic cough, choking after eating, hemoptysis or hematemesis or both, and hoarseness. Pain is an unusual symptom and indicates local extension.

DIAGNOSTIC STUDIES AND FINDINGS

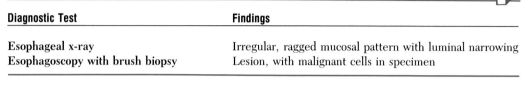

Diagnostic Test	Findings
Esophageal x-ray	Irregular, ragged mucosal pattern with luminal narrowing
Esophagoscopy with brush biopsy	Lesion, with malignant cells in specimen

MEDICAL MANAGEMENT

SURGERY

Esophagogastrectomy: Left chest for lesions in lower esophagus; laparotomy and right thoracotomy or transhiatal approach for higher lesions; transhiatal approach for lesions at thoracic inlet and cervical esophagus; stomach as esophageal replacement

RADIATION THERAPY

External beam for squamous cell lesions above aortic arch
Palliation for obstructive symptoms, pain control

CHEMOTHERAPY

Preoperative cisplatin-based chemotherapy alone or in combination with radiation therapy
Used alone for palliation with locally recurrent or metastatic disease
Used with radiation therapy (without surgery) for palliation of dysphagia

SURGERY

An aggressive approach provides excellent palliation, increased longevity, and a chance for a cure. Standard resection seems to give as good results as radical procedures. Complications include myocardial infarction, cerebrovascular accident, pulmonary embolus, mechanical obstruction or decreased gastric tone, and anastomotic strictures secondary to gastroesophageal reflux.

RADIATION THERAPY

Complications include esophageal perforation or hemorrhage, which may also occur as part of the natural history of the disease; stricture, which may be a late effect of radiation therapy; radiation fibrosis; or cardiomyopathy.

CHEMOTHERAPY

Symptoms that require nursing intervention stem from the myelosuppression of the agents as well as from mucositis and other gastrointestinal toxicities.

NURSING CARE OF THE PERSON WITH ESOPHAGEAL CANCER

NURSING DIAGNOSIS

Altered nutrition: less than body requirements related to obstruction of esophagus by tumor as evidenced by dysphagia, regurgitation and aspiration, odynophagia, GI reflux, weight loss

NURSING INTERVENTIONS AND RATIONALE

1. Assess patient to determine which foods patients can and cannot swallow, in order to select and prepare edible foods.
2. Provide a diet that omits alcohol, spicy food, or foods at extreme temperature, since they may irritate the esophageal mucosa, and include bland foods, which are less likely to irritate the mucosa.
3. Teach the patient to eat slowly, chew food thoroughly, and arch back while swallowing, to increase amount ingested.
4. Have patient eat sitting upright and remain sitting after meal to avoid regurgitation or aspiration.
5. Have patient avoid eating 1 to 2 hours before bedtime to avoid heartburn of reflux esophagitis.
6. Have patient sip half a glass of water after each meal to cleanse the esophagus.

NURSING DIAGNOSIS

Pain related to esophageal irritation by tumor as evidenced by odynophagia

NURSING INTERVENTIONS AND RATIONALE

1. Place the head of the patient's bed on 4 inch blocks to prevent reflux esophagitis.
2. Provide antacids at bedside so that patient can medicate self when indigestion occurs.
3. Assess patient for evidence of mouth filling with fluid refluxing from esophagus, dysphagia, and heartburn that increases when the patient lies down as evidence of esophagitis that requires aggressive medical management.
4. Administer solution of meat tenderizer to relieve food impaction, which may be a cause of pain.
5. Observe for evidence of GI bleeding such as hematemesis or melena, which indicate severe esophageal irritation.

Gastric Cancer

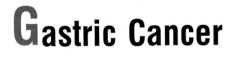

The incidence of **gastric cancer** has declined significantly in western Europe and the United States. Approximately 23,000 new cases (2.3% of all new cancer cases) will be diagnosed in 1991.

In the 1940s gastric cancer was the most common malignant disease in the United States. The incidence apparently has not changed in Japan, where gastric cancer accounts for 60% of all cancers in men and 40% of all cancers in women. In the gastrointestinal (GI) tract, gastric cancer is more common than cancer of the esophagus, small intestine, biliary tract, or liver but slightly less common than cancer of the pancreas.

EPIDEMIOLOGY

Gastric cancer is more common in people 50 to 70 years of age. It is predominantly a disease of men

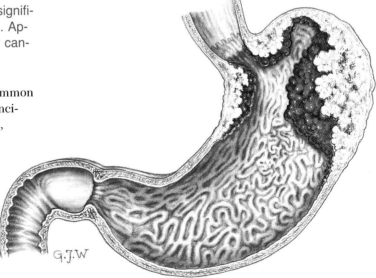

CARCINOMA OF STOMACH

worldwide in the ratio of 2:1. The incidence is greater in countries farther from the equator, for unknown reasons. Gastric cancer is also more common in lower socioeconomic groups. The incidence increases slightly in the direct relatives of people with gastric cancer, but this is less likely to be genetic than to be related to some exposure in early life. Gastric cancer is also more common in individuals with pernicious anemia, hypochlorhydria, or achlorhydria. The incidence is 15% to 20% higher in people of blood group A. The relationship of gastric cancer to benign gastric ulcer is unclear. Nitrosamines are also believed to be a carcinogen that may be a factor in the development of stomach cancer. In Japan, early screening of those at risk with x-ray studies and endoscopy has resulted in earlier diagnosis and increased survival rates.

PATHOPHYSIOLOGY

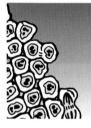 Of malignant lesions of the stomach, 90% are adenocarcinomas, most of which are found in the distal stomach on the lesser curvature. Less common lesions are primary lymphoma and leiomyosarcoma. Other rare types of gastric cancer include carcinoid and metastatic cancer. These lesions can spread through the gastric wall and directly involve contiguous anatomic structures such as the pancreas, spleen, esophagus, colon, duodenum, gallbladder, liver, or adjacent mesenteries. These tumors also spread via the lymphatics in approximately two thirds of patients. The nodes involved are determined to some extent by the location of the primary lesion in the stomach. Gastric cancer can also spread via the bloodstream to the liver and can spread directly to the peritoneum.

SIGNS AND SYMPTOMS

Benign lesions become manifest in such a way that cancer must be suspected, but there are no classic signs or symptoms of gastric cancer. Most patients have nonspecific gastrointestinal complaints such as vague epigastric discomfort or indigestion, vomiting, belching, or postprandial fullness. Ten percent have complaints similar to those of peptic ulcer, and 10% have nonspecific anemia, weakness, and weight loss. A smaller number have acute intraabdominal problems such as massive upper gastrointestinal bleeding, acute obstruction of the esophagus or pylorus, or gastric perforation. Signs of advanced disease include a palpable ovarian mass, hepatomegaly, an abdominal mass, ascites, jaundice, and cachexia. Lymphatic spread to the left supraclavicular nodes is a classic sign of inoperability.

DIAGNOSTIC STUDIES AND FINDINGS

Diagnostic Test	Findings
Stool occult blood test	Blood
Upper gastrointestinal x-ray	Suspicious lesion
Endoscopy with brush biopsy	Presence of lesion with malignant cells in specimen

MEDICAL MANAGEMENT

SURGERY

Exploratory celiotomy: initial intervention in all patients with gastric cancer except those with peritoneal metastases, documented liver metastases, or other distant metastases; if the tumor is regionally localized, the primary tumor is resected, as well as actual and potentially involved regional lymph nodes; postoperative staging of the tumor is completed, and further treatment decisions are made

Distal subtotal gastric resection

Proximal subtotal gastric resection

MEDICAL MANAGEMENT—cont'd

Total gastrectomy: includes resection of adjacent organs involved by local extension such as body and tail of pancreas, portion of liver, transverse colon, or duodenum and head of pancreas (See Figure 6-3).

Palliative resection

RADIATION THERAPY

Palliation of obstruction (particularly in the cardia) or chronic bleeding

CHEMOTHERAPY

Single-agent palliation with fluorouracil (5FU)

Combination chemotherapy: 5FU, nitrosoureas, mitomycin-C, doxorubicin; FAM (5FU, doxorubicin, mitomycin-C); 5FU and methyl lomustine (CCNU)

The prognosis for patients with gastric cancer is poor, since almost two thirds of them have findings at the time of diagnosis that limit the possibility of survival. Nodal involvement is a significant prognostic factor. Patients with a short history of symptoms have a poorer prognosis than do those with a longer history. Patients with ulcer syndrome do better than those with the more common symptoms of indigestion.

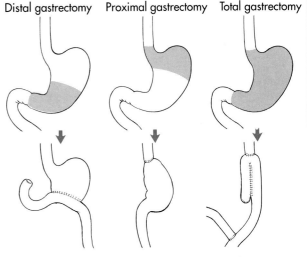

FIGURE 6-3
Operative resections used for gastric cancer. The method of reconstruction is shown below each procedure.

NURSING CARE OF THE PATIENT WITH GASTRIC CANCER

NURSING DIAGNOSIS

Altered nutrition: less than body requirements related to gastric obstruction by tumor as evidenced by vague epigastric discomfort or indigestion, vomiting, belching, or postprandial fullness, weight loss, weakness

NURSING INTERVENTIONS AND RATIONALE

1. Assess caloric intake—kinds and amounts, percentages of protein, carbohydrate, and fat—to determine needed changes in diet.
2. Observe the patient for evidence of weight loss and dehydration to intervene quickly with food, nutritional supplements, and fluids.
3. Ask patient if he is experiencing discomfort or indigestion, vomiting, belching, postprandial fullness, or weakness, as evidence of tumor pressure and obstruction.
4. Provide palpable meals based, as much as possible, on patient likes and dislikes to increase caloric consumption.
5. Offer dietary supplements as needed to maintain adequate nutritional balance.
6. Offer medications that relieve abdominal distention and flatulence, since these symptoms tend to adversely affect appetite.
7. Provide frequent small feedings each day.

NURSING DIAGNOSIS

Fluid volume deficit related to gastric obstruction or perforation as evidenced by massive GI bleeding, increasing severity and diffuseness of pain, rebound tenderness, abdominal guarding, melena, hematemesis

NURSING INTERVENTIONS AND RATIONALE

1. Observe characteristics and amount of emesis and stool to determine need for fluid and blood component therapy.
2. Monitor vital signs at frequent intervals during episodes of bleeding to detect shock early.
3. Monitor intake and output and urine specific gravity to detect renal dysfunction.
4. Administer IV fluids as prescribed to replace lost fluid volume.
5. Monitor lab reports to detect development of anemia.
6. Observe for signs and symptoms of worsening fluid volume deficit, including decreased urine output, concentrated urine, output greater than intake, weakness, change in mental status, blood in emesis or stool, severe or diffuse abdominal pain, rebound tenderness, and guarding, to determine need for large volumes of IV fluids and blood components at rapid rate of infusion.

Pancreatic Cancer

Pancreatic cancer is the second most common gastrointestinal cancer and the fourth leading cause of cancer death in the United States. The major obstacle to successful management of this cancer is the inability to establish the diagnosis at an early, curable stage.

EPIDEMIOLOGY

Carcinoma of the pancreas has increased more than 20% in recent years. The reason for this is unknown, although cigarette smoking and dietary fat may be causative factors. The incidence of pancreatic cancer increases with age, with a slight predominance among men, both white and nonwhite. It occurs more frequently in Jews in New York City and Israel. The incidence is lower among Mormons than among nonsmoking white men in both California and Utah. There does seem to be a dose-related association between pancreatic cancer and smoking. Other possible etiologic factors include alcoholism and organic chemicals such as coke, coal gas, betanaphthylamine, and benzidine. None of these factors is specific enough to define a population at risk.

SIGNS AND SYMPTOMS

Pancreatic cancer often is insidious in onset and frequently is diagnosed late in its course. Weight loss, often gradual and progressive, is one of the earliest symptoms. Pain is most likely to be midepigastric, steady, dull, boring, and usually worse at night. Pain in the left

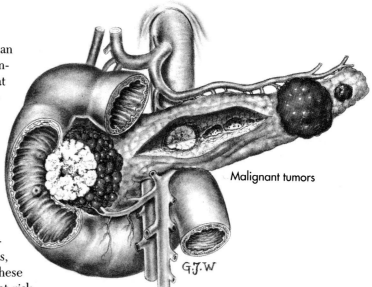

Malignant tumors

CARCINOMA OF PANCREAS

upper quadrant is more common with cancer in the body or tail of the pancreas. A small number of patients have lower abdominal pain, and 15% to 30% complain of back pain that is aggravated by lying flat and relieved by sitting up and bending forward or lying curled in a fetal position. Jaundice, the third most common symptom, usually is progressive and may occur late. It commonly is accompanied by pruritus of the arms, legs, and abdomen that typically is worse in the evening and at night. Nonspecific signs and symptoms include anorexia with weight loss. Constipation, bloating, and flatulence are nonspecific gastrointestinal complaints. Thrombophlebitis is most frequently seen with advanced disease. Many patients have recent-onset diabetes or deterioration of previously stable diabetes. Psychiatric symptoms, such as depression, may precede physical symptoms by a median interval of 6 months.

DIAGNOSTIC STUDIES AND FINDINGS

Diagnostic Test	Findings
Computed tomography (CT), ultrasound studies	Mass, liver metastases, perivascular invasion, lymphadenopathy, dilation of pancreatic duct
Fine-needle aspiration biopsy	Malignant cells
Endoscopic retrograde cholangiopancreatography (ERCP)	Irregular, eccentric, or "rat tail" termination of pancreatic duct; nodular or eccentric stenosis; "double duct" of tumor contiguous to both common bile and pancreatic ducts
Angiography	Arterial encasement, stenosis, or major venous involvement by avascular pancreatic tissue; localization of islet cell tumors; arterial displacement
Laparoscopy	Metastatic lesions
Cancer antigen (CA) 19-9	Elevated
Carcinoembryonic antigen (CEA)	Elevated

MEDICAL MANAGEMENT

SURGERY

Pancreatoduodenectomy (Whipple procedure)
Total pancreatectomy
Palliation to relieve jaundice and itching (e.g., anastomosis of jejunum to distended common bile duct)

RADIATION THERAPY

High-dose external beam
Interstitial seeds of iodine-125 (^{125}I) or iridium-192 (^{192}Ir), brachytherapy
Intraoperative radiation therapy
Adjuvant radiation therapy

CHEMOTHERAPY

5FU alone or with radiation therapy
Nitrosoureas, mitomycin C, doxorubicin

NURSING CARE OF THE PATIENT WITH PANCREATIC CANCER

NURSING DIAGNOSIS

Altered nutrition: less than body requirements related to anorexia with weight loss, constipation, bloating or flatulence, recent onset or unstable diabetes, weight loss

NURSING INTERVENTIONS AND RATIONALE

1. Assess caloric intake—kinds and amounts, percentages of protein, carbohydrate, and fat—to determine needed changes in or additions to diet.
2. Observe the patient for evidence of weight loss and dehydration to intervene quickly with foods, nutritional supplements, and fluids.
3. Ask patient if he is experiencing anorexia, constipation, bloating, flatulence, or other signs and symptoms of GI distress, as evidence of tumor pressure and possible disease progression.
4. Provide palatable meals based, as much as possible, on patient likes and dislikes to increase caloric intake.
5. Encourage the patient to eat frequent small meals in order to increase intake.
6. Offer medications that relieve abdominal distention and flatulence, since these symptoms tend to adversely affect appetite.

NURSING DIAGNOSIS

Pain related to tumor pressure and irritation of tissues in close proximity as evidenced by midepigastric pain that is steady, dull, boring, usually worse at night; or back pain aggravated by lying flat; pruritus

NURSING INTERVENTIONS AND RATIONALE

1. Assess location, onset, duration, radiation, and intensity of pain to determine appropriate interventions; for example, back pain is often relieved by sitting up and bending forward or lying curled in a fetal-type position.
2. Provide prescribed medications for pain as needed to decrease patient's discomfort.
3. Teach patient self-care strategies with which to manage pain, such as relaxation exercises, imagery, application of heat or cold.
4. Monitor diet to determine if certain foods increase or decrease patient pain or GI discomfort.
5. Offer patient frequent baths, lotions, and ointments to soothe skin and decrease itching.

CHAPTER 7

Genitourinary Cancers

Cancers of the genitourinary tract are among the most common malignancies. This organ system is the site of 32% of new cancers among men each year.

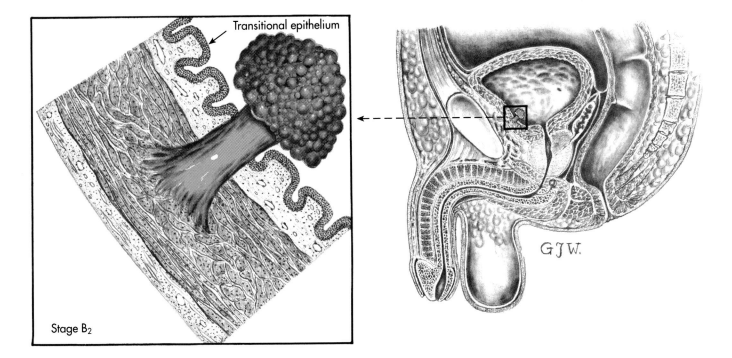

Stage B$_2$

Transitional epithelium

GJW.

TRANSITIONAL CELL CARCINOMA OF THE BLADDER (WITH STALK)

Bladder Cancer

The bladder is the most common site of urinary tract cancer. Although this type of cancer occurs most often in men between 50 and 70 years of age, particularly among white men, the incidences in younger men and in women have increased in recent years.

EPIDEMIOLOGY

Occupational exposure to dust or fumes of dyes, rubber, leather and its products, paint, and such organic chemicals as benzidine may be factors in the development of bladder cancer, with a 6- to 20-year latent period from the time of exposure to tumor transformation. This is believed to be true of as many as one third of these cancers. Cigarette smoking is associated with as much as a sixfold higher incidence of bladder cancer.

Table 7-1

CHARACTERISTICS AND TUMOR STAGING OF SUPERFICIAL VERSUS INVASIVE BLADDER CANCER

Characteristics	TNM* stage	Depth of invasion
Superficial		
In situ	T_{is}	Superficial
Confined to mucosa	T_a	Mucosa
Submucosa involved	T_1	Submucosa
Invasive		
Superficial muscle involved	T_2	Muscle
Deep muscle involved	T_{3a}	Deep muscle
Perivesical fat	T_{3b}	Fat
Adjacent organ invasion	T_4	Fat, adjacent organs
Nodal metastasis		
Pelvic lymph nodes	N_{1-3}	Nodes
Distant metastasis	N_4-M_1	Nodes, distant sites

From Held and Volpe.[31]
*Tumor, node, metastasis.

PATHOPHYSIOLOGY

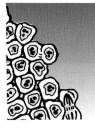 Most bladder tumors (90%) are transitional cell carcinomas, and the remaining 10% are squamous cell carcinomas and adenocarcinomas. The characteristics of transitional cell carcinoma are multicentricity and papillary growth into the bladder lumen, with the potential for local invasion into the bladder muscle and regional spread into surrounding nodes, the pelvis, and other pelvic structures. The cancer is spread by the blood to the lungs, bones, and liver. The depth of invasion is the most important factor in the prognosis (Table 7-1).

The bladder is also the site for contiguous spread of cancer from lesions of neighboring viscera, especially the uterine cervix and the prostate. These tumors may invade the bladder by direct extension. The bladder may also be invaded by cancer of the sigmoid colon, rectum, or uterine body.

Superficial tumors that are confined to the bladder mucosa may recur in 75% of patients. Although these patients have an excellent prognosis (the 5-year survival rate is 85% to 90%), they must accept bladder cancer as a chronic process that requires lifetime surveillance to diagnose and treat recurrent lesions. Approximately half of the patients who have muscle invasion die within 5 years as a result of recurrence and metastases.

SIGNS AND SYMPTOMS

The most common sign of bladder cancer is hematuria, although some patients are asymptomatic until urethral obstruction, hydronephrosis, and renal failure occur. Women with bladder cancer are more likely to have been treated for urinary tract infection with antibiotics (hematuria being attributed to hemorrhagic cystitis). Menstruating women may associate occasional spotting with vaginal bleeding rather than bleeding from the bladder.

The second most common symptom complex is marked urgency, dysuria, and frequency with small volumes of urine. Low back pain may indicate sacral or lumbar metastases. Lymphatic or venous obstruction may cause pelvic pain or leg edema.

DIAGNOSTIC STUDIES AND FINDINGS

Diagnostic Test	Findings
Urine culture	Sterile urine (in patient with symptoms of cystitis)
Excretory urography	Tumor or evidence of ureteral or urethral obstruction
Cystoscopy with selected bladder biopsies, urinary tract cytologic tests	Tumor visualization, malignant cells
Bimanual abdominal examination	Firm or hard nodularity
Cystoscopic retrograde ureteropyelography	Tumor visualization, evidence of obstruction
Flow cytometry	>15% of cells above diploid level or clearly aneuploid tumor cell line with more or less than half the number of chromosomes usually found
Renal arteriography	Evidence of obstruction or increased tumor vascularization
Renal ultrasound	Local extent of tumor and degree of bladder wall involvement
Computed tomography (CT) or magnetic resonance imaging (MRI) studies of abdomen and pelvis	Local extent of tumor, identification of pelvic lymph node metastases
Chest and skeletal x-rays, bone scan, liver function studies	Evidence of metastatic disease
Carcinoembryonic antigen (CEA)	Elevated
Autocrine motility factor (AMF)	Increased in widely metastatic disease

MEDICAL MANAGEMENT

SURGERY

Noninvasive bladder cancer: endoscopic resection and fulguration; laser therapy

Invasive bladder cancer: radical cystectomy with urinary diversion

RADIATION THERAPY

Preoperative regimen before radical cystectomy

For control of hemorrhage and bony metastases

CHEMOTHERAPY

Noninvasive bladder cancer: Intravesical instillation with bacille Calmette-Guérin (BCG), thiotepa, doxorubicin, mitomycin-C, and interferons

Invasive bladder cancers: CMDV (cisplatin, methotrexate, doxorubicin, vinblastine); MVC (methotrexate, vinblastine, cisplatin); single agents (methotrexate with or without leucovorin, doxorubicin, vinblastine)

Neoadjuvant (before radiation therapy)

SURGERY

The goal of surgery for noninvasive bladder cancer is to prevent the tumor from invading the bladder muscle wall. Endoscopic resection and fulguration are used to diagnose and treat superficial lesions, which have a slow recurrence rate. This treatment can also help control bleeding in patients who are poor operative risks or who have advanced disease. Transurethral resection may be used for low-grade, early-stage tumors. This procedure preserves the bladder and sexual functions and has low morbidity and mortality rates.

An Nd:YAG laser (neodymium:yttrium-aluminum-garnet) is used to treat superficial transitional cell cancer. The benefits of this procedure are the use of a local anesthetic, the minimal discomfort for the patient, the lack of bleeding, and the maintenance of bladder integrity. The use of hematoporphyrin derivatives (HPD) with tumor cells sensitized to light is also being studied. However, this treatment has drawbacks: because the patient is photosensitive for as long as a month after therapy, no body parts should be exposed to sunlight; also, some patients complain of irritable bladder symptoms. The need for special equipment and the high cost of this therapy have limited its availability to patients.

Radical cystectomy is the surgery of choice for invasive bladder cancer. In men it involves resection of the local pelvic nodes, prostatic seminal vesicles, and penile urethra. The newer nerve-sparing technique lessens the likelihood of postoperative impotence. In women the procedure involves resection of the urethra, uterus, ovaries, and fallopian tubes. The anterior third of the vagina is lost with this procedure, which may cause difficulty with penile insertion. Because the clitoris may be injured, the patient may also experience altered sensation.

When the tumor is invasive, high grade, and superficial without metastases in the pelvic area, the prognosis is good.

COMPLICATIONS

Ureterocutaneous fistula
Wound dehiscence
Partial small-bowel obstruction
Wound infection
Small-bowel fistula

Urinary diversion may involve an ileal loop (ileal conduit), colon loop, rectal bladder, or continent diversion. The ileal conduit is most commonly used (Figure 7-1). To create the conduit, a piece of terminal ileum is isolated, the proximal end is closed, and the distal end is

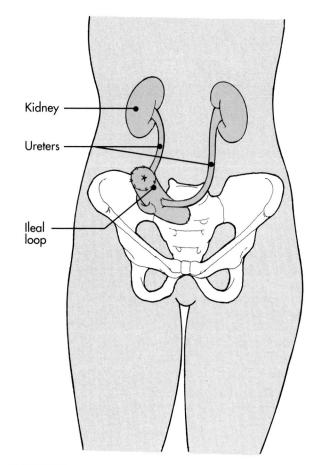

FIGURE 7-1
Urinary diversion (ileal conduit).

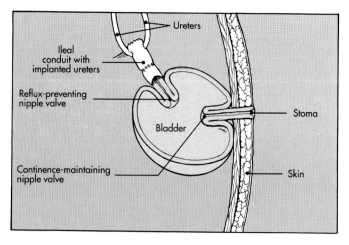

FIGURE 7-2
Kock pouch (continent ileal reservoir).

brought through an opening in the abdominal wall and sutured to it, creating a stoma. The ileal segment must reach from the retroperitoneum to the skin comfortably and without tension on the end of the stoma. The ureters are implanted into the ileal segment. Urine flows into the conduit, where it is propelled by peristalsis through the stoma. The stoma should be flush with the skin and recessed so that the appliance will fit properly. Urinary stents may be threaded into the ureters to prevent anastomosis in the early postoperative period. The stents are removed after 7 to 10 days.

Recently the continent diversion (Kock pouch procedure) has been used successfully in some men and women. A midportion of ileum is folded and opened onto itself to create a continent pouch with a nipple valve stoma, which usually is below the undergarment line. A small gauze pad may cover the stoma, which is the access for catheterization by the patient every 6 hours (Figure 7-2).

POSSIBLE COMPLICATIONS

Ileal conduit:
    Stomal stenosis with pain, stones, and potential
      pyelonephritis
    Ureteral reflux and ascending infection
Kock pouch:
    Leakage at stoma
    Difficult catheterization
    Electrolyte abnormalities
    Pyelonephrosis
    Stone formation

Preoperative Care

The nurse and enterostomal therapist should ensure the patient has the information he needs to choose the type of stoma and location best suited to his life-style and ability to care for himself. A stoma visitor may be invited to talk with the patient about these decisions as well as other fears and concerns. In preparation for surgery, the patient is given a low-residue diet for 2 days before surgery and clear liquids the day before surgery. Bowel preparation includes antibiotics and cathartics.

Postoperative Care

If the patient has the Kock pouch, it is intubated with a Medina Silastic catheter sutured to the skin line and connected to low-suction or gravity drainage. Three weeks after the surgery, the catheter and stents are removed. As the pouch heals, the patient develops a pattern of intubating and draining it every 3 to 4 hours.

If the patient has the ileal conduit, an appliance is placed on it after surgery. Some bleeding from the

CARE OF THE ILEAL CONDUIT

The appliance should be changed every 3 to 5 days.

The opening for the stoma is cut to allow ⅛ inch of space around the base.

The appliance's opening must fit securely to avoid maceration and denudation of the skin, as well as hypertrophic lesions (epitheliomatous hyperplasia).

The skin barrier may be on the appliance; if not, it should be applied to clean, dry skin before the appliance is placed over the stoma.

Cleansing of the skin includes removing alkaline encrustation, which can cause stoma stenosis.

Kidney function should be monitored through loopagraphy, excretory urography, and laboratory testing of urine and blood.

stoma may occur. A healthy stoma protrudes ½ to ¾ of an inch above the skin in the lower right quadrant; it has a deep pink to dark red color, may be edematous, and may have cloudy urine as a result of mucus being expelled. If the stoma is dusky in appearance (purple to black), circulation is impaired and further surgery may be necessary to avoid necrosis. The stoma shrinks over the first week or two and continues to shrink for several months to a year. Because excess mucus can clog the outlet of the appliance, the patient needs to increase fluid intake to 3 liters per day (see box on page 103 and Chapter 6 for other aspects of care).

RADIATION THERAPY

Patients with high-stage, high-grade tumors are commonly treated with radiation therapy. When used as the definitive treatment, radiation therapy can cure only 16% to 30% of patients with invasive bladder cancer. Preoperative radiation therapy is used to decrease pelvic recurrence and dissemination during radical cystectomy. The radiation is delivered to the pelvis, sometimes with a boost to the bladder alone. The dose most often is fractionated to reduce the severity of side effects. Radiation therapy can also improve hemorrhage control in advanced bladder cancer and is an important aspect of the treatment of bony metastases.

CHEMOTHERAPY

For noninvasive bladder cancer, patients may receive intravesical instillation of one of several agents. Thiotepa may be administered weekly for up to 8 weeks, with a mean complete response rate of 29% for definitive treatment or complete eradication of persistent lesions. The drug is well tolerated, with only 20% of patients developing bone marrow suppression. Treatment is delayed if the patient has a urinary tract infection, since this condition could increase absorption of the drug.

Doxorubicin decreases the incidence of bladder cancer recurrence, but it may cause diminished bladder capacity, chemical cystitis, hypersensitivity, and anaphylaxis. Mitomycin is also used for prophylaxis. This drug has minimum toxicity, but some patients develop chemical cystitis. To avoid contact dermatitis, patients are taught to wash their hands and genitalia when they urinate after treatment with mitomycin.

BCG (bacille Calmette-Guérin) is effective in 70% of cases of cancer in situ. Irritable bladder symptoms occur in 85% of patients, although the symptoms usually disappear after each treatment.

CMDV (cisplatin, methotrexate, doxorubicin, vinblastine) is used to stabilize the disease and to achieve partial to complete remission in invasive and metastatic bladder cancer. Patients treated with this regimen may develop alopecia, nausea and vomiting, bone marrow suppression, and mucositis. Adequate hydration decreases the incidence of renal and otologic toxicity.

Single-agent chemotherapy effects a subjective response and stabilizes the disease in 25% to 50% of patients. Intensive combination chemotherapy that includes cisplatin offers a higher complete response rate.

1 ASSESS

ASSESSMENT	OBSERVATIONS
Urinary function	Hematuria; urgency, frequency, and dysuria
Comfort	Low back or pelvic pain, leg edema
Psychosocial	Fear of incontinence, altered sexuality and fertility, pain, and death

2 DIAGNOSE

NURSING DIAGNOSIS	SUBJECTIVE FINDINGS	OBJECTIVE FINDINGS
Altered patterns of urinary elimination related to tumor in bladder	Complains of urgency, frequency, and dysuria	Hematuria; sterile urine
Pain related to pressure of tumor or metastases	Complains of low back or pelvic pain	Pained facial expression; leg edema; withdrawn demeanor; guarding of back or pelvic area

NURSING DIAGNOSIS	SUBJECTIVE FINDINGS	OBJECTIVE FINDINGS
Fear related to loss of control of urinary function, impotence, infertility, pain, and possible death	Expresses fear of incontinence, impotence, sterility, suffering, and death	Angry, withdrawn, and depressed demeanor

3 PLAN

Patient goals

1. The patient will have more normal urinary function.
2. The patient will have less pain or none at all.
3. The patient's fears will be alleviated.

4 IMPLEMENT

NURSING DIAGNOSIS	NURSING INTERVENTIONS	RATIONALE
Altered patterns of urinary elimination related to tumor in bladder	Measure intake and output.	To monitor adequacy of elimination.
	Inspect urine for blood; check with Hemastix.	To detect bleeding.
	Inspect abdomen for swelling and distention.	To assess for urinary retention.
	Encourage patient to get adequate rest and exercise.	To avoid stress-related distention.
	Increase patient's fluid intake.	To enhance renal circulation and flush bladder.
	Apply heating pad or hot water bottle to abdomen as ordered.	To relax abdominal muscles.
	Catheterize patient only if necessary.	To avoid infection associated with catheterization.
	Monitor blood studies: acid-base balance, hemoglobin (Hb), hematocrit (Hct), blood urea nitrogen (BUN), and creatinine. Also monitor urine studies: acid-base balance, creatinine, specific gravity, and protein.	To assess renal function.
Pain related to pressure of tumor or metastases	Change patient's position slowly.	To avoid injury or strain.
	Place patient in whirlpool bath, or apply heat.	To relax muscles.

NURSING DIAGNOSIS	NURSING INTERVENTIONS	RATIONALE
	Administer bladder antispasmodics as ordered.	To relieve bladder spasms.
	Discuss possible pain-relieving measures with patient; use those possible (e.g., heat, massage).	To promote self-care.
	Evaluate effectiveness of pain-relief measures.	To determine need for further intervention.
Fear related to loss of control of urinary function, impotence, infertility, pain, and possible death	Validate sources of fear with patient, and help him identify coping skills used successfully in the past.	This guides therapeutic intervention and facilitates problem solving.
	Encourage patient to ask questions and express feelings.	To try to relieve anxiety and help patient put thoughts into perspective.
	Provide accurate information about control of urinary function, sexuality, fertility, pain control, and prognosis (see section on prostate cancer).	To alleviate fears.
Knowledge deficit	See Patient Teaching.	

5 EVALUATE

PATIENT OUTCOME	DATA INDICATING THAT OUTCOME IS REACHED
Urinary function is normal.	Patient has no complaints of urgency, frequency, or dysuria, and there is no evidence of hematuria.
Patient's pain has been relieved.	Patient has no low back or pelvic pain and can carry out self-care activities.
Patient's fears have been alleviated.	Patient acknowledges his fear of loss of control of urinary function, impotence, sterility, pain, and death but has refocused his concerns on resuming activities of daily living.

PATIENT TEACHING

1. Emphasize the need for an adequate fluid intake, exercise, and rest.
2. Encourage oral fluids/foods that cause alkaline urine such as fruits, vegetables, and milk. Avoid tobacco and foods/fluids that irritate the bladder, such as alcohol, tea, and spices.
3. To reduce the incidence of urinary tract infections, female patients should: (a) void after sexual intercourse to reduce the number of bacteria that may be introduced into the urethra; (b) avoid bubble baths; (c) wear cotton undergarments.
4. Discuss pain-relieving measures (e.g., exercise, warmth, and medication).
5. Instruct the patient in self-care if he has a urinary diversion (see Patient Teaching Guide, page 251).
6. Provide the patient with information and referrals as needed for sperm banking, sexual counseling, and reconstructive or implant surgery.

Renal Cancer

Approximately 10,000 people die of renal cancer each year. However, because computed tomography (CT) and ultrasound are now widely used in health care practice, more unsuspected renal tumors are being diagnosed.

EPIDEMIOLOGY

Renal cancer usually occurs in people over 40 years of age; the average age at the time of diagnosis is 55 to 60. Renal cell carcinoma occurs in 80% of cases and is twice as common in men as in women. Ten percent of renal tumors are transitional cell or squamous cell tumors of the renal pelvis, which have an equal incidence in men and women.

The cause of renal cancer is unclear. Some studies have suggested a relationship between smoking and renal pelvis carcinoma. Individuals with acquired cystic disease caused by renal failure are also prone to renal cell cancer. The autosomal dominant, hereditary von Hippel-Lindau disease frequently is associated with this type of cancer. Some renal pelvic tumors may occur as a result of chronic inflammation and irritation secondary to renal calculi. Hormones and radiation may also play a role in the development of renal cancer.

PATHOPHYSIOLOGY

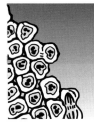

Hypernephroma, or adenocarcinoma of the renal parenchyma, is the most common renal tumor in adults. It grows slowly but may metastasize at any stage. Metastasis via the bloodstream results in spread to the lungs, bones, regional lymph nodes, liver, and other visceral organs. Parenchymal tumors infiltrate more rapidly than hypernephroma and have a poor prognosis. Papillary tumors of the renal pelvis (transitional cell, squamous cell, or adenocarcinoma) usually are multiple and involve the ureters, often the bladder, and the lymphatics.

Nephrotic carcinomas usually are large and encapsulated; as many as 50% may perforate the apparently intact capsule. Hematogenous metastasis results from early invasion of renal venules. The tumor often extends into the renal vein and vena cava. Distant metastases occur in the lungs, lymph nodes, liver, bones, adrenal gland, opposite kidney, brain, and heart.

The kidney more often is the site of metastatic rather than primary tumors. The most frequent sites of origin are the lungs and breasts.

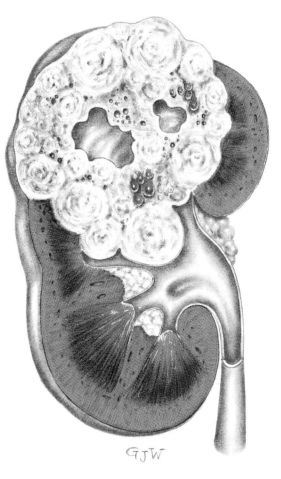

RENAL CELL CARCINOMA

SIGNS AND SYMPTOMS

Signs and symptoms develop late in the course of the disease. The most common sign is painless, intermittent hematuria; others include pain and a palpable abdominal mass. Fever, weight loss, an elevated erythrocyte sedimentation rate, or anemia may also be present. Paraneoplastic syndromes (e.g., hypercalcemia caused by parathyroid hormone overproduction and erythrocytosis caused by overproduction of erythropoietin) have also been observed.

Because of the long interval between the onset of signs and symptoms and the diagnosis of renal cancer, about one third of patients have metastases.

Improved survival rates for early hypernephroma have been attributed to thoracoabdominal nephrectomy with node dissection and earlier diagnosis of "incidental" carcinomas. Reports of spontaneous regression have prompted investigational therapy with biologic response modifiers.

DIAGNOSTIC STUDIES AND FINDINGS

Diagnostic Test	Findings
Urinalysis	Red blood cells
Excretory urography	Space-occupying mass with pelvocalyceal displacement and alteration of renal contour; filling defect in pelvocalyceal system
Nephrotomography	Solid tumor
Retrograde pyelogram	Filling defect
Renal ultrasound study	Solid tumor
Renal computed tomography (CT) scan	Solid tumor; enlarged regional lymph nodes
Renal magnetic resonance imaging (MRI) study	Renal vein or vena caval involvement
Selective renal arteriography	Neovasculature
Venacavography	Shows extent of lesion in renal vein or vena cava
Needle aspiration of avascular cystic masses, with cytologic testing and use of contrast materials	Malignant cells; space-occupying mass
Abdominal CT scan	Shows density and size of tumor, extent of local invasion, vena caval or renal vein involvement, and metastases

MEDICAL MANAGEMENT

SURGERY

Radical nephrectomy (abdominotransperitoneal or thoracoabdominal approaches)

Lymphadenectomy (controversial)

Palliative nephrectomy for bleeding and pain control

Resection of solitary metastatic site (e.g., in brain or liver)

Bilateral tumors
  Nephrectomy of larger tumor and partial nephrectomy for smaller lesion in bilateral disease
  Bilateral nephrectomies and chronic hemodialysis or peritoneal dialysis; later, transplantation

Nephroureterectomy for carcinomas of the renal pelvis

RADIATION THERAPY

Treatment for local recurrences or symptomatic bony tumor

Postoperative irradiation for residual or recurrent tumor

CHEMOTHERAPY

Hormonal therapy: Progesterone (Depo-Provera, Megace), testosterone, antiestrogens

Vinblastine

Biologic response modifiers: Interferon-alpha (IFN-α), interleukin-2 (IL-2) with lymphokine-activated killer (LAK) cells; autolymphocyte therapy with supernumerary lymphormones

NURSING CARE OF THE PERSON WITH RENAL CANCER

NURSING DIAGNOSIS

Fluid volume deficit related to renal irritation by tumor as evidenced by gross hematuria

NURSING INTERVENTIONS AND RATIONALE

1. Observe characteristics and amount of urine, particularly color, to determine need for fluid and blood component replacement.
2. Monitor vital signs at frequent intervals during episodes of gross hematuria to detect shock early.
3. Encourage patient to drink large volumes of fluid to prevent dehydration.
4. Monitor intake and output and urine specific gravity to detect renal function and to monitor its progression.
5. Administer IV fluids as prescribed to replace lost fluid volume.
6. Monitor lab reports to detect development of anemia.
7. Observe for signs and symptoms of worsening fluid volume deficit, including decreased urine output, concentrated urine, output greater than intake, weakness, and change in mental status, to determine need for large volumes of IV fluids and blood components at rapid rate.

NURSING DIAGNOSIS

Pain related to progressive disease in kidney, such as passage of blood clots or obstruction of the ureteropelvic junction as evidenced by complaints of flank pain, palpable mass

NURSING INTERVENTIONS AND RATIONALE

1. Assess patient's pain history, including analgesic use, to determine previously effective medications.
2. Assess location, onset, duration, radiation, and intensity of pain to determine appropriate interventions.
3. Provide prescribed medications for pain as needed to decrease patient's discomfort.
4. Teach patient self-care strategies with which to manage pain, such as relaxation exercises, imagery, application of heat or cold.
5. Demonstrate use of pillow to support flanks, exercises to relax muscles, and massage to relieve discomfort.

Prostate Cancer

The prostate is the most common site of cancer in men, and prostate tumors account for 21% of all male cancers. Approximately 106,000 cases of prostate cancer are diagnosed each year.

EPIDEMIOLOGY

The incidence and mortality of prostate cancer are increasing, especially among blacks. In men over 50 years of age, the incidence may be as high as 37%; in men over age 85, it may be as high as 89%. The influence of endogenous hormones, especially dihydrotestosterone, is the only factor clearly associated with the promotion and development of prostate cancer. Other possible etiologic factors are genetic influences; dietary fat; exposure to certain viruses, pathogens, or industrial chemicals; or urbanization.

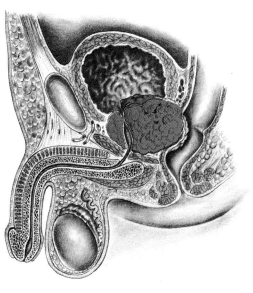

CARCINOMA OF PROSTATE

PATHOPHYSIOLOGY

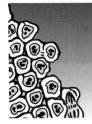 Most prostate cancers are adenocarcinomas. These slow-growing tumors arise in the posterior portion of the prostate, are usually multifocal, and eventually involve the entire gland. They spread via the lymphatics throughout the pelvic region and into the pelvic bones. Hematogenous spread involves the lungs, liver, kidneys, and bones (vertebrae, pelvis, femur, and ribs). By the time these tumors are diagnosed, most of them have already invaded the base of the bladder, seminal vesicles, or perivesicular fascia, or they have moved laterally into the levator ani muscles.

The rest of these tumors are of the ductal type (transitional cell and squamous cell carcinoma, endometrioid cancer, and sarcoma). Acinar dysplasia has been characterized as prostatic intraepithelial neoplasia (PIN), a premalignant lesion.

Grading of the tumors (i.e., well, moderately, or poorly differentiated) correlates with the prognosis; the more poorly differentiated the tumor, the poorer the prognosis.

SIGNS AND SYMPTOMS

Early symptoms resemble those of benign prostate hypertrophy; they include weak urinary stream, urinary frequency, dysuria, and difficulty in starting and stopping urination. Some patients initially report pain in the lower back, pelvis, or upper thighs. Bilateral ureteral obstruction with renal insufficiency is not uncommon at the time of diagnosis.

DIAGNOSTIC STUDIES AND FINDINGS

Diagnostic Test	Findings
Digital rectal examination	50% of palpable prostatic nodules are cancerous
Excretory urogram	Bladder outlet involvement; ureteral obstruction or displacement
Closed or open needle biopsy via perineal or transrectal route	Malignant cells
Transrectal ultrasonography	Prostate lesions are hypoechoic
Pelvic computed tomography (CT) scan	Local extensions; nodal involvement
Magnetic resonance imaging (MRI) study	Capsular penetration; seminal vesicle involvement
Lymphangiography	Paraaortic and pelvic node involvement
Prostate-specific antigen	Elevated in localized disease; clinical recurrence
Prostatic acid phosphatase	Elevated in localized disease

MEDICAL MANAGEMENT

SURGERY

Transurethral resection

Radical prostatectomy

Bilateral orchiectomy

RADIATION THERAPY

External beam radiation

Interstitial implant

MEDICAL MANAGEMENT—cont'd

CHEMOTHERAPY

Single agents: Cyclophosphamide, 5FU, doxorubicin, methotrexate, cisplatin, mitomycin, dacarbazine (DTIC)

Hormonal therapy: Diethylstilbestrol (DES), Premarin, estradiol, Stilphostrol, estramustine phosphate
    Medical adrenalectomy: Aminoglutethimide, ketoconazole, spironolactone, glucocorticoids
    Antiandrogens: Cyproterone acetate, flutamide, megesterol acetate
    Gonadotropin-releasing hormone (GnRH) agonists: Leuprolide, Zoladex, Buserelin

SURGERY

Transurethral Resection

Transurethral resection is used for a solitary lesion of the prostate. A resectoscope is inserted through the urethra, and the prostate tissue is scraped out with a movable metal loop that cuts tissue with a high-frequency current. The competence of the internal bladder sphincter is destroyed, allowing seminal fluid to pass back into the bladder rather than out through the penis. Transurethral resection often is followed by external radiation beam therapy. (See Figure 7-3.)

COMPLICATIONS

Retrograde ejaculation
Psychologic impotence

Radical Prostatectomy

Radical prostatectomy by the perineal approach is used in patients with early-stage clinical disease and is considered one of the most effective ways of eradicating the tumor. This procedure involves removing the entire prostate, including the true prostatic capsule, seminal vesicles, and a portion of the bladder neck. The remaining portion of the bladder neck is reanastomosed to the urethra. The retropubic approach often is used first, since it provides access to the regional lymph nodes in the pelvis (pelvic lymphadenectomy) and affords more urinary control and less stricture formation.

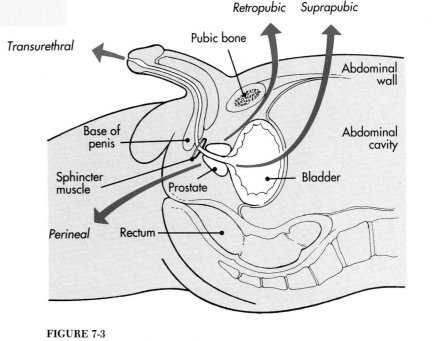

FIGURE 7-3
Surgical approaches to prostatectomy.

COMPLICATIONS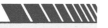

Infection
Fecal incontinence from sphincter injury
Thromboembolism
Lymphedema (rare)
Sexual dysfunction

Bilateral Orchiectomy

Bilateral orchiectomy may be used to eliminate 95% of testosterone production, a step that is useful in managing metastatic disease. Removing the testes effects an immediate response and avoids the cardiac complications of hormone therapy, without adversely affecting secondary sex characteristics such as body hair and distribution of fat.

COMPLICATIONS (RARE)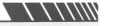

Incontinence
Urethral stricture
Sexual dysfunction (absence of emission and ejaculation, loss of ability to achieve erection)

Preoperative Preparation

The patient should be encouraged to express his concerns about sexual function and urinary continence. Plans for sperm banking, sexual counseling, and penile implants can be discussed at this time. The patient should also be taught turning, coughing, deep breathing, and leg exercises, and he should be fitted for anti-embolic stockings.

Preoperative bowel preparation is completed, and a Foley catheter is inserted if the patient has renal or bladder problems. Coexisting problems such as hypertension, cardiovascular disease, pulmonary disease, and diabetes should be stabilized if possible.

Postoperative Care

The patient who has undergone a transurethral resection will have a three-way catheter in place, which is removed 3 to 5 days after surgery. The urine should be observed for amount and color. Bladder irrigation, either continuous or intermittent, may be ordered to prevent clots and promote drainage. Aseptic technique should be used to prevent infection. Catheter obstruction, whether caused by a kinked tube, mucous plugs, or clots, will cause bladder distention and spasms if not diagnosed and treated early. Bladder spasms should be treated with antispasmodics, and stool softeners are given to prevent constipation caused by the narcotic in the antispasmodic. Once the catheter has been removed, the patient should be assessed frequently for problems with voiding, incontinence, and urethral stricture. Patients may have dribbling and urgency for several weeks.

The patient who has undergone a radical prostatectomy will also have a three-way indwelling catheter with the same needs for assessment and intervention as noted above. This patient may also have a suprapubic cystotomy catheter for 2 to 3 days after surgery. A retropubic incision will have a Penrose-type rubber drain, which is covered with a sterile dressing and removed 5 days after surgery. A perineal wound requires cleaning, heat lamp treatments, and a T-binder to stabilize the dressing. The patient is given a low-residue diet to prevent fecal contamination.

Ninety percent of men who have a radical prostatectomy are impotent. Either pharmacologic erection or surgical implantation of a prosthesis may be offered to these patients. Sympathomimetic agents such as ephedrine or imipramine may be helpful to some patients. The two major types of penile implants are the inflatable penile prosthesis and the rod prosthesis (Figure 7-4). The rod prosthesis is a malleable, semirigid, plastic rod placed in the bodies of the corpora cavernosa. This prosthesis gives the man a permanent semierection that is not painful and does not interfere with activities of daily living. With the inflatable prosthesis, the man squeezes and releases a pump bulb in the scrotum to pump fluid from the reservoir into both of the penile cylinders until he has an erection. Finger pressure on the valve that holds the fluid under pressure deflates the device.

Although the patient who undergoes bilateral orchiectomy may not have erection problems, his body image may be altered to such an extent that he has psychologic impotence. Implanting a testicular prosthesis at the time of surgery may prevent this.

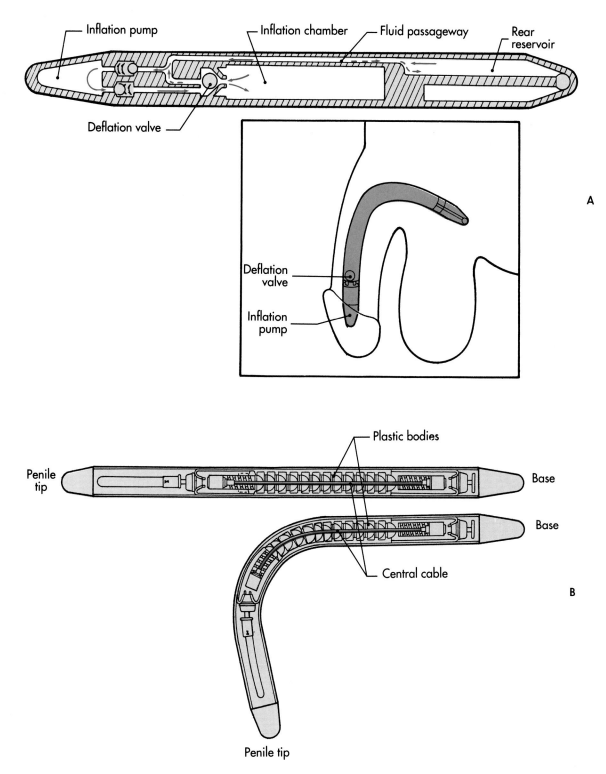

FIGURE 7-4
A, One-piece inflatable penile prosthesis. **B,** One-piece prosthesis with central cable.

RADIATION THERAPY

Radiation therapy may be the primary treatment of choice, particularly if the patient has a low performance status (as measured by the Karnofsky Performance Status scale [see Chapter 14, Table 14-2]) or other chronic medical conditions or if he prefers radiation therapy over surgery. External beam therapy of 6,000 to 7,000 rad may be given for cure.

COMPLICATIONS

Skin reaction
Urethral stricture
Incontinence, urinary frequency
Proctitis
Erectile dysfunction (20% to 40%)
Cystitis

Preprocedural Care

A patient who is to receive interstitial radiation must be told why health care providers spend limited amounts of time with him, stay away from the source of the radiation, and monitor his urine and bed linens for loss of radioactive materials. It should be emphasized to the patient that he is not radioactive.

Postprocedural Care

The patient who develops proctitis should be given an antidiarrheal drug and should be encouraged to follow a low-residue diet. Some patients may benefit from steroid enemas or suppositories.

Cystitis, which often develops during the first 1 to 3 weeks of treatment, is best managed by increasing oral fluids and administering antispasmodics and analgesics.

The care of patients receiving interstitial radioactive gold (^{198}Au) or iodine (^{125}I) should be governed by the principles of time, distance, and shielding. If radioactive iodine is used, problems such as symptoms of delayed irritative voiding, proctitis, rectal ulceration, or fistulas may develop, requiring treatment.

CHEMOTHERAPY

About 80% of prostate cancers are androgen dependent. Approximately half of patients with prostate cancer have metastases at diagnosis, and the mainstay of treatment for these patients is to decrease circulating androgens. Bilateral orchiectomy is one ablative procedure (see Surgery, page 112). Exogenous hormones such as diethylstilbestrol (DES) profoundly inhibit se-

cretion of pituitary luteinizing hormone, reduce circulating testosterone to castration level, increase sex steroid–binding globulin, and promote secretion of prolactin. DES usually is given in dosages of 1 to 3 mg per day orally. DES causes sodium retention, which may require diuretic therapy.

COMPLICATIONS

Cardiac failure
Gynecomastia
Loss of libido
Impotence
Thrombophlebitis, pulmonary embolus, cerebro-
vascular accident (with high dosages)
Hypercalcemia
Edema

Surgical adrenalectomy is no longer commonly used. Medical adrenalectomy can be induced with aminoglutethimide, which blocks adrenal steroidogenesis and synthesis of mineralocorticoid, glucocorticoid, and sex steroids. High-dose ketoconazole (an antifungal agent) affects the gonadal and adrenal androgens; however, it is expensive and presents problems of gastrointestinal intolerance or potent hepatotoxicity or both for some patients. Ketoconazole is given on an 8-hour schedule. It has been used in combination with orchiectomy, estrogens, and gonadotropin-releasing hormone (GnRH) analogs. Spironolactone inhibits adrenal and testicular precursors. Glucocorticoids suppress adrenocorticotropic hormone (ACTH).

Antiandrogens such as cyproterone acetate, flutamide, and megestrol acetate peripherally inhibit the action of dehydrotestosterone by interfering with the receptor steroid binding at the intracellular level.

GnRH agonists used for advanced prostate cancer inhibit prostatic growth and reduce the serum testosterone to castration level. High-intensity therapy may cause hot flashes, decreased libido, and erectile impotence.

Eighty percent of patients respond to hormonal manipulation with regression in tumor size, decreased urinary obstruction, decreased bone pain, and weight gain. The response lasts 1 to 3 years.

Single-agent chemotherapy, which has palliative benefit in men with hormone-resistant tumors, is as effective as combination therapy. Drugs used in combination include doxorubicin, 5FU, and mitomycin-C. Some agents have been combined with a hormonal agent such as estramustine phosphate and used in protocols with cyclophosphamide.

1 ASSESS

ASSESSMENT	OBSERVATIONS
Urinary function	Weak urinary stream, frequency, dysuria, difficulty starting and stopping urination; renal insufficiency, as evidenced by decreased output
Comfort	Pain in lower back, pelvis, or upper thighs
Psychosocial	Expressed fears of incontinence, altered sexuality, pain, and death

2 DIAGNOSE

NURSING DIAGNOSIS	SUBJECTIVE FINDINGS	OBJECTIVE FINDINGS
Altered patterns of urinary elimination related to presence of tumor surrounding urethra	Complains of urgency, frequency, dysuria, and difficulty starting and stopping urination	Weak stream; decreased output
Pain related to metastases to spine or pelvis	Complains of pain in lower back, pelvis, or upper thighs	Pained facial expression; guarding; withdrawn demeanor; impaired mobility
Fear related to incontinence, altered sexuality, pain, and death	Expresses fear of loss of bladder control, impotence, pain, and death	Angry; withdrawn; depressed

3 PLAN

Patient goals
1. The patient will have more normal urinary function.
2. The patient will have less or no pain.
3. The patient's fears will be alleviated.

4 IMPLEMENT

NURSING DIAGNOSIS	NURSING INTERVENTIONS	RATIONALE
Altered patterns of urinary elimination related to presence of tumor surrounding urethra	Weigh patient daily, and measure intake and output.	To monitor renal function and adequacy of elimination.
	Monitor blood studies: blood urea nitrogen (BUN), creatinine, acid-base balance, hemoglobin (Hb), and hematocrit (Hct). Also monitor urine studies: acid-base balance, creatinine, and specific gravity; test urine for protein.	To monitor renal function.

→ › ›

NURSING DIAGNOSIS	NURSING INTERVENTIONS	RATIONALE
	Assess for edema.	Edema is an indication of fluid retention.
	Monitor blood pressure.	Elevated blood pressure is an indication of fluid retention.
	Be alert for complaints of frequency, pain, and urination difficulties.	These signs may indicate infection or obstruction.
	Encourage patient to get adequate rest and exercise.	To decrease stress on urinary system.
	Increase patient's fluid intake.	To flush renal system.
	Catheterize patient only if necessary.	To eliminate urine retention.
Pain related to metastases to spine or pelvis	Change patient's position slowly.	To avoid injury and strain.
	Place patient in whirlpool bath, or apply heat.	To relax muscles.
	Provide safety measures such as use of walker or other assistive devices.	To prevent injury.
	Administer analgesics as needed.	To relieve pain.
	Offer massage.	To achieve muscle relaxation.
	Evaluate effectiveness of pain-relief measures.	To determine need for further intervention.
Fear related to incontinence, altered sexuality, pain, and death	Validate sources of fear with patient.	This guides therapeutic interventions.
	Help patient identify coping skills used successfully in the past.	To facilitate problem solving.
	Encourage patient to ask questions and express his feelings.	To try to relieve anxiety and help patient put thoughts into perspective.
	Provide accurate information about control of urinary function, sexuality, pain control, and prognosis.	To alleviate fears.
Knowledge deficit	See Patient Teaching.	

5 EVALUATE

PATIENT OUTCOME	DATA INDICATING THAT OUTCOME IS REACHED
Urinary function is normal.	Patient has no complaints of urgency, frequency, or dysuria and can start and stop stream.
Patient's pain has been relieved.	Patient has no pain in the lower back, pelvis, or upper thighs and can carry out self-care activities.
The patient's fears have been alleviated.	Patient acknowledges his fear of loss of control of urinary function, impotence, pain, and death but has refocused his concerns on resuming activities of daily living.

PATIENT TEACHING

1. Emphasize the need for an adequate fluid intake, exercise, and rest.
2. Instruct the patient in pain-relieving measures (e.g., exercise, warmth, and medication).
3. Tell the patient to notify the physician or nurse if signs and symptoms of renal insufficiency appear.
4. Discuss alternate expressions of sexuality, the value of sexual counseling, and the possibility of recovering some or all of sexual function after treatment ends.

Testicular Cancer

Testicular cancer is a rare form of cancer, but it is the most common cancer in young men between 15 and 35 years of age. With the advent of tumor markers (which indicate the presence of disease and enable the physician to monitor its response to treatment), refined surgery, and effective chemotherapy, the cure rate is as high as 90%.

EPIDEMIOLOGY

The cause of testicular cancer is unknown, although the incidence is higher in men with cryptorchism (undescended testes) or atrophic testis. Men with either of these conditions have a 40 times greater likelihood of developing cancer than do those with normal testes. When orchiopexy (surgical descent of a cryptorchid testis) is performed on boys before age 2, the likelihood of cancer developing is virtually eliminated. Testicular cancer is more common in whites than in blacks in the United States. The incidence is also higher in the higher socioeconomic

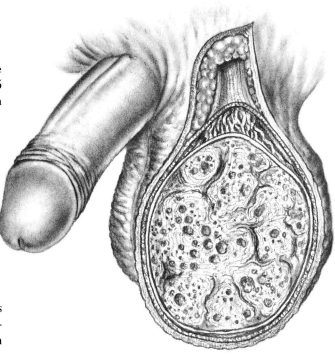

G.J.W.

classes. Men whose mothers took exogenous hormones during pregnancy also have a higher incidence of testicular cancer.

As recommended by the American Cancer Society, young men from puberty through age 40 should be taught and encouraged to perform monthly testicular self-examination (TSE). After a warm bath or shower, the index and middle fingers are placed on one side of the testicle and the thumbs on the other side. Digital separation of the anterior testis from the posterior elements, including the epididymis and cord, must be done with care so that the intrascrotal contents can be palpated. A gentle, rolling motion enables the man to palpate each testicle completely. One testicle may be larger than the other. Any lump or change in either testicle should be reported to the nurse or physician. (See Patient Teaching Guide, page 240.)

PATHOPHYSIOLOGY

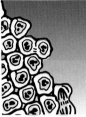

Most testicular tumors are of germ cell origin and are malignant. The basic categories are the seminoma and the heterogeneous, nonseminomatous germ cell tumor. Three percent of testicular tumors arise from stromal tissue.

Some testicular tumors first become apparent in extragonadal tissues, primarily the mediastinum. Paraaortic lymph node involvement, ureteral obstruction, and pulmonary metastases may be present at diagnosis.

SIGNS AND SYMPTOMS

The first sign of the disease usually is a small, hard, painless lump in the testicle. Symptoms include a sensation of heaviness in the testicle, sudden fluid accumulation in the scrotum, and perineal pain or discomfort.

Some men report a history of trauma, mumps, or orchitis; episodic testicular pain; low back, groin, or abdominal ache; and breast enlargement or tenderness. If these symptoms persist after antibiotic therapy for suspected epididymitis, the physician should suspect testicular cancer.

DIAGNOSTIC STUDIES AND FINDINGS

Diagnostic Test	Findings
Palpation of testes	Mass
Transillumination	Intrascrotal lesion
Excretory urography	Displacement of ureters or kidney
Abdominal computed tomography (CT) and ultrasound studies, lymphangiography	Areas of abnormality
Serum alpha-fetoprotein (AFP)	Elevated
Human chorionic gonadotropin (HCG)	Elevated
Chest x-ray, CT scan, and whole lung tomography	Evidence of metastatic disease
Radical inguinal orchiectomy (biopsy)	Malignant cells

MEDICAL MANAGEMENT

SURGERY

Inguinal exploration and orchiectomy

Bilateral retroperitoneal lymph node dissection

RADIATION THERAPY

External beam radiation

CHEMOTHERAPY

Seminomas: Cyclophosphamide

Nonseminomas: PVB (cisplatin, vinblastine, bleomycin)

SURGERY

Radical inguinal orchiectomy is the removal of the testis, epididymis, a portion of the vas deferens, and a portion of the gonadal lymphatics and their blood supply. Hyperplasia of the remaining testis will provide enough testosterone to maintain the man's sexual characteristics. He may have a lower sperm count or decreased sperm motility.

Retroperitoneal lymphadenectomy is the removal of all perivascular tissue from the area bounded superiorly by the renal arteries and veins, inferiorly by the common iliac arteries to the bifurcation, and laterally by the ureters. This procedure usually is unilateral. After surgery the patient may be able to achieve an erection, but his ability to ejaculate may be diminished.

Preoperative Preparation

Sexuality and fertility counseling should be offered to the patient after reviewing the impact of the surgery on his anatomy and function. Other aspects of preoperative care include measures taken with all patients undergoing general anesthesia.

Postoperative Care

The patient who has an orchiectomy will have a high inguinal incision. Nursing care focuses on relieving pain, maintaining a dry, sterile dressing on the wound, and reassuring the patient that his altered body image does not affect his fertility.

The patient who has a retroperitoneal lymphadenectomy usually has a transabdominal incision. A nasogastric tube is attached to suction and maintained until bowel sounds return. The patient may have a Foley catheter to facilitate urinary drainage during the early postoperative period. The vital signs should be monitored for early diagnosis of hemorrhage and shock. The dressing should be checked for amount and type of drainage and should be changed using sterile technique. The patient will need to adjust to his diminished ejaculatory ability.

Instead of treating nonseminomas with radical retroperitoneal lymph node dissection, the patient may be placed on a surveillance program with monthly follow-up for 12 months (physical examination, tumor markers, chest x-ray). If the patient remains negative after 1 year, he will go to follow-up every 2 months for the second year and then every 6 months for life. This surveillance program avoids unnecessary node dissections, but patient compliance is critical. Patients who relapse receive salvage combination chemotherapy.

RADIATION THERAPY

External beam therapy is used for seminomas, which are very radiosensitive. The retroperitoneal area receives a dose of 2,000 to 3,500 rad. A lead cup is used to shield the remaining testis.

COMPLICATIONS

Fatigue
Bone marrow suppression
Diarrhea
Decreased sperm count (recovery is dose related)

CHEMOTHERAPY

Chemotherapy may be used before surgery in the management of advanced, unresectable, retroperitoneal disease. This therapy frequently converts an unresectable tumor into a tumor that can be safely resected by means of radical retroperitoneal lymph node dissection. Salvage chemotherapy may be prescribed if elevated tumor markers are seen in disseminated disease caused by nonseminomatous tumors.

The use of PVB (cisplatin, vinblastine, bleomycin) leads to a 10% long-term survival rate. Patient problems include leukopenia, sepsis, nausea, vomiting, and cisplatin-induced nephrotoxicity and neurotoxicity. PVB or doxorubicin (Adriamycin) may be used before irradiation to treat metastases to retroperitoneal nodes or other sites.

With regard to sterility, there is a high degree of recovery of spermatogenesis 2 to 3 years after chemotherapy is begun. There is no increase in the incidence of fetal abnormalities.

1 ASSESS

ASSESSMENT	OBSERVATIONS
Scrotum	Small, hard painless lump in testis; sensation of heaviness, swelling
Breasts	Enlargement or tenderness
Comfort	Perineal pain or discomfort; low back, groin, or abdominal ache
Psychosocial	Fear of altered sexuality, infertility, pain, and death

2 DIAGNOSE

NURSING DIAGNOSIS	SUBJECTIVE FINDINGS	OBJECTIVE FINDINGS
Body image disturbance related to changes in scrotum and/or breasts	Complains of sensation of heaviness in scrotum, tenderness in breasts	Small, hard, painless lump in testis; breast enlargement
Pain related to pressure of tumor or metastases on perineum, groin, or abdomen	Complains of perineal pain or discomfort and low back, groin, or abdominal pain	Pained facial expression; withdrawn demeanor; guarding; restlessness
Fear related to altered sexuality, infertility, pain, or death	Expresses fear of impotence, sterility, pain, or death	Angry; withdrawn; depressed

3 PLAN

Patient goals
1. The patient will accept the change in his body and integrate it into a positive self-concept.
2. The patient will be free of pain.
3. The patient's fears will be alleviated.

4 IMPLEMENT

NURSING DIAGNOSIS	NURSING INTERVENTIONS	RATIONALE
Body image disturbance related to changes in scrotum and/or breasts	Assess patient's perception of impact of scrotal mass and/or breast enlargement on spouse or partner.	To clarify patient's perception of severity of problem.
	Respect patient's need for period of denial and his individual coping style.	Denial can be an effective defense mechanism.
	Help patient express feelings as anger.	May defuse some anxiety.
	Encourage patient to talk about changes.	To help patient see problem realistically.

NURSING DIAGNOSIS	NURSING INTERVENTIONS	RATIONALE
	Explore patient's feelings about impact of change on his appearance.	To determine need for disguising the change.
	Provide information about treatment options.	To enable patient to make realistic decisions.
Pain related to pressure of tumor or metastases on perineal, groin, or abdominal regions	Handle patient gently.	To prevent further discomfort.
	Apply heat as ordered with heating pad; hot water bottle; warm, moist compress; or warm water bath.	To promote circulation and decrease swelling and irritation.
	Discuss pain-relieving measures such as scrotal support, analgesics, and massage.	To enhance patient's comfort.
	Evaluate effectiveness of pain-relieving measures.	To determine need for further intervention.
Fear related to altered sexuality, infertility, pain, or death	Validate sources of fear with patient.	This guides therapeutic interventions.
	Help patient identify coping skills used successfully in the past.	To facilitate problem solving.
	Encourage patient to ask questions and express feelings.	To try to relieve anxiety and help patient put thoughts into perspective.
	Provide accurate information about sexuality, pain control, and prognosis.	To alleviate fears.
Knowledge deficit	See Patient Teaching.	

5 EVALUATE

PATIENT OUTCOME	DATA INDICATING THAT OUTCOME IS REACHED
Patient has a healthy body image.	Patient can look at and touch his scrotum and can describe himself as a person with a unique body configuration.
Patient's pain has been relieved.	Patient has no perineal, groin, or abdominal pain.
Patient's fears have been alleviated.	Patient acknowledges his fears, but has refocused his concerns on resuming activities of daily living.

PATIENT TEACHING

1. Inform the patient about testicular implants.
2. Discuss the ability of a healthy testis to compensate for loss of function in the other, so that male characteristics are not adversely affected.
3. Provide information about sperm banking and sexual counseling.
4. Stress importance of lifelong follow-up evaluations.

CHAPTER 8

Gynecologic Cancers

The incidence of gynecologic cancers is increasing in the United States; these cancers account for 15% of all cancer diagnoses in women. Gynecologic cancers are linked to life-style habits such as smoking, obesity, sexually transmitted diseases, and early age at the time of initial intercourse. On the positive side, the survival rate for these cancers is also increasing.

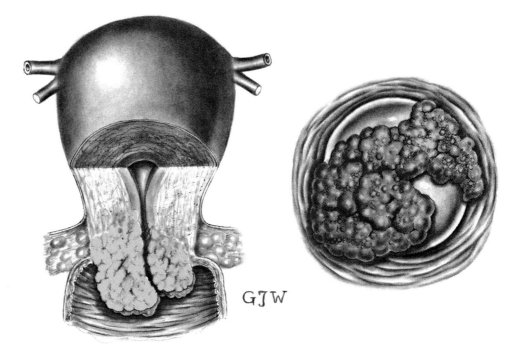

GJW

ADVANCED CERVICAL CANCER

Cervical Cancer

Cancer of the cervix is more common among women of lower socioeconomic status, many of whom are black or Hispanic, but all women are at high risk for developing it. The incidence of invasive cervical cancer is steadily decreasing, but that of carcinoma in situ is increasing and affecting younger women.

EPIDEMIOLOGY

The most important risk factor is initial intercourse at an early age, particularly in the 15- to 17-year-old age group. This is because the biologic change in the cervical epithelium renders it more susceptible to carcinogens. Other risk factors are multiple sex partners; sexually transmitted diseases (particularly human papilloma virus and possibly herpes simplex virus); pregnancies in the teen years; and smoking.

Beta-carotene or some related aspect of a diet rich in carrots and green vegetables is believed to help protect against invasive cervical cancer. Vitamins C and A, barrier-type contraception, and vasectomy in sexual partners are also protective. Some researchers believe that cervical cancer may be a venereal disease.

The Papanicolaou (Pap) smear (Figure 8-1) is highly effective when used for secondary prevention, although there is some question as to when women should begin having this test. Current guidelines recommend a yearly Pap smear with pelvic examination after age 20 or whenever sexual activity begins. Primary prevention guidelines include abstaining from intercourse during adolescence and eating adequate amounts of carrots and green vegetables.

PATHOPHYSIOLOGY

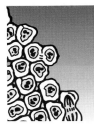

Cervical cancers are predominantly the squamous cell type (85% to 90%); the remaining 10% to 15% are adenocarcinomas. Adenocarcinomas, especially clear cell tumors, are related to in utero exposure to diethylstilbestrol (DES). They are seen more often in younger women and are increasing in incidence.

Cervical cancer begins as a neoplastic change in the squamocolumnar junction. Over time abnormal cells progress to involve the full thickness of this epithelium. These changes are called *cervical intraepithelial neoplasia* (CIN).

Three types of lesions can be seen with cervical cancer:

Exophytic lesion: cauliflower-like, fungating, friable, bleeds easily, may be small or extensive

Excavating or ulcerative-necrotic lesion: replaces upper vagina and cervix with ulcer or crater that bleeds easily

Endophytic lesion: develops within the endocervical canal, manifests no visible tumor or ulcer, and renders the cervix hard to the touch

Cervical cancer spreads by means of direct extension (most common route), via the lymphatics, or by the hematogenous route.

Staging of the disease is useful for making treatment decisions and determining the prognosis (Table 8-1).

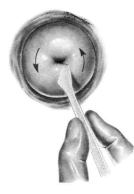

FIGURE 8-1
A Papanicolaou smear. The cervix is scraped with the bifid end of the spatula. (From Seidel et al.[53])

The cure rate for cervical cancer at each stage is as follows:

Ia: nearly 100%
Ib and IIa: (for 5 years) 65% to 90%
IIb: 50% to 50%
III: 30% to 40%
IV: 5% to 10%

Adenocarcinoma has a poor prognosis. Thorough follow-up after initial treatment of cervical cancer is essential, because the disease persists or recurs in one third of women with invasive cancer. These patients should have a pelvic examination every 3 months for 1 year, then every 6 months for the rest of their lives. Seventy-five percent of recurrence is local, and 25% is distant metastases to the liver, bones, and mediastinal or supraclavicular nodes.

SIGNS AND SYMPTOMS

Abnormal bleeding is the most common sign of cervical cancer. The bleeding at first may be a thin, watery, blood-tinged vaginal discharge, which progresses to spotting and frank bleeding. Other signs and symptoms include a prolonged menstrual period or intermittent periods, "contact" bleeding after intercourse, and anemia caused by chronic blood loss. Advanced disease is marked by odor or possibly pain in the lower back, legs, and groin; leg edema; difficulty voiding, urgency, and hematuria (as a result of invasion of the bladder); and rectal tenesmus and bleeding (as a result of invasion of the rectum). Cervical cancer rarely occurs during pregnancy, but it should be ruled out if the patient has unexplained bleeding.

Table 8-1 _____

INTERNATIONAL STAGING OF CANCER OF THE CERVIX

Stage	Description and features
0	Carcinoma in situ, intraepithelial carcinoma (cases of stage 0 should not be included in any therapeutic statistics for invasive carcinoma)
I	Carcinoma strictly confined to the cervix; extension to the corpus should be disregarded
	a. Preclinical carcinomas of the cervix; i.e., those diagnosed only by microscopy
	Ia1. Minimal microscopically evident stromal invasion
	Ia2. Lesions detected microscopically that can be measured; the upper limit of the measurement should not show a depth of invasion of more than 5 mm taken from the base of the epithelium, either surface or glandular, from which it originates, and a second dimension, the horizontal spread, must not exceed 7 mm; larger lesions should be staged as Ib
	Ib. Lesions of greater dimension than stage Ia2, whether seen clinically or not; space involvement should not alter the staging but should be specifically recorded so as to determine whether it should affect treatment decisions in the future
II	Carcinoma extending beyond the cervix but not onto the pelvic wall; involves the vagina but not the lower one third
	a. No obvious parametrial involvement
	b. Obvious parametrial involvement
III	Carcinoma extending onto the pelvic wall (on rectal examination, there is no cancer-free space between the tumor and the pelvic wall; the tumor involves the lower third of the vagina; all cases with a hydronephrosis or nonfunctioning kidney)
	a. No extension onto the pelvic wall
	b. Extension onto the pelvic wall; urinary obstruction of one or both ureters on intravenous pyelogram (IVP) without the other criteria for stage III disease
IV	Carcinoma extending beyond the true pelvis or clinically involving the mucosa of the bladder or rectum (a bullous edema, as such, does not permit a case to be allotted to stage IV)
	a. Spread to adjacent organs
	b. Spread to distant organs

From American Cancer Society.[1]

DIAGNOSTIC STUDIES AND FINDINGS

Diagnostic Test	Findings
Cervical examination and biopsy by means of colposcopy	Visible mass or malignant cells, or both
Computed tomography (CT) scan of the abdomen	Involvement of retroperitoneal lymph nodes
Magnetic resonance imaging (MRI) study	Estimated tumor volume
Lymphangiography followed by fine needle aspiration	Involvement of lymph channels
Supraclavicular node biopsy	Malignant cells
Chest x-ray, excretory urography, cystoscopy, proctosigmoidoscopy	Evidence of spread of tumor
Complete blood count	Anemia

MEDICAL MANAGEMENT

SURGERY

Conization

Cryotherapy or laser ablation

Abdominal or vaginal radical hysterectomy and pelvic node dissection

Pelvic exenteration

RADIATION THERAPY

External beam radiation

Intracavity therapy

CHEMOTHERAPY

Cisplatin, carboplatin, cyclophosphamide, melphalan, 5FU, vincristine, methotrexate, hydroxyurea

SURGERY

Cervical Conization/Cryotherapy

Cervical conization may be used as a conservative measure to treat carcinoma in situ in women of childbearing age. The procedure maintains the integrity of the internal os. **Cryotherapy** (freezing of the malignant lesion with portable cautery) or laser ablation may be selected instead. The use of any of these treatments requires a lesion that is visible by means of colposcopy and a negative endocervical curettage.

COMPLICATIONS

Immediate:
  Hemorrhage
  Uterine perforation
  Complications of anesthesia
Delayed:
  Cervical stenosis
  Infertility
  Cervical incompetence
  Increased incidence of preterm (low birth weight) delivery

Hysterectomy

Abdominal or vaginal radical hysterectomy with pelvic node dissection may be the treatment of choice for patients with cancer in stage Ia, Ib, or IIa. The decision to use surgery rather than radiation therapy in stages Ib and IIa is based on preserving ovarian function, which is easier to accomplish with surgery, although the ovaries can be protected from the irradiated field if radiation therapy is used alone or with surgery. The decision is based on the tumor's size, location, and involvement and on the patient's health status.

COMPLICATIONS

Ureteral fistulas
Bladder dysfunction
Pulmonary embolus
Pelvic infection
Bowel obstruction
Rectovaginal fistulas
Hemorrhage

Pelvic Exenteration

Pelvic exenteration usually includes nodal dissection and removal of the bladder, urethra, uterus, cervix, vagina, rectum, and all lateral supporting tissues. The patient will have a permanent colostomy and ileal conduit. An anterior exenteration involves removal of all pelvic viscera except the rectosigmoid, with creation of an ileal conduit. A posterior exenteration involves removal of all pelvic viscera except the bladder, with creation of a permanent colostomy. Vaginal reconstruction may be done at the time of the surgery or as a later procedure.

IMMEDIATE POSTOPERATIVE COMPLICATIONS

Pulmonary embolus	Myocardial infarction
Pulmonary edema	Sepsis
Cerebrovascular accident	Small-bowel
Hemorrhage	obstruction

Preoperative Care

The patient receives the preoperative preparation given to all patients undergoing abdominal surgery. In addition, she usually receives a douche with an antiseptic solution the evening before or the morning of surgery, or both. The extent of the procedure, as well as the patient's perception of the impact of the surgery on her body image and sexuality, determine the teaching and counseling she needs.

The patient and her significant other may find it helpful to discuss their concerns with the health care provider, a sexual counselor, or a former patient trained in addressing issues related to sexuality. If the patient is to undergo a pelvic exenteration, she may wish to have an ostomy visitor before the surgery.

Postoperative Care

The patient should be encouraged to turn, cough, and deep breathe at regular intervals, splinting her abdomen with her arms or a pillow to avoid tension on the incision. The dressing should be evaluated frequently and changed as needed. Early ambulation is encouraged to prevent circulatory and respiratory complications.

If the patient has one or more stomas, she should be guided in the care of them as her physical recovery from the surgery permits (see page 85 for care of bowel stomas and page 103 for care of urinary stomas). The dramatic change in the patient's body image resulting from exenteration will require the nurse's patience, sensitivity, and support as the patient adjusts to the change and its impact on her self-concept and self-confidence.

The patient having cervical conization by dilation and curettage should be told to expect spotting and bleeding for as long as a week after the procedure. Cramping may also occur and usually can be controlled with oral analgesics. Coitus and douching should be avoided for 2 to 3 weeks after the procedure.

The patient undergoing abdominal surgery should be instructed to avoid coitus or douching for 6 weeks or as indicated by the physician; to walk at regular intervals and to avoid sitting for prolonged periods at home or when traveling; to inspect the incision site and report abnormalities to the health care provider; and to avoid heavy lifting and vigorous activity for 6 to 8 weeks after surgery.

RADIATION THERAPY

Radiation therapy is the primary treatment for cervical cancer in stages IIb, IIIa, IIIb, and IV. In stage I disease, radiation therapy and radical surgery achieve similar cure rates, but radiation may cause delayed complications and secondary sexual dysfunction. Radiation therapy may also be used to treat a recurrence of cervical cancer.

The radiation field includes one chain of lymph nodes above the site of the malignancy. The larger the tumor, the more likely the patient is to respond positively to external beam rather than intracavity therapy. Brachytherapy is directed toward the primary tumor and its paracervical and vaginal extensions. An applicator with colpostats approximated to the vaginal fornices is inserted into the uterine cavity so that high doses of radiation are delivered directly to the cervix. If the vagina is distorted by advanced cancer, a group of 18-gauge, hollow, steel needles may be inserted into the parametrium; however, this technique may increase morbidity and needs further study.

External beam therapy is used to treat extension of the tumor into the extrauterine pelvic soft tissue and lymph nodes. The beam is aimed so as to reach the upper end of the fifth lumbar vertebra.

External beam therapy and brachytherapy may be used in combination, for example, to shrink an invasive tumor and prepare the area for placement of an intracavity device.

COMPLICATIONS

Acute:
  Skin reactions
  Acute radiation cystitis
  Proctosigmoiditis
  Enteritis
Delayed:
  Retrovaginal or vesicovaginal fistula
  Sigmoid perforation or stricture
  Rectal ulcer or proctitis
  Intestinal obstruction
  Ureteral stricture
  Severe cystitis
  Bladder ulcer
  Pulmonary embolus
  Pelvic hemorrhage, abscess
  Sexual dysfunction secondary to vaginal stenosis

CHEMOTHERAPY

Chemotherapy is used to treat stage III and stage IV disease. However, the results with this treatment have not been favorable, with an increased survival time of only 4 to 9 months.

Thirty-five percent of patients with cervical cancer have a recurrence, with a higher incidence in the later stages of the disease. The recurrence usually develops within 2 years of initial treatment. The patient often has unexplained weight loss; leg edema; pelvic, thigh, or buttock pain; serosanguineous vaginal bleeding; ureteral obstruction; and/or enlarged left supraclavicular nodes. As noted above, radiation therapy may be used for palliation with some degree of symptomatic relief.

1 ASSESS

ASSESSMENT	OBSERVATION
Perineal area	Unusual bleeding or vaginal discharge; prolonged or intermittent menstrual periods; "contact" bleeding after intercourse; malodorous discharge
Hematologic	Anemia
Renal	Difficulty voiding, urgency, hematuria
Intestinal	Rectal tenesmus, bleeding
Comfort	Pain in lower back, legs, and groin; leg edema

2 DIAGNOSE

NURSING DIAGNOSIS	SUBJECTIVE FINDINGS	OBJECTIVE FINDINGS
Impaired skin integrity related to vaginal discharge	Complains of pruritus	Vaginal bleeding or discharge; redness or swelling, warmth of perineal area; odor
Pain related to pressure of tumor on adjacent structures	Complains of pain in lower back, legs, and groin; rectal tenesmus	Grimacing; impaired mobility; leg edema
Fatigue related to blood loss and anemia	Complains of being tired, lacking energy	Anemia
Altered patterns of urinary elimination related to pressure of tumor on urethra	Complains of difficulty voiding, urgency	Hematuria

→ › ›

NURSING DIAGNOSIS	SUBJECTIVE FINDINGS	OBJECTIVE FINDINGS
Body image disturbance related to actual or potential alterations in anatomic structure	Expresses concern about effect of tumor and its treatment on her appearance and sexuality	Anxious; withdrawn; depressed

3 PLAN

Patient goals

1. The patient's perineal area will be clean and odor free.
2. The patient will be free of pain.
3. The patient will have the energy she needs for activities of daily living and recreational activities.
4. The patient will have normal urinary elimination.
5. The patient will have a positive self-image and self-concept as a person and a woman.

4 IMPLEMENT

NURSING DIAGNOSIS	NURSING INTERVENTIONS	RATIONALE
Impaired skin integrity related to vaginal discharge	Change dressings or pads frequently; maintain dry, clean linen and dry skin; provide clean clothing.	To maintain cleanliness and enhance patient's comfort.
	Observe skin for irritation.	To determine need for further intervention.
	Observe quality and quantity of drainage.	To determine status of infection.
	Administer antibiotics as ordered.	To combat infection.
	Administer perineal care as indicated.	To promote comfort and remove drainage from skin.
Pain related to pressure of tumor on adjacent structures	*For abdominal pressure:*	
	Change patient's position frequently, and remove constrictive clothing.	To relieve pressure.
	Give small, frequent feedings.	To avoid abdominal distention.
	Place patient in sitting position.	To relieve abdominal pressure.
	Insert rectal tube as indicated.	To relieve flatus.
	Auscultate abdomen for abnormal bowel sounds.	To assess gastrointestinal status.

NURSING DIAGNOSIS	NURSING INTERVENTIONS	RATIONALE
	For back pain, leg pain, or lymphedema:	
	Position patient comfortably, and change position slowly.	To avoid injury and increased pain.
	Maintain body alignment.	To avoid injury or muscular stretching.
	Apply heating pad, hot water bottle, or warm, moist compress.	To relax muscles and increase circulation.
	Bathe patient in warm water.	To relax muscles.
	Massage gently.	To promote circulation and relax muscles.
	Encourage adequate rest.	To decrease energy expenditure.
	Provide pain-relief measure of patient's choice.	To promote self-care.
	Be alert for complaints of pain, and assess duration and radiation of pain.	To determine need for further intervention.
Fatigue related to blood loss and anemia	Help patient and significant others understand the physiologic basis for fatigue and that it will diminish upon improvement or correction of the anemia.	Understanding nature of fatigue helps patient better tolerate it.
	Encourage patient to discuss feelings related to fatigue.	Expression of strong feelings often relieves anxiety and thus fatigue.
	Encourage patient to identify behavior associated with fatigue (e.g., emotional lability and irritability).	Behaviors are temporary, caused by anemic condition.
	Help patient plan periods of rest and activity.	To achieve adequate levels of energy for activities of daily living (ADL).
Altered patterns of urinary elimination related to pressure of tumor on urethra	Measure intake and output.	To monitor fluid balance.
	Inspect urine for bleeding; check with Hemastix.	To detect urinary tract bleeding.
	Encourage patient to get adequate rest and exercise.	To maintain general well-being.
	Ambulate patient often.	To promote renal circulation and urinary elimination.
	Apply heating pad or hot water bottle.	To relax bladder musculature.
	Catheterize only if necessary.	To avoid infection.

NURSING DIAGNOSIS	NURSING INTERVENTIONS	RATIONALE
Body image disturbance related to actual or potential alterations in anatomic structures	Encourage patient to discuss feelings and concerns with health care providers and significant others.	Articulating feelings may decrease anxiety.
	Help patient identify, label, and express feelings about significance of female genitals, treatment modalities, and anticipated prognosis.	Patient can then deal with specific issues.
	Involve other disciplines in planning and managing patient care.	Varied perspectives are helpful in addressing complex psychosocial needs.
	Promote acceptance of a positive, realistic body image.	So patient can resume preillness life-style.
Knowledge deficit	See Patient Teaching.	

5 EVALUATE

PATIENT OUTCOME	DATA INDICATING THAT OUTCOME IS REACHED
Patient's perineal area is clean and odor free.	Perineal area is clean, free of odor, and normal in color; patient reports feeling clean and comfortable in perineal area.
Patient's pain has been relieved.	Patient's facial expression is calm and relaxed; her body appears relaxed, and she says she has no pain.
Patient's fatigue is gone.	Patient can coordinate rest and activity so that she can carry out ADL and enjoy recreational activities.
Patient's urinary function is normal.	Patient maintains a balance between intake and output and voids without difficulty.
Patient's body image is realistic.	Patient shows realistic sense of self and body.

PATIENT TEACHING ■■■■■■■■■■■■■■■■■■■■■■■■■■■■■■■■■

1. Emphasize the need to maintain perineal hygiene.
2. Teach the patient nonpharmacologic comfort measures (e.g., heat, positioning, relaxation exercises, guided imagery, and distraction).
3. Help the patient plan periods of activity and rest, which will enable her to accomplish activities of daily living and recreational activities.
4. Teach the patient to drink large quantities of water and nonacidic fluids, to void when she feels the urge, and to use warmth and other individually effective techniques to stimulate voiding.
5. Refer the patient to support groups, sexual counselors, and other community programs that will help her to maintain a positive self-image.

Endometrial Cancer

Endometrial cancer, the most common gynecologic malignancy, is found primarily in postmenopausal women, with the largest number of cases in women between 55 and 60 years of age. As many as 80% of all women are diagnosed after menopause. Because of early diagnosis and treatment, only 13% of patients die of the disease. The increasing prevalence of this type of cancer may be related to the fact that women are living longer.

EPIDEMIOLOGY

Risk factors for endometrial cancer include obesity (more than 15% over normal weight); never having had a child (nulliparity); endometrial hyperplasia; polycystic ovarian disease; late menopause (after age 52); a history of irregular menses; failure of ovulation; a history of breast, colon, or ovarian cancer; diabetes; hypertension; and prolonged use of exogenous estrogen therapy (unopposed estrogen). The incidence is higher among urban, white, and Jewish women.

Unopposed estrogen (without progestational influence), whether exogenous or endogenous, can cause varying degrees of cystic and adenomatous hyperplasia, which is a precursor to endometrial cancer. Estrogen stored in the fat of obese women and released in a slow manner can cause increased unopposed estrogen. Obesity is also linked with diabetes and hypertension. Obese postmenopausal women have depressed secretion of serum sex hormone–binding globulin (SHBG), leaving higher concentrations of free estradiol in the blood. Using cyclic progesterone with estrogen as replacement therapy can decrease the risk of endometrial cancer.

Prevention focuses on healthier eating habits, weight control, and regular health examinations. There is no test for premalignant conditions of the uterus, although malignant endometrial cells are occasionally found in a cervical Pap smear.

Stage I tumors have the highest 5-year survival rate (about 77%). Other prognostic factors include the depth of myometrial invasion, lymph node involvement, the histologic grade of the cells, uterine size, peritoneal cytologic findings, and the patient's age.

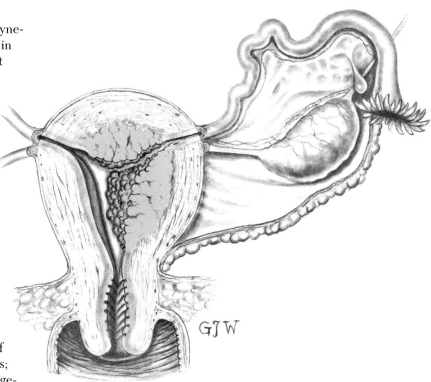

ENDOMETRIAL CANCER

PATHOPHYSIOLOGY

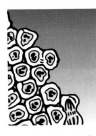

Most endometrial cancers (90%) are adenocarcinomas. Other types seen are adenoacanthoma, clear cell, and squamous cell tumors. Although rare, squamous cell carcinomas are aggressive; they arise from the endometrial stroma and myometrium and affect younger women (median age is 43 to 56).

Adenocarcinomas usually start in the fundus and may spread to involve the entire endometrium. The tumor may infiltrate the myometrium, extend through the serosa into the endocervical canal, and involve the entire cervix. It also may extend into the parametrium, fallopian tubes, and ovaries.

Metastatic spread most commonly is to the pelvic and paraaortic lymph nodes (Figure 8-2). Spread has been positively correlated with tumor differentiation, stage of disease, and amount of myometrial invasion. Hematogenous spread, seen most often in sarcomas, involves the lungs, liver, bones, and brain.

SIGNS AND SYMPTOMS

Any postmenopausal bleeding should be evaluated as endometrial cancer, as should prolonged and excessive bleeding at any point in time. Another presenting symptom is pain in the lumbosacral, hypogastric, and pelvic areas. Advanced disease causes bowel obstruction, jaundice, ascites, and respiratory difficulty.

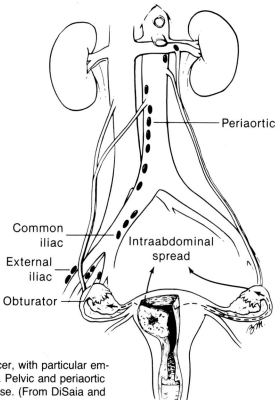

Periaortic

Common iliac

External iliac

Obturator

Intraabdominal spread

FIGURE 8-2
The spread pattern of endometrial cancer, with particular emphasis on potential lymph node spread. Pelvic and periaortic nodes are at risk, even in stage I disease. (From DiSaia and Creasman.[17])

DIAGNOSTIC STUDIES AND FINDINGS

Diagnostic Test	Findings
Pap smear	May indicate presence of malignant endometrial cells
Endometrial biopsy or fractional dilation and curettage (D & C)	Malignant cells
Laparotomy with sampling of peritoneal fluid or washings	Malignant cells

MEDICAL MANAGEMENT

SURGERY

Total abdominal hysterectomy with bilateral salpingo-oophorectomy with pelvic and paraaortic lymph node biopsies

RADIATION THERAPY

Preoperative intracavity therapy

Postoperative external beam radiation

CHEMOTHERAPY

Progesterone: Megace and/or hydroxyprogesterone or medroxyprogesterone acetate

Single-agent chemotherapy: Cisplatin, doxorubicin, hexamethylmelamine, cyclophosphamide

SURGERY

Total abdominal hysterectomy with bilateral salpingo-oophorectomy and pelvic and paraaortic lymph node biopsies is the treatment of choice for most cases of endometrial cancer. The procedure usually includes peritoneal washings and exploration of the abdomen for evidence of disease beyond the uterus. (See pages 125-126 for care of the patient undergoing total abdominal hysterectomy.)

RADIATION THERAPY

Radiation therapy may be combined with surgery (i.e., an intracavity radium or cesium implant may be placed in the uterus, endocervical canal, and vaginal fornices). When done before surgery, this form of radiation therapy decreases the likelihood of viable tumor cells being seeded into the operative field, thus providing the basis for local recurrence or distant dissemination of the tumor. Areas of nodal involvement may also be irradiated at this time. External beam radiation therapy may be used after surgery to meet the same goals.

CHEMOTHERAPY

Chemotherapy is used in endometrial cancer to manage metastatic or recurrent disease. The treatment of choice is hormonal manipulation with such progestational agents as oral megestrol acetate (Megace) and/or hydroxyprogesterone or intramuscular medroxyprogesterone (Depo-Provera). This therapy is most effective with well-differentiated estrogen and/or progesterone receptor–positive tumors with a long disease-free interval after initial treatment.

Studies are continuing on the role of estrogen and progesterone receptors in endometrial cancer, the advisability of adjunctive systemic hormonal therapy, and the use of hormonal therapy after initial treatment of the cancer.

Single-agent chemotherapy with cisplatin, doxorubicin, hexamethylmelamine, and cyclophosphamide has shown some therapeutic effect, particularly with doxorubicin as the standard to which new agents or combinations of agents are compared. High-dose cisplatin in women who have had no prior chemotherapy has been shown to produce a high response rate.

NURSING CARE OF THE PATIENT WITH ENDOMETRIAL CANCER

NURSING DIAGNOSIS

Fluid volume loss related to postmenopausal bleeding as evidenced by serosanguineous discharge to frank bleeding; there may be irregular or heavy menstrual flow in premenopausal woman

NURSING INTERVENTIONS AND RATIONALE

1. Observe characteristics and amount of blood loss to determine need for fluid and blood component replacement.
2. Monitor vital signs at frequent intervals during episodes of heavy bleeding to detect shock early.
3. Encourage patient to drink large volumes of fluid to prevent dehydration.
4. Monitor intake and output and urine specific gravity to detect renal dysfunction.
5. Administer IV fluids as prescribed to replace lost fluid volume.
6. Monitor lab reports to detect development of anemia.
7. Observe for signs and symptoms of worsening fluid volume deficit, including decreased urine output, concentrated urine, output greater than intake, weakness, and change in mental status, to determine need for large volumes of IV fluids and blood components at rapid rate.

NURSING DIAGNOSIS

Pain related to pressure of tumor on lumbosacral, hypogastric, and/or pelvic areas, as evidenced by patient complaints of pain, facial grimacing, guarding of abdominal or pelvic area, limited mobility

NURSING INTERVENTIONS AND RATIONALE

1. Assess patient's pain history, including analgesic use, to determine previously effective medications.
2. Assess location, onset, duration, radiation, and intensity of pain to determine appropriate interventions.
3. Provide prescribed medications for pain as needed to decrease patient's discomfort.
4. Teach patient self-care strategies with which to manage pain, such as relaxation exercises, imagery, application of heat or cold.
5. Demonstrate use of pillow to splint abdomen, exercises to relax back and pelvic muscles.

NURSING DIAGNOSIS

Fear related to diagnosis, anticipated treatment, impact of disease and treatment on sexuality, and prognosis, as evidenced by depression, anger, withdrawal, expressions of fear

NURSING INTERVENTIONS AND RATIONALE

1. Assess appetite, weight loss, sleep patterns, activity level to detect signs and symptoms of depression.
2. Assess presence and quality of support system to determine if persons are available to assist patient.
3. Monitor changes in communication with others, since silence or withdrawal may indicate anger or depression.
4. Encourage patient to use physical expression of fears, since physical activity can be a way of expressing fears and anger.
5. Assist patient in identifying information, support groups, and other resources of value in solving problems that cause her to be fearful.

Ovarian Cancer

Ovarian cancer is the fourth leading cause of death from cancer in women. Its incidence is increasing faster than the survival rate.

EPIDEMIOLOGY

The increasing incidence of ovarian cancer among nulliparous and single women suggests that uninterrupted ovulation may be a predisposing factor. More than 60% of women with the disease are diagnosed with advanced disease. This insidious cancer often is discovered late in its natural history. Although the cause is unknown, women over 50 years of age (postmenopausal) show an increasing likelihood of developing the disease, and the increase is steady up to age 70. Other risk factors are nulliparity, celibacy, infertility, a long history of menstrual irregularity, higher socioeconomic status, a high-fat diet, and exposure to industrial chemicals such as asbestos and talc. Other variables under study are age at menopause, history of such childhood diseases as rubella and mumps, family history of ovarian cancer, family size, and ovarian malfunctions.

The endocrine dysfunctions associated with the development of ovarian cancer have led to the following observations: use of oral contraceptives seems to de-

CANCER OF THE OVARIES

crease the risk of developing this cancer; pregnancy may be protective by inhibiting incessant ovulation or by inducing permanent changes in the pituitary gland that affect secretion of tropic hormones; early age at pregnancy may be protective, as may breast-feeding.

It is believed that the free communication between the external environment and the ovaries and peritoneal cavity may account for the relationship between talc or diaphragms and the development of ovarian cancer.

Women should continue to have annual pelvic examinations after menopause so that changes indicative of ovarian cancer can be found at an early and potentially curable stage.

PATHOPHYSIOLOGY

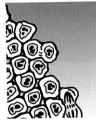

Seventy to eighty percent of ovarian cancers are epithelial in origin. The most common type is serous cystadenocarcinoma, and most of these tumors arise from the germinal epithelium or outer cortex. Other types seen are mucinous, endometrioid, and clear cell tumors. Only 5% to 10% of ovarian tumors arise from a primary source in another part of the body, usually the breast.

Dissemination of the tumor occurs through implantation of cells into the surfaces of the pelvic peritoneum, sigmoid colon, cecum, and terminal ileum and omentum, as well as via the submesothelial lymphatics.

Ovarian cancer is staged as follows:

Stage I   Growth limited to the ovaries
Stage II   Growth involving one or both ovaries with pelvic extension
Stage III Growth involving one or both ovaries with intraperitoneal metastases outside the pelvis and/or involvement of the retroperitoneal nodes
Stage IV   Growth involving one or both ovaries with distant metastases

The 5-year survival rate for stage I tumors is 55% to 90%; for stage II tumors, 0 to 40%; it is poor for stages III and IV tumors.

SIGNS AND SYMPTOMS

Women usually manifest the signs and symptoms of late disease, such as ascites, abdominal or pelvic pain or fullness, abnormal uterine bleeding, a palpable mass in the abdomen, persistent gastrointestinal complaints, urinary complaints, or a change in respiratory status. Many women seek health care for menstrual irregularities.

DIAGNOSTIC STUDIES AND FINDINGS

Diagnostic test	Findings
Pelvic examination with bimanual manipulation	Enlarged or irregular ovary
Laparoscopy with biopsy	Abnormal ovary and malignant cells in specimens
Lymphangiography	Involvement of retroperitoneal nodes
Cancer antigen 125 (CA-125)	Elevated

MEDICAL MANAGEMENT

SURGERY

Simple salpingo-oophorectomy

Total abdominal hysterectomy with bilateral salpingo-oophorectomy and partial or complete omentectomy

RADIATION THERAPY

Intracavity radiation

External beam radiation

CHEMOTHERAPY

Single agent: Chlorambucil, melphalan, doxorubicin, cyclophosphamide, 5FU, methotrexate, vinblastine, bleomycin, cisplatin, nitrogen mustard, thiotepa, tetracycline

Combination therapy (containing cisplatin)

SURGERY

Conservative treatment is used with stage I tumors if the woman has low parity and wants more children. However, several conditions must obtain: (1) the tumor must show borderline morphologic findings; (2) it must be intracystic, unruptured, and free of adhesions; (3) the pelvis must be normal and show no invasion of the lymphatic capsule or mesovarium; and (4) the biopsy findings for the omentum and opposite ovary must be negative. The treatment of choice in this situation is a simple salpingo-oophorectomy. Women with stage I disease who are not concerned about having more children and women with stage II or stage III disease usually undergo a total abdominal hysterectomy, bilateral salpingo-oophorectomy, and partial or complete omentectomy. If the tumor is grossly visible, debulking and estimation of the extent and location of residual masses are done. In stage IV disease more aggressive surgery is called for, including appendectomy and removal of the omentum.

RADIATION THERAPY

Radiation therapy is used after surgery in stage II and stage III disease. Chromic phosphate (^{32}P) may be injected intraabdominally immediately after surgery by means of a peritoneal catheter. Patients with stage II disease may also receive external beam therapy for 5 to 7 weeks, beginning no later than 4 weeks after surgery. The liver and kidneys are shielded after 1,500 to 2,000 rad.

COMPLICATIONS

Cramps, diarrhea, anorexia, vomiting
Bone marrow depression
Adhesions
Severe radiation enteritis
Intestinal obstruction, fistula, necrosis

CHEMOTHERAPY

Patients with stage I, II, or III disease may receive such alkylating agents as chlorambucil or melphalan. Patients with stage IV disease receive chemotherapy as definitive treatment. The drugs used are doxorubicin, cyclophosphamide, 5FU, methotrexate, vinblastine, bleomycin, and cisplatin. Combination regimens include cisplatin.

Intraperitoneal administration of chemotherapeutic agents has proved quite effective in women with ovarian cancer. It is believed to be particularly helpful to patients with microscopic or minimum residual disease. In addition, the technique decreases general toxicity, because the drug is not administered systemically (see page 216 and Patient Teaching Guide, page 245).

A second-look laparotomy often is performed 6 to 24 months after chemotherapy has ended, to detect evidence of recurrent disease.

■ ■ ■

Patients with advanced disease often have peritoneal or pleural effusion, as evidenced by a firm, tense abdomen; a dull ache in the abdomen; shortness of breath; coughing; dyspnea; and/or chest pain. Treatment may include intracavity isotope radiation therapy, external beam therapy, and chemotherapy.

These patients must be observed for hemorrhage, pain, urinary or bowel obstruction, and malnutrition. Gastrointestinal complications often are the immediate cause of death.

NURSING CARE OF THE PERSON WITH OVARIAN CANCER

NURSING DIAGNOSIS

Altered nutrition: less than body requirements related to pressure of tumor on gastrointestinal tract, as evidenced by abdominal discomfort, dyspepsia, indigestion, flatulence, eructations, loss of appetite, and nausea

NURSING INTERVENTIONS AND RATIONALE

1. Assess caloric intake—kinds and amounts, percentages of protein, carbohydrate, and fat—to determine needed changes in diet.
2. Observe the patient for evidence of weight loss and dehydration to intervene quickly with foods, nutritional supplements, and fluids.
3. Ask patient if she is experiencing abdominal discomfort, dyspepsia, indigestion, flatulence, loss of appetite, nausea, as evidence of tumor pressure and possible disease progression.

4. Provide palpable meals based, as much as possible, on patient likes and dislikes to increase caloric consumption.
5. Offer dietary supplements as needed to maintain adequate nutritional balance.
6. Offer medications that relieve abdominal distention and flatulence, since these symptoms tend to adversely affect appetite.

NURSING DIAGNOSIS

Altered patterns of urinary elimination related to pressure of tumor on bladder, as evidenced by urinary frequency, dysuria, incontinence, infection, and/or retention

NURSING INTERVENTIONS AND RATIONALE

1. Measure intake and output to monitor for fluid balance.
2. Inspect urine for bleeding to detect evidence of infection or bladder wall irritation.
3. Inspect abdomen for distention to determine effectiveness of bladder emptying.
4. Ambulate patient as tolerated to promote urinary elimination.

5. Apply heating pad or hot water bottle to abdomen to relax bladder.
6. Catheterize only as necessary to avoid infection.

NURSING DIAGNOSIS

Fear related to diagnosis, anticipated treatment, impact on sexuality, and prognosis, as evidenced by depression, anger, withdrawal, expressions of fear

NURSING INTERVENTIONS AND RATIONALE

1. Assess sleep patterns and activity level to detect signs and symptoms of depression.
2. Assess presence and quality of support system to determine if persons are available to assist patient.
3. Monitor changes in communication with others, since silence or withdrawal may indicate anger or depression.
4. Encourage patient to use physical expression of fears, since physical activity can be a way of expressing anger or depression.
5. Assist patient in identifying information, support groups, and other resources of value in solving problems that cause her to be fearful.

Vaginal Cancer

Vaginal cancer accounts for approximately 2% of all gynecologic cancers.

EPIDEMIOLOGY

The median age for noninvasive vaginal cancer is in the fifth decade of life; for invasive cancer it is in the sixth decade. Women 18 to 20 years of age who have been diagnosed with vaginal cancer generally had mothers who took diethylstilbestrol (DES) during pregnancy. Other risk factors are previous radiation therapy for invasive cervical cancer and tumors of the rectum.

All women over age 20, or when they become sexually active, should have an annual bimanual pelvic examination with Pap smear and thorough inspection of the vagina, vulva, and perineal area. Those whose mothers took DES should start having checkups at an earlier age. As with all women, they should be taught prudent genital hygiene and to report promptly any abnormal or suspicious signs and symptoms to the health care provider.

PATHOPHYSIOLOGY

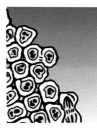

The most common site of vaginal cancer is the posterior wall of the upper third of the vagina. The tumor may spread along the vaginal wall to involve the cervix or vulva. Anterior vaginal lesions penetrate into the vesicovaginal septum in an early stage. Posterior lesions can invade the rectum, but this usually occurs in the later stages. The tumor spreads by direct extension into the obturator fossa, cardinal ligaments, lateral pelvic wall, and ureterosacral ligament. Metastasis is to the lungs or supraclavicular nodes in squamous cell cancer, which tends to occur in more advanced stages.

SIGNS AND SYMPTOMS

Abnormal vaginal bleeding is the most common symptom of vaginal cancer. Other symptoms that patients may report are postcoital bleeding or intermenstrual bleeding, and vaginal discharge. Pain or other symptoms referable to the bladder or rectum indicate advanced disease, although the proximity of the tumor to the bladder neck can result in compression of the urethra at an earlier stage of disease.

DIAGNOSTIC STUDIES AND FINDINGS

Diagnostic test	Findings
Colposcopy with biopsy	Malignant cells

MEDICAL MANAGEMENT

SURGERY

Local excision

Total vaginectomy with reconstruction

Radical hysterectomy, partial vaginectomy, and pelvic lymphadenectomy

RADIATION THERAPY

External beam radiation

Brachytherapy (intravaginal radium and cesium)

CARBON DIOXIDE LASER

CHEMOTHERAPY

Topical 5FU

SURGERY

Surgical management of vaginal cancer is based on the lesion's location and size and whether it is single focus or multiple foci. Local excision is the treatment of choice for single lesions or for several lesions in a single part of the vagina. Total vaginectomy with reconstruction is reserved for women in whom more conservative therapy has failed. With invasive disease, it is recommended that the patient undergo a radical hysterectomy, partial vaginectomy, and pelvic lymphadenectomy. Lesions in the middle or lower vagina may require either anterior or posterior exenteration as the primary surgical intervention. Pelvic recurrences within 2 years of the initial therapy may be treated surgically with procedures ranging from wide excision to a total pelvic exenteration.

RADIATION THERAPY

Stage II vaginal cancer is treated with external beam radiation therapy and brachytherapy. Radium or cesium may be inserted intravaginally by means of cylinders, intrauterine tandems with vaginal colpostat, needles, or applicators with perineal templates. However, this treatment has been disappointing because of the frequency of recurrence and the residual vaginal stenosis.

CARBON DIOXIDE LASER

Excision with a carbon dioxide laser often is the treatment of choice for early stage vaginal cancer (see Chapter 14).

CHEMOTHERAPY

Topical application of 5FU cream every night for 5 days, repeated for 6 to 12 weeks until the lesion has been eradicated, is being investigated for its therapeutic value.

■ ■ ■

The overall survival rate for all stages of squamous cell vaginal carcinoma is 51%: 65% for stage I, 60% for stage II, 35% for stage III, and 39% for stage IV. The rate climbs to 80% for adenocarcinoma, because it can be detected early with annual pelvic examinations and Pap smears.

NURSING CARE OF THE PERSON WITH VAGINAL CANCER

NURSING DIAGNOSIS

Fluid volume loss related to abnormal vaginal bleeding, as evidenced by vaginal discharge, postcoital bleeding, intermenstrual bleeding

NURSING INTERVENTIONS AND RATIONALE

1. Observe characteristics and amount of discharge to determine need for fluid and blood component replacement.
2. Monitor vital signs at frequent intervals during episodes of heavy bleeding to detect shock early.
3. Encourage patient to drink large volume of fluid to prevent dehydration.
4. Monitor intake and output and urine specific gravity to detect renal dysfunction.
5. Administer IV fluids as prescribed to replace lost fluid volume.
6. Monitor lab reports to detect development of anemia.
7. Observe for signs and symptoms of worsening fluid volume deficit, including decreased urine output, concentrated urine, output greater than intake, weakness, and change in mental status, to determine need for large volumes of IV fluids and blood components at rapid rate.

NURSING DIAGNOSIS

Altered sexuality patterns related to anatomic and functional changes caused by disease and/or treatment.

NURSING INTERVENTIONS AND RATIONALE

1. Assist patient to identify current and potential changes in sexual structure and function.
2. Encourage identification and use of support systems for exchange of thoughts and feelings with significant other and other women having the same or similar experiences.
3. Encourage the patient to express her feelings about potential loss of uterus and resultant sexual dysfunction.
4. Assess the patient's understanding and level of comprehension regarding the function of the uterus in relation to sexual response cycle and potential impact of therapy on sexual function.

NURSING DIAGNOSIS

Fear related to diagnosis, anticipated treatment, impact of disease and treatment on sexuality, and prognosis, as evidenced by depression, anger, withdrawal, expressions of fear

NURSING INTERVENTIONS AND RATIONALE

See nursing care of the person with endometrial cancer, p. 133.

Vulvar Cancer

The incidence of vulvar intraepithelial neoplasia (VIN) and carcinoma in situ is increasing in older women, which necessitates greater attention to this particular gynecologic cancer.

EPIDEMIOLOGY

Cancer of the vulva is a disease of older women, with the peak incidence in the seventh decade of life. The cause is unknown, although obesity, hypertension, diabetes, early menopause, cervical cancer, and sexually transmitted diseases have been suggested as risk factors. Long-term pruritus seems to increase the risk of developing vulvar cancer.

Because no specific tests are available for screening and detection, all women 40 years of age or older should have an annual checkup that includes a bimanual pelvic examination with careful inspection of the vulvar area. Women should also learn vulvar self-examination. (See patient teaching guide, p. 242.) As with other gynecologic cancers, early detection and treatment improve the survival rate at all stages of disease.

PATHOPHYSIOLOGY

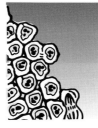

Invasive squamous cell carcinomas account for 90% of vulvar cancers. Other cell types include malignant melanoma, basal cell carcinoma, and adenocarcinoma of Bartholin's and Skene's glands. These cancers usually develop slowly and spread by direct contact to adjacent tissues or by way of the lymphatics to the inguinal lymph nodes (Figure 8-3).

Lesions are found on the labia majora three times more often than on the labia minora. The least common site for lesions is the clitoris. When the lesion is smaller than 2 cm, the incidence of positive nodes is approximately 15%. If the lesion is larger than 2 cm, the rate of

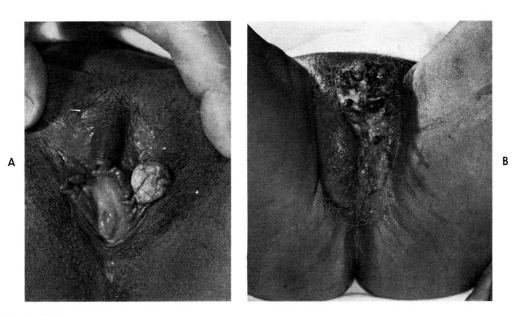

FIGURE 8-3
A, Well-differentiated carcinoma of the vulva. **B,** Advanced carcinoma of the vulva, involving the entire vagina, urethra, and rectum. (From Willson et al.: *Obstetrics and gynecology,* ed 8, St Louis, 1987, Mosby–Year Book.)

nodal involvement is three times higher. When the lesions are confined to the vulva, approximately 30% of patients have metastases to the nodes.

The survival rates are 80% to 85% for patients with no involvement of the lymph nodes and 40% to 50% for those with involvement of the inguinal nodes.

SIGNS AND SYMPTOMS

Approximately half of the patients with vulvar cancer have already had symptoms of pruritus, pain, and a lump or mass in the vulvar area when they seek medical attention. Other, less common signs and symptoms are vaginal bleeding or discharge, or dysuria of 2 to 16 months' duration.

DIAGNOSTIC STUDIES AND FINDINGS

Diagnostic test	Findings
Biopsy of atypical areas with Keyes dermatologic punch	Red, white, warty, or other atypical pigmentation; malignant cells
Colposcopy with Pap smear	Cervical metastases; definition of limits of vulvar lesion
Magnetic resonance imaging (MRI) study	Involvement of retroperitoneal nodes

MEDICAL MANAGEMENT

SURGERY

Limited wide local excision

Simple vulvectomy

Skinning vulvectomy

Radical vulvectomy with bilateral inguinal lymphadenectomy

ELECTROCAUTERY, CRYOSURGERY, OR LASER TREATMENT

RADIATION THERAPY

External beam

Internal implant

Radiation therapy with hyperthermia

CHEMOTHERAPY

Topical chemotherapy with 5FU, dinitrochlorobenzene (DNCB)

Preoperative chemotherapy with mitomycin-C and 5FU

SURGERY

Surgery is the treatment of choice for more than 80% of patients with vulvar cancer. Limited wide local excision using either primary-closure skin flaps or skin graft with close follow-up is recommended for patients with carcinoma in situ.

For multicentric lesions, skinning vulvectomy is used. The vulvar skin is excised (conserving fat, muscle, and glands below the skin), and a split-thickness skin graft is applied. This technique produces excellent cosmetic and functional results. A simple vulvectomy may be indicated in elderly women with chronic medical problems, because the healing of the skin graft after a skinning vulvectomy requires prolonged bed rest.

A radical vulvectomy with bilateral inguinal lymphadenectomy is the removal of external genital and bilateral groin lymph nodes, both superficial and deep. The urethra usually is left intact but can be excised to half of its length without affecting function. A "butterfly" incision is made to remove the vulva and lymph nodes. This incision extends from the iliac spine across the lower abdomen to the inguinal ligament and ends slightly above the rectum (Figure 8-4).

COMPLICATIONS

Wound breakdown
Lymphedema
Sexual dysfunction

ELECTROCAUTERY, CRYOSURGERY, OR LASER TREATMENT

Depending on the size of the lesion and the area of involvement, wide local excision may be done by electrocautery, cryosurgery, or laser treatment. The problem with all these methods is that they create painful ulcers that may take up to 3 months to heal.

RADIATION THERAPY

Both external beam and internal implant modes of radiation therapy are controversial as treatments for vulvar cancer. They are used primarily as palliative therapy for patients in whom surgical resection is not indicated. Hyperthermia combined with radiation therapy has shown some promise in managing locally advanced disease.

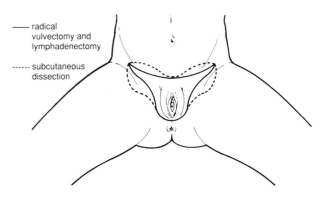

radical vulvectomy and lymphadenectomy

subcutaneous dissection

FIGURE 8-4
Skin incision for a radical vulvectomy and lymphadenectomy *(solid line)*; boundaries for subcutaneous dissection *(broken line)*. (From Otto.[48])

CHEMOTHERAPY

Topical chemotherapy with 5FU or dinitrochlorobenzene (DNCB) has been used with some patients. Combination treatment has involved using topical chemotherapy for 1 week before surgical excision of the vulvar lesion. Other studies report that preoperative chemotherapy with mitomycin-C and 5FU followed by pelvic irradiation is helpful in treating advanced vulvar cancer. Chemotherapy alone is not very helpful but may provide palliation in advanced disease.

• • •

Further study is needed to determine the feasibility of less radical surgery and the therapeutic effects of combined treatment with surgery, chemotherapy, and radiation therapy.

NURSING CARE OF THE PERSON WITH VULVAR CANCER

NURSING DIAGNOSIS

Impaired skin integrity related to pruritus, presence of a lump or mass, bleeding, or discharge

NURSING INTERVENTIONS AND RATIONALE

1. Cleanse skin to prevent infection.
2. Apply warm, moist compress to promote circulation and drainage.
3. Apply antibiotic ointment and sterile dressing, if indicated, to prevent or treat infection.

4. Expose draining area to air, if possible, to promote healing.
5. Observe for increased discharge, skin changes, swelling, and lesions to detect complications early.

NURSING DIAGNOSIS

Fear related to diagnosis, anticipated treatment, possible impact of disease and treatment on sexuality and body image, and prognosis, as evidenced by depression, anger, withdrawal, expressions of fear

NURSING INTERVENTIONS AND RATIONALE

1. Assess appetite, weight loss, sleep patterns, and activity level to detect signs and symptoms of depression.
2. Assess presence and quality of support system to determine if persons are available to assist patient.
3. Monitor changes in communication with others, since silence or withdrawal may indicate anger or depression.
4. Encourage patient to use physical expression of fears, since physical activity can be a way of expressing fears and anger.
5. Assist patient in identifying information, support groups, and other resources of value in solving problems that cause her to be fearful.

CHAPTER 9

Skin Cancers

Skin cancer is the most common malignancy found in humans. An estimated 600,000 cases are discovered each year. Most involve the highly curable basal cell and squamous cell carcinomas. Malignant melanoma, the most serious skin cancer, is diagnosed in about 32,000 people annually, and the incidence is increasing by 4% per year. The reason for the increasing incidence of all skin cancers is believed to be a widespread change in life-style, with greater exposure of successive generations to sunlight—specifically, ultraviolet radiation.

For close-ups of skin cancers, see Color Plates 1 through 11, pages x and xi.

Other less common but clinically significant skin cancers include Bowen's disease (squamous cell carcinoma in situ), Kaposi's sarcoma, lymphangiosarcoma, dermatofibrosarcoma protuberans, leiomyosarcoma, and mycosis fungoides.

Basal Cell and Squamous Cell Carcinomas

EPIDEMIOLOGY

Basal cell and squamous cell cancers are more common among people with lightly pigmented skin and those at latitudes near the equator. Basal cell carcinoma is more common in men than in women and occurs more often in people over 40 years of age. Squamous cell carcinoma also is more common in men, with the average age of onset at 60 years. Other risk factors are excessive exposure to the sun and occupational exposure to coal, tar, pitch, creosote, arsenic compounds, and radium. Blacks, because of their heavy skin pigmentation, are at low risk of developing these skin cancers.

Prevention and detection focus on decreasing exposure to the sun and finding the cancer early through skin self-assessment (see Patient Teaching Guide). Protecting the cutaneous surfaces of the skin from excessive exposure to the sun would alone significantly reduce the current high incidence of skin cancer. General guidelines for such protection are outlined in the box on page 145.

PATHOPHYSIOLOGY

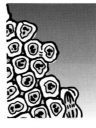

A **basal cell carcinoma** often appears as a single, small, firm, dome-shaped, flesh-colored nodule with raised edges and pearly white borders. Small, red, focal lesions (telangiectatic vessels) are often prominent and can be seen through the thin epidermis. The lesion may resemble a pimple that has not healed, with an ulcerated, bleeding center. The most common form, noduloulcerative cancer, frequently occurs on the face, especially the cheeks, forehead, eyelids, and nasolabial folds. Invasion usually is local, although metastatic disease does occur in rare cases. Left untreated, the tumor will invade such vital structures as blood vessels, lymph nodes, nerve sheaths, cartilage, bone, lungs, and the dura mater. The histologic appearance of the tumor is that of small, undifferentiated basal cells with minimum nuclear atypia. Recurrence indicates that initial treatment did not completely eradicate the tumor; however, 90% to 95% of patients are considered cured after surgery or radiation therapy.

GUIDELINES FOR PROTECTING THE SKIN AGAINST EXCESSIVE EXPOSURE TO THE SUN

- Avoid intense sunlight between 10 AM and 3 PM, when ultraviolet rays are the strongest.
- Plan such outdoor activities as walking, gardening, and other hobbies for early morning or late afternoon.
- Wear protective clothing such as hats and long-sleeved shirts.
- Use a sunscreen with a sun protection factor (SPF) of 15 or higher. The sunscreen should be applied 15 to 30 minutes before going out into the sunlight and every 2 to 3 hours during exposure (it may need to be applied more often because of heat, humidity, and sweating). Sunscreen should be applied liberally to the head and neck, with special attention to the nose, rims of the ears, cheeks, and forehead.

A **squamous cell carcinoma** is a scaly, slightly elevated lesion with or without a cutaneous horn. This tumor frequently occurs on the hands and forearms, as well as on the head and neck (especially the ears, lower lip, scalp, and upper face). It is found most often in sun-damaged skin previously affected by actinic keratoses, which are erythematous, scaly lesions found especially on the face, shoulders, and dorsa of the hands. With complete tumor eradication, the prognosis is excellent. Tumors more difficult to treat are those arising in an old, unstable thermal burn scar (Marjolin's ulcer); a chronically ulcerated area at the site of a chronic sinus tract (such as that caused by osteomyelitis); or a site of previous radiation damage. Squamous cell carcinoma can metastasize, with 2% to 3% of tumors spreading to regional lymph nodes or to the lungs. Primary tumors of the lip metastasize at a rate greater than 10%. The cure rate for this type of cancer is 75% to 80% when it is treated with surgery or radiation therapy.

SIGNS AND SYMPTOMS

The clinical characteristics of superficial basal cell cancer include barely elevated, moderately firm plaques, usually with crusted and erythematous centers and raised, threadlike, pearly borders. Noduloulcerative basal cell cancer is characterized by moderately firm, elevated lesions with umbilicated, ulcerated centers and raised, waxy or pearly borders.

The appearance of squamous cell carcinoma varies. It may look like an elevated nodular mass; a punched-out, ulcerated lesion; or a fungating mass. Unlike basal cell carcinomas, these lesions are opaque.

DIAGNOSTIC STUDIES AND FINDINGS

Diagnostic Test	Findings
Incisional or total excisional biopsy	Malignant cells

MEDICAL MANAGEMENT

SURGERY

Excisional surgery

Cryosurgery

Electrodesiccation and curettage

Mohs chemosurgery

RADIATION THERAPY

External beam radiation

CHEMOTHERAPY

Topical 5-fluorouracil

Biologic response modifiers

SURGERY

Excisional surgery is the treatment of choice in 90% of basal cell cancers, including large tumors or those with poorly defined margins on the cheeks, forehead, trunk, and legs. Along with the lesion, a 3 mm margin is removed. Excision may also be indicated when metastatic spread is present. With squamous cell carcinoma, the margin should be slightly larger. It is also important to examine the regional lymph nodes in individuals with evidence of nodal involvement because of the greater likelihood of metastases with this cancer. When immediate coverage of the surgical wound is required, a free full-thickness skin graft is used.

Cryosurgery (the destruction of tissue by freezing) is used only in small-to-large nodular and superficial basal cell carcinomas. Electrodesiccation and curettage (the application of heat to destroy cancerous tissue) is used with small-to-medium nodular and superficial basal cell carcinomas with well-defined margins. This procedure may be performed using electrocautery or a carbon dioxide laser.

Mohs chemosurgery is the removal of the tumor layer by layer until all margins are free of tumor, as verified by microscopic examination. This is the treatment of choice in recurrent basal cell lesions or those without well-defined margins. This procedure is also indicated when the basal cell carcinoma occurs in a cosmetic or functional area such as the eyelid or nose.

COMPLICATIONS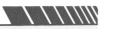

Wound infection
Pain and immobility related to grafting
Disfigurement

Preoperative Care

In addition to the usual preparation for surgery, the patient must be informed and reassured about the healing phases of the surgical wound and the plans for cosmetic surgery, such as grafting or later reconstruction.

Postoperative Care

Postoperative care focuses on keeping the surgical wound clean and dry while observing for signs and symptoms of infection. If skin grafting is required, the nurse must help the patient keep the grafted area immobile to prevent stress on the edges of the wound. The graft site must also be kept clean and free of clots. Patients often have pain at the donor site and may need analgesics and heat applied to the site.

Disfigurement, real or perceived, requires reassurance and planning for reconstructive surgery when possible. Patients often find comfort in speaking with a plastic surgeon or specialist in nonsurgical reconstructive procedures such as individually prepared makeup and clothing.

RADIATION THERAPY

External beam therapy may be the treatment of choice for elderly or debilitated individuals who cannot tolerate surgery. One of the benefits of radiation therapy is tissue conservation, especially when treating lesions on the nose, eyelid, or lips. Extensive tumors may require a combination of preoperative and postoperative radiation, and surgery. Treatment failures, which usually are seen within 1 year of primary intervention, are best treated by surgery, since the skin and subcutaneous tissues will be poorly vascularized as a result of the earlier radiation therapy.

CHEMOTHERAPY

Topical 5FU is recommended for treating premalignant actinic keratosis. Systemic retinoids have produced response rates greater than 70% in individuals with advanced squamous cell carcinoma; topical and systemic retinoids have shown some activity against basal cell carcinoma. 5FU may be used in nevoid basal cell carcinoma syndrome but is contraindicated in other types, because it destroys the surface tumor without affecting deeper malignant cells.

Biologic response modifiers, especially interferon-alpha (IFN-α), have produced a response rate as high as 75% in recurrent or advanced local, regional, or metastatic basal cell carcinoma.

NURSING CARE

See pages 150-151.

Malignant Melanoma

Although a relatively uncommon cancer, malignant melanoma is a more serious problem than other skin cancers because it can spread quickly and insidiously, thus becoming life-threatening at an earlier stage of development.

EPIDEMIOLOGY

Malignant melanoma is much more common in whites. When it does occur in dark-skinned people, the most common sites are the palms, soles, nail beds, fingers, toes, and mucous membranes. Melanoma may occur in individuals in their teens and early twenties and thirties, although the highest incidence is in those over 60 years of age. The incidence is equal in men and women; the upper back is the most common site in men, whereas the back and lower extremities are the most common sites in women.

Exposure to the sun and geographic latitude are important environmental factors. The risk of melanoma is increased for fair-skinned individuals who have intense, intermittent exposure to the sun, especially during childhood and adolescence. Countries with areas of high solar exposure (i.e., those close to the equator) have the highest incidence of melanoma.

People who burn easily and do not tan well are at greater risk of developing melanoma, as are those with intermittent heavy sun exposure. A personal or family history of dysplastic nevus syndrome, congenital nevi, or melanoma also increases the risk.

The key to diagnosing malignant melanoma is early detection. Monthly skin self-examination is essential, especially for those at high risk (see Patient Teaching Guide). The early warning signs of melanoma are identified in the acronym ABCD (see box on page 148).

The key prognostic factor in malignant melanoma is the thickness of the lesion. Individuals with lesions less than 0.76 mm thick have a survival rate nearing 100%, whereas those with lesions 3 mm thick or thicker have survival rates of less than 50%.

Even though more people are using more effective sunscreens, the incidence of melanoma will continue to rise in the years ahead because there is a delay of 10 to 20 years from the time damage is inflicted by ultraviolet radiation until the cancer appears.

PATHOPHYSIOLOGY

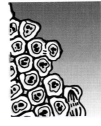

Malignant melanomas arise from three distinct types of moles, or nevi: common acquired nevi, dysplastic nevi, and congenital melanocytic nevi. The most common pigmented lesion is the common acquired nevus, which is not present at birth. Nevus production begins in childhood and tapers off at about 35 to 40 years of age. Most adults have about 20 to 40 nevi on their bodies. Common acquired nevi usually are small and uniform in color, surface, symmetry, and regularity of borders. The risk of this type of nevus developing into a melanoma is small.

Dysplastic nevi are considered precursors of melanoma, as well as markers of those at risk for melanoma. Dysplastic nevus syndrome usually becomes apparent during young adulthood, with the individual having more than 100 nevi on the body. Dysplastic nevi are larger than common acquired nevi and have irregular borders and variegated colors. They can occur anywhere on the body but are found more often on the trunk, back, breasts, buttocks, genitals, and scalp. Those with dysplastic nevi who have two or more first-degree relatives with melanoma have almost a 100% chance of developing melanoma, whereas people with sporadic dysplastic nevus syndrome have a 5% to 25% greater risk of developing melanoma than does the general population.

Congenital melanocytic nevi are raised, dark brown to black, oval or round macules that may have coarse hairs. They are present at birth and usually are small (under 1.5 cm) or medium-sized (1.5 to 19.9 cm). People with congenital nevi larger than 3 to 5 cm are thought to be at greatest risk for developing melanoma, although those with small and medium-sized nevi may have a risk as high as 22 times that of the general population.

The four distinct forms of malignant melanoma, in order of decreasing incidence, are:

Superficial spreading melanoma (70%), which occurs anywhere on the body surface. The lesion has a haphazard combination of colors and an irregular shape. It occurs more often in women 40 to 50 years of age. Common sites are the lower extremities and back.

Nodular melanoma (15%) also occurs anywhere on the body surface. It occurs twice as often in men 50 to 60 years of age. Common sites are the head, neck, and trunk.

ABCD RULE FOR EARLY DETECTION OF MELANOMA

A=Asymmetry

Most true moles tend to be symmetric. Melanomas tend to be asymmetric (one half does not match the other).

B=Border

Most true moles have a clear-cut border. Melanomas tend to have a notched, scalloped, or indistinct border.

C=Color

True moles may be dark or light, but they usually are uniform in color. Early melanomas have an uneven or variegated color (may range from various hues of tan and brown to black, with red and white intermingled).

D=Diameter

Once they have the A, B, and C characteristics, most melanomas are larger than 6 mm in diameter. Moles tend to be smaller. A sudden or progressive increase in the size of a mole should be reported.

DANGER SIGNALS SUGGESTING MALIGNANT TRANSFORMATION IN PIGMENTED LESIONS

Change in color

Especially sudden darkening, mottled and variegated shades of tan, brown, and black; red, white, and blue

Change in diameter

Especially a sudden increase

Change in outline

Especially development of irregular margins

Change in surface characteristics

Especially scaliness, erosion, oozing, crusting, bleeding, ulceration, or development of a mushrooming mass on the surface of the lesion

Change in consistency

Especially softening or friability

Change of symptomatology

Especially a sense of pruritus

Change in shape

Especially irregular elevation from a previously flat condition

Change in the surrounding skin

Especially "leaking" of pigment from lesion into surrounding skin or pigmented "satellite" lesions

From the American Cancer Society.[1]

Lentigo maligna melanoma (5% to 10%) occurs on exposed surfaces, especially the face, lower legs, and hands. It usually undergoes many color changes.

Acral lentiginous melanoma (less than 10%) tends to occur on the palms, soles, nail beds, fingers, toes, and mucous membranes. It is the most common type of melanoma in blacks, Orientals, and Hispanics.

Malignant melanoma may spread to any organ or remote viscera, although common sites are the skin (intracutaneous or subcutaneous metastasis), bones, brain, liver, and lungs.

All melanomas except the nodular type have an initial radial growth phase (spreading outward from a common center) that may last longer than 10 years, during which time the melanoma cells remain confined to the epidermis. The tumor expands horizontally with only a slight increase in depth. During the vertical phase dermal penetration occurs, and the melanoma cells invade the dermis and subcutaneous tissue. The tumor may then metastasize by vascular or lymphatic spread, with rapid movement of melanoma cells to other parts of the body. This accounts for the high mortality rate of malignant melanoma. When these tumors progress into the dermis or subcutaneous fat, "leaking" pigment or "satellite" nodules may appear around the periphery. Nodular malignant melanomas usually are convex and are palpable because of the tumor's growth elevation above the level of the epidermis.

SIGNS AND SYMPTOMS

The signs of melanoma include any unusual skin condition; scaliness, oozing, and/or bleeding of a nevus or other pigmented lesion; spread of the pigment beyond the normal border; a change in sensation, itchiness, tenderness, or pain; and development of a new nodule (see box on page 148).

DIAGNOSTIC STUDIES AND FINDINGS

Diagnostic Test	Findings
Excisional biopsy and measurement of maximum thickness of tumor	Malignant cells

---

MEDICAL MANAGEMENT

SURGERY

Wide excision

Regional lymph node dissection

RADIATION THERAPY

External beam radiation

CHEMOTHERAPY

Dacarbazine (DTIC), nitrosoureas (BCNU), cisplatin, and methotrexate

Biologic response modifiers: Interferon, interleukin

Hormonal therapy: Tamoxifen, diethylstilbestrol (DES)

SURGERY

Wide excision of the primary lesion is the treatment of choice. The surgeon makes an excision of at least 2 cm around a lesion less than 1.5 mm thick; for lesions more than 1.5 mm thick, the margin of 5 cm includes the underlying fascia. Surgery may also be used for palliation if metastatic disease is present.

Regional lymph node dissection is somewhat controversial, with some surgeons recommending the procedure only if there is a significant possibility of node involvement without evidence of metastatic disease. If this exploration is done, postoperative lymphedema can be minimized by elevating the limb above the level of the heart (see the section on basal cell and squamous cell carcinomas for other aspects of preoperative and postoperative care).

RADIATION THERAPY

Because melanoma tends to be radioresistant, radiation therapy is not recommended as primary treatment. It is useful for alleviating the signs and symptoms of metastatic disease to the bones, brain, and gastrointestinal tract.

CHEMOTHERAPY

Agents with some value against melanoma are dacarbazine, nitrosoureas, cisplatin, and methotrexate. Hyperthermic regional perfusions may be used to administer such drugs so that large doses can be delivered to the extremity affected by the malignant melanoma with minimum systemic toxicity. This procedure often is combined with wide local excision and regional lymph node dissection.

Biologic response modifiers such as interferon and interleukin are being investigated for their therapeutic value. Hormonal therapy with agents such as tamoxifen and diethylstilbestrol is also under study.

1 ASSESS

ASSESSMENT	OBSERVATIONS
Skin	Scaliness, oozing, and/or bleeding of a nevus or other pigmented lesion; spread of pigment beyond normal border; change in sensation, itchiness, tenderness, or pain
Psychosocial	Fear

2 DIAGNOSE

NURSING DIAGNOSIS	SUBJECTIVE FINDINGS	OBJECTIVE FINDINGS
Impaired skin integrity related to presence of lesion	Complains of change in sensation, itchiness, tenderness, or pain	Scaliness, oozing, or bleeding; spread of pigment beyond normal border
Fear related to cancer, its treatment, and prognosis	Expresses fear of disease, treatment, and possibility of disfigurement and death	Appears sad, withdrawn, angry, and depressed

3 PLAN

1. The patient's skin will be free of infection or ulceration.

2. The patient will be less fearful about the diagnosis, treatment, and prognosis.

4 IMPLEMENT

NURSING DIAGNOSIS	NURSING INTERVENTIONS	RATIONALE
Impaired skin integrity related to presence of lesion	Bathe patient in warm water, or apply warm, moist compresses.	To maintain cleanliness.
	Apply sterile dressings with antibiotic ointments as prescribed.	To prevent infection.
	Observe lesion or lesions for change in shape, size, and color and for bleeding.	To detect progressive disease.

NURSING DIAGNOSIS	NURSING INTERVENTIONS	RATIONALE
Fear related to cancer, its treatment, and prognosis	Assess appetite, weight loss, sleep patterns, mobility, and bowel activity.	May indicate depression.
	Assess presence and quality of support system.	To determine need for other sources of support.
	Listen to and accept expression of anger, sadness, and helplessness.	To foster expression of strong emotions.
	Encourage patient to identify fears, obtain needed information, generate alternative solutions, and focus on actions to be taken.	To support coping and problem solving.
Knowledge deficit	See Patient Teaching.	

5 EVALUATE

PATIENT OUTCOME	DATA INDICATING THAT OUTCOME IS REACHED
Patient's skin has healed.	Skin integrity is maintained without evidence of infection or ulceration.
Patient shows progress in lessening fear.	Patient talks about diagnosis and treatment options and realistic plans for reconstructive procedures.

PATIENT TEACHING

1. Explain to the patient the need for regular physical examinations and regular skin self-assessment (see Patient Teaching Guide, page 241).
2. Encourage the patient to protect skin from the sun by using sunscreens and protective clothing and by limiting exposure.
3. Instruct the patient and family to notify the health care provider if there are changes in the skin or other signs and symptoms indicating recurrent or metastatic disease.

CHAPTER 10

Lymphomas

The malignant lymphomas are a heterogeneous group of cancers that arise from the lymphoreticular system. They include lymphosarcoma, reticulum cell sarcoma, Burkitt's lymphoma, T cell cutaneous lymphoma, and Hodgkin's disease. Even though they are only the seventh most common cancer in the United States, they account for more years of life lost than do many of the more common cancers because they affect a relatively younger age group.

Malignant lymphomas are among the most curable of all cancers, and as researchers' understanding of the pathogenesis and therapy of lymphomas advances, even higher cure rates should be seen.

Hodgkin's Disease

Hodgkin's disease is responsible for about 14% of all malignant lymphomas. For 1991 it was estimated that 7,400 new cases would be diagnosed and that 1,600 people would die of the disease.

EPIDEMIOLOGY

Hodgkin's disease has a bimodal age-incidence distribution, meaning that the incidence rises sharply after 10 years of age, peaks in the late 20s, and then declines until age 45. After age 45 the incidence again increases steadily with age. Men are affected twice as often as women, and boys five times more often than girls.

The clinical symptoms of Hodgkin's disease suggest an infectious cause. The childhood social environment has been implicated as influencing risk of the disease in young adulthood. The risk of acquiring the disease is increased by factors that diminish or delay exposure to infectious agents, such as higher social class, more education, small family size, and early birth order position.

Epstein-Barr virus (EBV) is a possible causative agent, as suggested by the virus' ability to transform lymphocytes and by the presence of Reed-Sternberg–like cells in the lymphoid tissue of patients with infectious mononucleosis. Hodgkin's disease is also associated with some of the prodromal manifestations seen in acquired immunodeficiency syndrome (AIDS) when it presents in advanced stages with a higher incidence of bone marrow involvement.

Brothers and sisters of a patient with Hodgkin's disease have a sevenfold greater risk than the general public of developing the disease, and other first-degree relatives have a threefold greater risk; this suggests the important role genetic factors play in the development of the disease.

PATHOPHYSIOLOGY

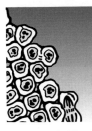

The Reed-Sternberg cell, which is present in Hodgkin's disease but not in other lymphomas, is believed to be derived from the monocyte-macrophage cell line. These cells have been shown to secrete the monokine interleukin-1, which causes proliferation of T lymphocytes and fibroblasts and acts as an endogenous pyrogen, two common histologic features of Hodgkin's disease.

Abnormalities in cellular immunity have been demonstrated in batteries of skin tests. Lymphocyte depletion is seen in 40% to 50% of patients and is more common in advanced stages of the disease. These lymphocytes proliferate poorly when stimulated. Macrophages adhere poorly to foreign surfaces and have abnormal antigen processing.

The histologic pattern and anatomic distribution of the disease vary with age. The nodular sclerosis form predominates in young adults, whereas the mixed cellularity form is most common in the older age group. Among elderly patients 25% have only subdiaphragmatic disease at the time of diagnosis, compared with fewer than 5% of young adult patients. More than half of young patients have mediastinal involvement, compared with fewer than 25% of elderly patients.

Hodgkin's disease initially affects one lymph node and then travels through the lymphatic channels to nodes throughout the body; it may also appear in the liver and spleen, vertebrae, ureters, and bronchi. Staging of the disease is based on the microscopic appearance of the lymph nodes, the extent and severity of the disease, and the prognosis. Both clinical staging and pathologic staging are recommended. The clinical stage is determined by means of a thorough history and physical examination, blood counts and chemistry findings, a chest x-ray, an abdominal computed tomography (CT) scan, and bipedal lymphangiography. The pathologic stage is based on the clinical stage and information gained by histologic review of tissue obtained through a bone marrow biopsy or a laparotomy or from other sites.

The **Ann Arbor staging system** (Figure 10-1) is as follows:

Stage I: involvement of a single lymph node region or a single extranodal side
Stage II: involvement of two or more lymph node regions on the same side of the diaphragm, or localized involvement of an extranodal site and one or more lymph node regions on the same side of the diaphragm

Stage III: involvement of lymph node regions on both sides of the diaphragm and possibly of a single extranodal site or the spleen, or both (now subdivided into lymphatic involvement of the upper abdomen in the spleen and in splenic, celiac, and portal nodes, and involvement of the lower abdominal nodes in the periaortic, mesenteric, and iliac regions)
Stage IV: diffuse or disseminated disease of one or more extralymphatic organs or tissues with or without associated lymph node involvement; the extranodal site is identified as H (hepatic), L (lung), P (pleura), M (marrow), D (dermal), or O (osseous)

The patient's symptoms are also indicated in this system, with "A" referring to patients without certain general symptoms and "B" referring to those with certain general symptoms, including unexplained fever with an oral temperature above 38° C (100.4° F), night sweats, and unexplained weight loss of more than 10% of body weight during the previous 6 months.

The **Rye classification system** is used by pathologists and physicians to subclassify the histology of Hodgkin's disease into four subtypes (Table 10-1).

The **lymphocyte-predominant** subtype accounts for 5% to 10% of patients. In this form of the disease mature lymphocytes diffusely infiltrate the abnormal lymph nodes. The prognosis for patients with this subtype is excellent (i.e., a 5-year survival rate of 90%).

The **nodular sclerosis** subtype accounts for 30% to 60% of cases. Interlacing bands of collagen that divide the cellular infiltrate into discrete islands produce the lymph node's nodular appearance. This subtype is seen most often in young women, and at the time of diagnosis the disease most often is localized in the cervical nodes and mediastinum. The prognosis is good, with a high 5-year survival rate.

The **mixed cellularity** subtype is the second most common of the four, making up about 33% of cases. With this subtype the nodes contain a pleomorphic infiltrate of eosinophils, normal lymphocytes, and readily identifiable Reed-Sternberg cells. The 5-year survival rate of all stages is 50% to 60%.

The **lymphocyte-depleted** subtype is the least common. With this form the Reed-Sternberg cells predominate, and mature lymphocytes are virtually absent in affected lymph nodes. This pattern occurs primarily in older patients and is associated with B symptoms and an advanced stage at presentation. The 5-year survival rate is less than 50%.

Table 10-1

HISTOPATHOLOGIC CLASSIFICATION OF HODGKIN'S DISEASE (RYE CLASSIFICATION)

Histologic subtype	Relative frequency
Lymphocyte predominant	5% to 10%
Nodular sclerosis	30% to 60%
Mixed cellularity	20% to 40%
Lymphocyte depleted	5% to 10%

From American Cancer Society.[1]

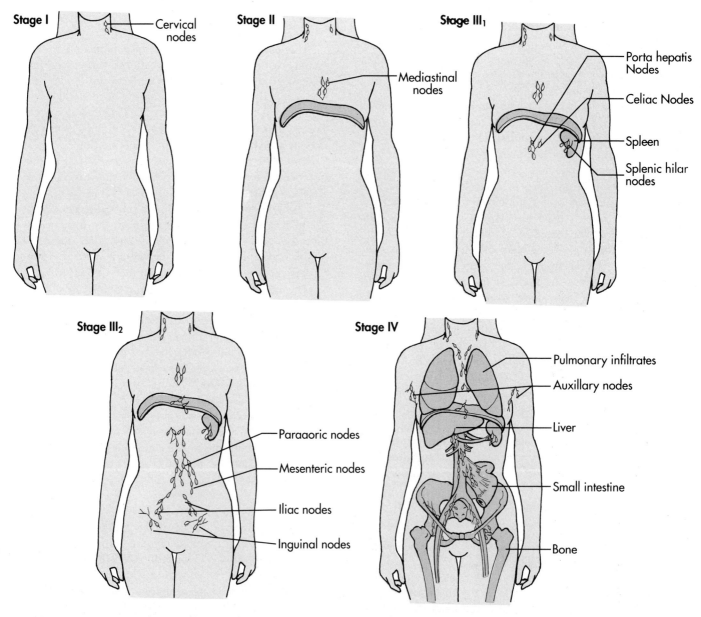

FIGURE 10-1
Nodal involvement by stage in Hodgkin's disease. (Based on modified Ann Arbor staging system.)

SIGNS AND SYMPTOMS

Young adults with Hodgkin's disease typically come to the health care provider with painless lymphadenopathy, although associated symptoms of malaise, fever, night sweats, pruritus, and weight loss may also be present. The enlarged lymph node usually is supradiaphragmatic (90%) and frequently is in the cervical region (60% to 80%). Axillary or mediastinal lymphadenopathy is less common. Massive mediastinal lymph nodes may cause such symptoms as coughing, wheezing, dyspnea, or superior vena cava syndrome. Subdiaphragmatic symptoms are uncommon in young patients, but this area is the only site of disease in 25% of older patients. Involvement of the retroperitoneal nodes, liver, spleen, and bone marrow usually occurs after the disease becomes generalized. Mesenteric lymph nodes are rarely involved, although in advanced disease any organ can be involved.

DIAGNOSTIC STUDIES AND FINDINGS

Diagnostic Test	Findings
Lymph node biopsy of largest, most central node in an involved group (preferably cervical node)	Reed-Sternberg cells
Complete blood count	Mild normochromic, normocytic anemia; neutrophilic leukocytosis; lymphopenia; eosinophilia; hemolytic anemia (advanced disease); elevated erythrocyte sedimentation rate
Blood chemistry	Elevated serum alkaline phosphatase; hypergammaglobulinemia (early disease; Ig levels may drop in advanced disease or during treatment); elevated serum copper and ceruloplasmin
Posteroanterior and lateral chest x-ray; chest computed tomography (CT) scan	Lung or pleural involvement
Bipedal lymphangiography	Abnormal nodes
Abdominal CT scan	Suspicious and enlarged nodes
Bilateral bone marrow biopsy	Abnormal cells
Laparotomy with splenectomy	Nodal and extranodal sites of disease

MEDICAL MANAGEMENT

SURGERY

Therapeutic splenectomy

RADIATION THERAPY

External beam radiation

CHEMOTHERAPY

Multiagent chemotherapy: MOPP (nitrogen mustard, vincristine, procarbazine, prednisone); ABVD (doxorubicin, bleomycin, vinblastine, dacarbazine)

Single-agent chemotherapy

SURGERY

In Hodgkin's disease surgery is primarily used to obtain biopsy specimens and to perform a staging laparotomy (see box). Therapeutic excision of enlarged nodes in early-stage disease is not done; removal of bulky masses after therapy usually reveals fibrosis.

A therapeutic splenectomy may be done to treat an enlarged spleen, to increase the patient's tolerance to chemotherapy, or to reduce the size of the radiation field.

RADIATION THERAPY

Radiation therapy can achieve a cure in most patients with stage I or stage II disease and in some cases of stage IIIA disease. Chemotherapy may be added to the radiation therapy protocol in patients with such adverse prognostic factors as B symptoms, bulky disease, and stage III disease.

Megavoltage radiation therapy is used to treat opposed fields in tumoricidal doses, with careful field simulation and verification and close follow-up of all patients.

Using extended fields to include the adjacent clinically negative nodal sites is essential for high cure rates. Total nodal irradiation sequentially treats a mantle field above the diaphragm. Subtotal nodal irradiation involves treating a mantle field and then irradiating the periaortic nodes and splenic pedicle. Carefully constructed field shapes and blocks for shielding are used to protect the lungs, heart, spinal cord, larynx, kidneys, gonads, and iliac crests (Figure 10-2).

The tumoricidal dose level is approximately 4,000 to 4,500 rad, delivered at the rate of 1,000 rad per week; this dose may be reduced when used in combination with chemotherapy.

Using an opposed-field technique to treat deep-lying tissues, usually anterior and posterior, provides a homogenous dose distribution throughout the treatment area and decreases the chance of radiation damage to structures such as the heart and liver.

Consolidation radiation therapy involves lower doses given to areas of known involvement in individuals with advanced stage IIIB or stage IV disease after a complete response to chemotherapy.

COMPLICATIONS

Radiation pneumonitis	Hypothyroidism
Pericarditis	Transverse myelitis

STAGING LAPAROTOMY

A staging laparotomy should be performed only when the information to be gained is deemed to affect both therapy and outcome. It should include *all* the following procedures:
1. Inspection
2. Splenectomy
3. Liver biopsies
   Wedge biopsy of left lobe
   Needle biopsies of right and left lobes
4. Lymph node biopsies
   Splenic hilar
   Celiac
   Porta hepatis
   Mesenteric
   Periaortic
   Iliac
5. Placement of clips at biopsy site
6. Oophoropexy in women who want to avoid sterilization

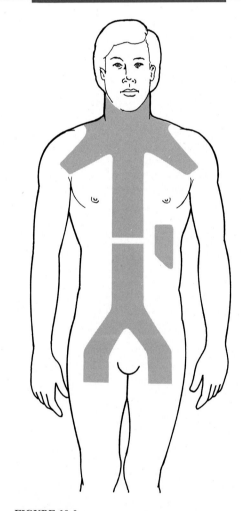

FIGURE 10-2
Radiation therapy ports used for total nodal irradiation.

Table 10-2

CHEMOTHERAPEUTIC AGENTS USEFUL WITH LYMPHOMAS

Alkylating agents	Nitrogen mustard (mechlorethamine)
	Chlorambucil
	Cyclophosphamide
	Carmustine (BCNU)
	Lomustine (CCNU)
Vinca alkaloids	Vincristine (Oncovin)
	Vinblastine
Antibiotics	Doxorubicin (Adriamycin)
	Bleomycin
Other	Prednisone
	Procarbazine
	Methotrexate
	Dacarbazine (DTIC)

From American Cancer Society.[1]

CHEMOTHERAPY

Multiagent chemotherapy of advanced Hodgkin's disease can produce a complete remission and a 5-year disease-free interval in most patients. Single-agent chemotherapy can produce complete and partial responses in 50% to 70% of patients, although the remissions last only a few months and complete responses are unusual. Single agents are useful in palliating advanced disease in older patients or for patients who are heavily pretreated with radiation therapy and, as a result of severe myelosuppression, cannot tolerate combined therapy (Table 10-2).

The MOPP regimen (nitrogen mustard, vincristine, procarbazine, and prednisone) has produced a high complete response rate and a durable remission. Numerous other drugs have been added or substituted by researchers in an effort to reduce toxicity and improve results. For example, ABVD has a similar complete response rate and can salvage MOPP failures. ABVD (doxorubicin, bleomycin, vinblastine, and dacarbazine) is often considered a second-line regimen because of potential cardiac and pulmonary toxicity; however, recent research demonstrated no increased cardiopulmonary toxicity and less risk of secondary leukemia.

Certain groups of patients benefit from combinations of radiation therapy and chemotherapy, such as those showing localized disease with masses exceeding one-third the diameter of the thoracic cavity (stage I or stage II disease with massive mediastinum); patients with stage IIIA disease with bulky sites; patients with stage IIIB or stage IV disease who achieve only partial remission with chemotherapy who are converted to complete remission with added radiation therapy; and children in whom combination chemotherapy will allow for reduced doses of radiation therapy, thus sparing bone growth.

COMPLICATIONS

Increased risk of secondary malignancies, particularly acute leukemia
Non-Hodgkin's lymphomas

1   ASSESS

ASSESSMENT	OBSERVATIONS
Skin	Painless swelling of lymph nodes
Comfort	Bone pain, nerve pain
Respiratory	Cough, wheezing, dyspnea
Immunologic	Increased susceptibility to infection
Gastrointestinal	Abdominal distention and discomfort; weight loss; anorexia
Energy	Malaise
Psychosocial	Fear of disease's impact on fertility

2   DIAGNOSE

NURSING DIAGNOSIS	SUBJECTIVE FINDINGS	OBJECTIVE FINDINGS
Impaired skin integrity related to swelling of lymph nodes and impaired function	Complains of pruritus and night sweats	Swollen lymph nodes
Pain related to disease progression to bones, nerves	Complains of bone pain, nerve pain, and numbness and tingling	Grimacing; limited movement; splinting
Ineffective breathing pattern related to disease progression to lungs and mediastinum	Complains of dyspnea	Cough; wheezing
Potential for infection related to impaired immunologic function	Complains of upper respiratory infections, urinary tract infections, painful itching, general malaise	Cough, sneezing, "runny" nose; frequency, urgency, dysuria; herpes zoster
Altered nutrition: less than body requirements related to disease progression to gastrointestinal tract	Reports anorexia and nausea	Decreased intake; abdominal distention; weight loss
Fear related to possible infertility and altered body image	Expresses fear about changes in body and sexual function	Appears sad, withdrawn, angry, and depressed

3 PLAN

Patient goals

1. The patient will have normal skin integrity.
2. The patient will be comfortable.
3. The patient will not have difficulty breathing.
4. The patient will be free of infection.
5. The patient will have adequate nutrition.
6. The patient will be less fearful about perceived and potential changes in body image and fertility.

4 IMPLEMENT

NURSING DIAGNOSIS	NURSING INTERVENTIONS	RATIONALE
Impaired skin integrity related to swelling of lymph nodes and impaired function	Bathe patient in cool water or apply cool, moist compresses; apply calamine lotion, cornstarch, sodium bicarbonate, and medicated powder.	To enhance comfort and relieve itching.
	Use a bed cradle and lightweight blankets and clothing.	To relieve pressure.
	Lubricate skin with baby oil, bath oil, body lotion, or petrolatum.	To enhance comfort.
	Maintain adequate humidity and cool room.	To decrease itching.
	Avoid adhesives, alkaline soap, and local heat.	They irritate skin.
Pain related to disease progression to bones, nerves	Position patient comfortably, change position gradually, and handle patient gently in an unhurried manner.	To avoid trauma (for bone pain).
	Support affected body part.	To prevent pressure.
	Encourage adequate rest.	To reduce incidence of pain related to activity.
	Provide pain-relief measures patient prefers, and give analgesics as ordered.	To relieve pain and to involve patient in self-care.
	Provide safety measures such as assistive devices for ambulation and pads for elbows and feet.	To prevent trauma related to numbness and tingling.
Ineffective breathing pattern related to disease progression to lungs and mediastinum	Place patient in sitting position.	To increase chest expansion.
	Remove constrictive clothing.	To relieve pressure on chest.
	Encourage deep breathing.	To assist alveolar expansion.
	Administer oxygen as needed.	To provide tissue oxygenation.

NURSING DIAGNOSIS	NURSING INTERVENTIONS	RATIONALE
	Keep emergency equipment nearby.	In case of airway obstruction.
	Inspect chest for respiratory rate, rhythm, and symmetric expansion.	To monitor changes from baseline.
	Auscultate lungs for abnormal breath sounds, aeration, rales, and rhonchi.	To detect development of infection or progression of disease.
	Observe for hoarseness, cough, stridor, pain, and change in skin color (cyanosis).	To detect evidence of complications.
	Monitor blood studies.	To detect abnormal gas exchange.
	Plan rest periods.	To prevent hyperventilation.
Potential for infection related to impaired immunologic function	Have the patient turn, cough, and deep breathe at regular intervals.	To prevent respiratory tract infection.
	Encourage patient to drink fluids and eat a balanced diet.	To maintain general well-being.
	Maintain reverse isolation.	To protect patient from microorganisms.
	Observe patient for "sniffles," sore throat, anorexia, pain on urination, and increase in temperature, pulse, and respiration.	These signs indicate infection.
	Administer antibiotics as ordered.	To treat infection.
	Assess patient's skin for development of herpes zoster, and notify physician of need for appropriate medication.	To detect infection early and treat appropriately.
Altered nutrition: less than body requirements related to disease progression to gastrointestinal tract	Provide small feedings of high-calorie, high-protein foods and fluids.	To increase nutritional intake.
	Assist with oral care, general hygiene, environmental control (temperature, appearance, odors).	To enhance appetite.
	Identify food preferences, and provide them as often as possible.	To promote adequate nutritional intake.
	Place patient in a sitting position after meals.	To decrease feeling of fullness.
Fear related to possible infertility and altered body image	Assess appetite, weight loss, sleep patterns, and activity level.	Depression may be manifested by changes in these areas.
	Assess presence and quality of support system.	To determine if someone is available and helpful to patient.

NURSING DIAGNOSIS	NURSING INTERVENTIONS	RATIONALE
	Monitor changes in communication with others.	Withdrawal or silence may indicate anger or depression.
	Listen to and accept patient's fears and anger.	To foster constructive expression of negative feelings and fears.
	Encourage patient to discuss specific fears with other patients, support group, or sexual counselor.	Talking with one who has had these experiences can validate fears and stimulate problem solving, such as sperm banking.
Knowledge deficit	See Patient Teaching.	

5 EVALUATE

PATIENT OUTCOME	DATA INDICATING THAT OUTCOME IS REACHED
Patient's skin is intact.	There is no evidence of irritation, and the patient has no complaints of pruritus.
Patient is comfortable.	Patient has no complaints of bone or nerve pain.
Patient's breathing is normal.	Patient has no complaints of dyspnea, and no cough or wheezing is observed.
Patient is free of infection.	There is no evidence of respiratory, urinary, or skin infection, and patient's temperature is within normal limits.
Patient's nutrition is adequate.	Patient's weight is normal and he has no complaints of anorexia, nausea, or abdominal distention.
Patient's fears are being dealt with.	Patient discusses plans for sperm banking or other methods of retaining ability to have children; patient plans realistically for possible changes in body image.

PATIENT TEACHING

1. Explain the need to avoid scratching and to care for the skin correctly to reduce susceptibility to infection and mechanical skin damage.
2. Teach correct maintenance of body alignment, use of body mechanics and ambulatory aids, and the early symptoms of vertebral compression and paralysis to report to the physician or nurse.
3. Teach ways to relieve pain without using medications as often as possible; bone, nerve, and abdominal pain is chronic and increases with pressure of disseminated disease.
4. Emphasize the importance of respiratory therapy to prevent or decrease the severity of symptoms of mediastinal lymph node enlargement, involvement of lung parenchyma, and invasion of pleura.
5. Teach the need for adequate rest and exercise and a balanced diet.
6. Help the patient make use of coping methods after exploring these with the patient and family.

Non-Hodgkin's Lymphoma

The American Cancer Society estimated that 37,200 people would be diagnosed as having non-Hodgkin's lymphoma in 1991, including 19,600 men and 17,600 women. It was estimated that 18,700 people would die of the disease. Higher age-adjusted incidence rates have been attributed to increases among older people, with lesser increases in the 35-to-64 age group and relatively unchanged rates among young adults. Among older people the incidence of diffuse large cell lymphoma is rising.

EPIDEMIOLOGY

A viral cause has been implicated in such non-Hodgkin's lymphomas (NHLs) as Burkitt's lymphoma, Mediterranean lymphoma, and T-cell leukemia/lymphoma, which is associated with human T-cell lymphotropic virus type 1 (HTLV-1). Non-Hodgkin's lymphomas (particularly central nervous system NHL) have been seen with increasing frequency in patients with acquired immunodeficiency syndrome (AIDS) and in individuals who are immunosuppressed following kidney and heart transplants. The risk of non-Hodgkin's lymphoma is also increased with Wiskott-Aldrich syndrome, X-linked immunodeficiency, ataxia-telangiectasia, and possibly Sjögren's syndrome.

PATHOPHYSIOLOGY

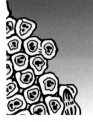

Cytogenetic abnormalities are seen in most non-Hodgkin's lymphomas. In Burkitt's lymphoma, chromosome 8 and chromosome 14 often are translocated. Other translocations have been observed.

Non-Hodgkin's lymphomas are now characterized as cancers of the immune system. Subclasses of lymphoma manifest similarities in immunologic phenotype to stages in the normal differentiation of T and B lymphocytes.

Histologic classifications for non-Hodgkin's lymphomas include low grade (B-cell tumors), intermediate grade (B-cell and some T-cell lymphomas), high grade (immunoblastic lymphomas/predominantly B-cell; lymphoblastic/T-cell tumors; Burkitt's and non-Burkitt's small noncleaved cell tumors/predominantly B-cell), and miscellaneous histiocytic (mycosis fungoides and others). All low-grade tumors and some intermediate-grade ones with long natural histories have a good prognosis; the prognosis is poor for the rapidly progressive high-grade tumors and some from the intermediate-grade group.

The histologic features of the most common subgroups of non-Hodgkin's lymphomas are as follows:

Follicular small cleaved cell lymphoma (most common type): patients usually manifest stage III or stage IV disease and have a high incidence of bone marrow involvement

Follicular mixed small cleaved and large cell lymphomas (second most common type): marrow involvement is common and most patients have stage III or stage IV disease at the time of diagnosis

Diffuse large cell lymphoma: these tumors frequently appear in extranodal as well as nodal sites and disseminate rapidly; they involve unusual areas such as the central nervous system, bones, and gastrointestinal tract

Immunoblastic lymphomas: high-grade tumors composed of cells commonly exhibiting a high mitotic rate

The staging for non-Hodgkin's lymphoma is the same as that for Hodgkin's lymphoma; however, because the former disease frequently is disseminated at the time of diagnosis, surgical staging is not commonly done. Current knowledge about the predictability and spread of non-Hodgkin's lymphoma is less certain than with Hodgkin's disease.

SIGNS AND SYMPTOMS

The presenting symptom of non-Hodgkin's lymphoma is an enlarged node or an abnormal chest x-ray (i.e., pleural effusion). The patient may also have superior vena cava syndrome. Gastrointestinal involvement may manifest itself as jaundice, abdominal cramping, bloody diarrhea, or signs and symptoms of total colonic obstruction. Ascites may be evident. The patient may also have hydronephrosis as a result of ureteral obstruction by retroperitoneal masses. Cord compression may occur in the rare incidence of neurologic involvement. Later in the course of the disease, hemolytic or unexplained anemia may be detected.

Immunodeficiencies are more pronounced in diffuse disease and include marked impairment of recall, reduced serum IgA, and lymphopenia, resulting in infections.

DIAGNOSTIC STUDIES AND FINDINGS

Diagnostic Test	Findings
Surgical biopsy	Malignant cells
Bilateral bone marrow biopsy	Malignant cells
Posteroanterior and lateral chest x-rays, computed tomography (CT) chest scan	Evidence of pleural effusion
Abdominal CT scan	Involvement of upper retroperitoneal and mesenteric nodes, liver, and spleen
Bipedal lymphangiography	Borderline lymphadenopathy
Staging laparotomy (see box, p. 156)	Evidence of hepatic, mesenteric, and gastrointestinal involvement
Peritoneoscopy with directed biopsies	Liver involvement
Bone scans	Bone involvement

MEDICAL MANAGEMENT

SURGERY

Resection of extranodal gastrointestinal involvement

Splenectomy

RADIATION THERAPY

External beam radiation

CHEMOTHERAPY

COP (cyclophosphamide, vincristine, prednisone)

CHOP (cyclophosphamide, doxorubicin, vincristine, prednisone)

BACOP (bleomycin, doxorubicin, cyclophosphamide, vincristine, prednisone)

MACOP-B (methotrexate with leucovorin rescue, doxorubicin, cyclophosphamide, vincristine, prednisone, bleomycin)

m-BACOD (cyclophosphamide, doxorubicin, vincristine, bleomycin, dexamethasone, methotrexate with leucovorin rescue)

ProMACE-CytaBOM (cyclophosphamide, doxorubicin, etoposide, prednisone, cytarabine, bleomycin, vincristine, methotrexate with leucovorin rescue)

SURGERY

Resection of areas of extranodal gastrointestinal involvement with staging at the time the affected nodes are removed lessens the risk of perforation or bleeding (or both) stemming from radiation therapy or chemotherapy. Splenectomy enables patients with hypersplenism to undergo more extensive chemotherapy.

RADIATION THERAPY

The goal of radiation therapy in non-Hodgkin's lymphoma is to control the disease in the area where it is clinically evident and not to irradiate adjacent areas. Low-grade lymphomas generally are highly responsive to irradiation, with local control rates exceeding 90%. Long-term follow-up of patients treated for stage I and stage II lymphomas indicates a 10-year survival and 50% freedom from relapse, particularly among younger patients. Total lymphoid irradiation, given alone or in combination with chemotherapy, and whole-body irradiation have been used to treat patients with stage III and stage IV disease, with a high remission rate.

Intermediate- and high-grade lymphomas present with almost equal frequency in localized stage I and stage II disease versus disseminated stage III and stage IV disease, as well as arising more commonly in such extranodal sites as the gastrointestinal tract, bone marrow, central nervous system, and skin. Current trials for these tumors combine chemotherapy with radiation therapy.

Radiation therapy has to be tailored to the site of origin of the localized NHL tumor; for example, Waldeyer's ring is treated in patients with disease in the nasopharynx, tonsillar area, or base of the tongue; low-dose, whole-abdominal radiation therapy with shielding of the kidneys, followed by a boost to adjacent nodes, is used for gastrointestinal involvement; radiation of the bone with local node treatment is done for primary bone lymphomas; and the thyroid bed on both sides of the neck and the superior mediastinum are irradiated for thyroid-localized disease. Radiation is important in the treatment of primary central nervous system non-Hodgkin's lymphoma and is effective for palliation of symptoms in individuals with advanced disease such as superior vena cava obstruction, spinal cord compression, ureter occlusion, and painful tumor masses.

CHEMOTHERAPY

Chemotherapy is the primary treatment for disseminated non-Hodgkin's lymphoma. The choice of agents is based on the tumor's histology and stage and on such general information as the patient's age and performance status. The quality of life usually is good, with long periods in which the patient has no symptoms.

Such combinations as COP, CHOP, BACOP, MACOP-B, m-BACOD, and ProMACE-CytaBOM (see page 163 for specific drugs) have been used. Although the remission rate is high with these regimens, the average remission lasts only 2 to 3 years. After successive relapses, the remissions induced with second courses of therapy generally are shorter. There is little evidence of curability for stage III and stage IV disease.

Research is focused on using progressive chemotherapy earlier in the course of the disease and/or biologic response modifiers in combination with chemotherapy or during maintenance. In addition, initial chemotherapy followed by radiation therapy for patients with incomplete responses is being studied in patients with stage I and stage II disease.

Because increasing central nervous system involvement has been observed, especially with diffuse large cell lymphomas and extensive marrow involvement, the cerebrospinal fluid should be evaluated for presence of lymphoma. If such involvement exists, the patient should be given either systemic agents at a dosage known to penetrate the cerebrospinal fluid or prophylactic intrathecal chemotherapy; these approaches appear to be warranted in most cases of children with non-Hodgkin's lymphoma.

NURSING CARE

See pages 158-161.

CHAPTER 11

Head and Neck Cancer

Although fewer than 5% of all cancers are neoplasms of the head and neck, they assume particular importance for people with these diagnoses because surgical treatment may result in extensive cosmetic deformities and may impair such vital functions as eating and speaking. The most common site of head and neck cancer is the larynx; other sites are the oral cavity, oropharynx, hypopharynx, and nasopharynx.

The incidence of these cancers is increasing, despite the fact that 90% of epidermoid head and neck malignancies are related to life-style or environmental risk factors that are amenable to primary prevention.

Cancer of the Larynx

The glottic larynx (true vocal cords) is the site of 60% to 65% of laryngeal carcinomas; carcinoma of the supraglottic larynx (epiglottis, arytenoid cartilages, and false cords) is less common.

EPIDEMIOLOGY

Ninety percent of laryngeal cancers occur in men, with the highest incidence in those between 60 and 70 years of age. The death rate for blacks is higher than that for whites. Squamous cell carcinoma of the glottic larynx is the classic smoker's cancer of the head and neck and generally occurs after many decades of cigarette smoking. It is extremely unusual in nonsmokers. Alcohol is not as significant a factor in this cancer as it is in those of the oral cavity or hypopharynx, although many patients diagnosed with laryngeal carcinoma have a history of heavy alcohol consumption.

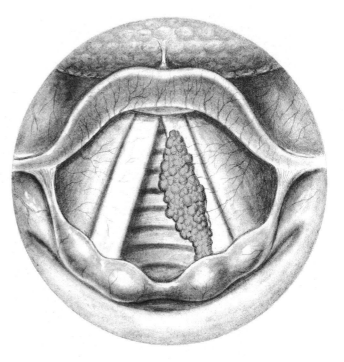

CANCER OF THE LARYNX

PATHOPHYSIOLOGY

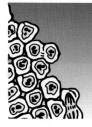

Squamous cell carcinoma is the most common type of laryngeal carcinoma. The glottic larynx, with the primary functions of phonation, airway protection during swallowing, and coughing, often is the site of inflammatory and premalignant changes. Carcinoma in situ may exist alone or in association with invasive disease. Because the symptoms of cancer in this area occur early, early diagnosis is also possible. There are few lymphatics, so nodal metastasis is rare, occurs late, and usually is seen only with long-standing and advanced local disease. The relative prognosis is good; however, limited vocal cord mobility resulting from deep muscle invasion and thyroid invasion indicates a poor prognosis.

The supraglottis functions not only as an air passage but also as a shield and sphincter to protect the airway. Malignancies in the supraglottic larynx can be silent and usually are diagnosed at a more advanced stage. Because this portion of the larynx interfaces superiorly with the oropharynx and laterally and posteriorly with the hypopharynx, the likelihood of occult or palpable nodal metastases is greater, and there are few barriers to primary-site extension.

The subglottic larynx, the airway below the true vocal cords and above the first tracheal ring, rarely develops a malignancy. More often subglottic involvement occurs through extension of a glottic or supraglottic tumor. The area's rich lymphatic network makes surgical treatment less feasible than in other locations.

Vocal cord fixation or clinically perceptible nodal metastases almost halve the 95% cure rate achievable in T_1 disease and the 80% to 85% cure rate achievable in T_2 glottic cancers (see page 53 for staging classifications). T_3 and T_4 lesions with nodal metastases have 5-year survival rates of less than 30%. Supraglottic laryngeal cancer is more lethal, stage for stage, for both early and more advanced lesions, with or without positive lymph nodes. The prognosis in primary subglottic cancer usually is poor.

SIGNS AND SYMPTOMS

Hoarseness and other vocal complaints are common symptoms. Signs and symptoms of a supraglottic tumor may include aspiration on swallowing, dysphagia, a foreign body sensation, a unilateral sore throat, earache, or a neck mass. Patients with a tumor on the vocal cord usually have hoarseness, dyspnea, difficulty swallowing, and a unilateral sore throat or earache, but these usually are late symptoms indicating a large tumor. Patients with infraglottic or subglottic tumors do not usually show symptoms until the tumor extends upward to the glottis or enlarges, causing dyspnea from encroachment on the airway.

DIAGNOSTIC STUDIES AND FINDINGS

Diagnostic test	Findings
Indirect mirror examination	Lesion on the larynx
Direct laryngoscopy and biopsy	Tumor; vocal cord fixation; occult extension; malignant cells
Anteroposterior laryngeal tomography	Subglottic extension of the disease
Pulmonary function studies	To assess preoperative pulmonary status
Chest x-ray	To identify associated pulmonary functional disease and coexistent lung cancer

MEDICAL MANAGEMENT

SURGERY

Endoscopic laser excision

Partial laryngectomy

Total laryngectomy with radical neck dissection

RADIATION THERAPY

External beam radiation

CHEMOTHERAPY

Cisplatin

5-Fluorouracil (5FU)

Adjuvant chemotherapy with methotrexate and 5FU

SURGERY

When treating laryngeal cancer, the goal is to achieve better results with less therapy or at least the same result with fewer side effects. Thus surgery that spares portions of the functional laryngeal anatomy is constantly being refined.

If no nodal disease is involved, early lesions usually can be treated successfully, so that the use of surgery or radiation therapy is determined by the probable morbidity in the glottic area. Limited surgery may be preferable, provided the functional integrity of the larynx can be preserved.

Small glottic lesions involving only one vocal cord can be excised using the endoscopic carbon dioxide laser technique. Larger glottic lesions are better treated with either partial laryngectomy or radiation.

Partial laryngectomy procedures include supraglottic laryngectomy; epiglottidectomy; cordectomy; anterior commissure resection; vertical hemilaryngectomy; frontolateral and extended frontolateral partial laryngectomy; and near-total laryngectomy. Evaluation of the patient's pulmonary function is important, because partial laryngectomy temporarily compromises pulmonary function, often resulting in aspiration.

Accurate pretreatment clinical staging is critical, since underestimating local extension of the disease could result in inappropriate treatment if intraoperative findings necessitate more extensive surgery.

Early supraglottic lesions are amenable to more conservative surgery, but the possibility of occult local extension, nodal metastasis, or both requires treatment that includes the primary site and the neck; this treatment often is external beam radiation therapy. Supraglottic laryngectomy is used for a more extensive T_2 lesion and is followed by postoperative radiation therapy. If nodal disease is present, neck dissection would be included.

Advanced lesions (T_3 or T_4) of the glottic or supraglottic larynx usually require total laryngectomy and postoperative radiation therapy to both the neck and larynx. Nodes positive for metastases require neck dissection.

Treatment of recurrent disease after radiation therapy, whether glottic or supraglottic, has required total laryngectomy with ipsilateral neck dissection. With unilateral endolaryngeal involvement, conservation surgery may be possible, but the obstacles include postradiation healing complications and persistent edema or fibrosis, which compromises laryngeal function and monitoring for future recurrence.

PREOPERATIVE PREPARATION

The patient and family must be taught about temporary and/or permanent changes in the airway. Both the patient and family need to be prepared for postoperative suctioning of the oral cavity and tracheostomy tube, intravenous therapy, wound care, drainage tubes, and the nasogastric tube. The patient should also be given the opportunity to express his fears, especially about the loss of verbal communication. The nurse should review the use of a magic slate or paper and pencil, flash cards, or a communication board. The patient may also be afraid of the expected change in body image and its impact on his self-concept and social acceptability.

POSTOPERATIVE CARE
Maintenance of Airway

The patient initially should be placed in a high Fowler's position to minimize edema, maximize coughing and deep breathing, facilitate suctioning, and provide comfort. Maintaining a patent airway is the priority for nursing care. The patient will have a tracheostomy tube in place; a cuffed tube is used to minimize aspiration and facilitate assisted or controlled ventilation. Because the cuffed tubes currently used exert only minimal pressure on the tracheal mucosa, they need not be routinely deflated. However, the cuff should be deflated at least once per shift to remove accumulated secretions. The tube is suctioned as often as necessary (using sterile technique) to remove excess secretions. Once the patient begins self-care, a clean technique can be used. The inner cannula should be removed and cleaned before the tracheostomy tube is suctioned. Removal of the entire tube usually is delayed until edema of the upper airway has subsided. Because the patient with a total laryngectomy has a permanent tracheostoma, daily tube changes can be instituted after 5 days.

Supplemental humidification is essential and may be supplied by means of a tracheostomy mask or a universal adapter attached to the tracheostomy tube.

Pressure dressings and neck drainage tubes are used in most patients after surgery to minimize the possibility of hematoma or seroma formation. The dressing should not be removed for several days after surgery until wound healing is under way.

Maintenance of Nutrition

A nasogastric tube may be used to maintain nutrition for the patient. Tube feedings are begun when bowel sounds return, usually on the first or second day after surgery. When the patient is alert and cooperative, he can be taught this procedure. The type of tube feedings used depends on the patient's ability to tolerate the feedings, which may include both blenderized diets and commercially prepared nutritional supplements. If the patient cannot tolerate bolus feedings several times a day, continuous-drip feeding can be administered.

OTHER ASPECTS OF CARE

Because the patient's history of smoking makes pulmonary complications more likely, early ambulation is important. Deep breathing and coughing, as well as suctioning of the tracheostomy tube, should be done frequently. Intermittent positive-pressure breathing (IPPB) devices and ultrasonic nebulization treatments may also help. Aspiration and pneumonia can be common occurrences in a patient with a temporary tracheostomy tube, so the patient should be assessed frequently.

Most patients have little pain; because many of the sensory nerves are cut, there is a sense of numbness and discomfort rather than pain. This discomfort, as well as that caused by position, dressings, and tubes, can be relieved with mild analgesics.

Depression is not uncommon and can be minimized by frequent explanations of the patient's progress and reassurance by the health care team. The family should be included in these discussions.

Self-care should begin as soon as possible after surgery. If the patient has had a partial laryngectomy, the tracheostomy tube is removed after the edema has subsided, and swallowing rehabilitation is instituted. The process of decannulation begins with deflating the cuff of the tracheostomy tube to determine if the patient can protect his airway from secretions. If no aspiration is observed, the tube can be changed to an uncuffed model that allows the patient to breathe around it when it is occluded.

The patient with a supraglottic laryngectomy may have difficulty swallowing as a result of removal of the epiglottis. It generally is believed that swallowing should not be instituted until the tracheostoma has closed; foods of a thick consistency are introduced gradually, with liquids saved until the patient can swallow. Standard instructions for supraglottic swallow are to take a deep breath, bear down to close the vocal cords, swallow, cough to rid the vocal cords of any food that may have collected, swallow, and breathe.

The patient with a total laryngectomy usually has a shorter hospital stay and can begin swallowing about 7 days after surgery. He begins on liquids and advances to a general diet before discharge. All patients should maintain a high calorie–high protein diet.

COMPLICATIONS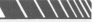

Hemorrhage
Airway obstruction
Infection
Thoracic duct leakage
Nerve injury

Thoracic duct leakage may occur as a result of resection of lymph nodes in the neck. The loss of fluid and protein may occur if a chyle leak exists; the depletion of lymphocytes may be significant. A chyle leak appears as a milky white liquid that often is mixed with serous fluid as it exits the wound-drainage site through tubes in the inferior aspect of the wound. A chyle fistula usually closes spontaneously; if it does not, surgical closure may be necessary.

Nerve Damage

Nerves may be sacrificed as part of the surgical resection, or they may be accidentally severed. The consequences are as follows:

Superior laryngeal nerve—Damage causes some interference in the patient's ability to swallow, but this loss usually is compensated for over a month's time. Severing both nerves results in severe impairment, and a laryngectomy may be necessary.

Vagus nerve—Severing this nerve at a high level in the neck can cause unilateral palatal and pharyngeal paralysis, supraglottic anesthesia, and glottic incompetence as a result of unilateral vocal cord paralysis. If the nerve is severed unilaterally, an ipsilateral laryngeal paralysis results; if the cord is in the abducted (open) position, the patient has a poor, raspy voice and frequent aspiration, and cannot perform an adequate cough. Injecting Teflon into the paralyzed cord adds bulk to the cord and improves closure.

Recurrent laryngeal nerve—Damage causes bilateral paralysis, which requires an immediate tracheostomy, since this nerve is responsible for adduction and abduction of the vocal cords.

Phrenic nerve—If this nerve is severed on only one side, paralysis of the hemidiaphragm results.

Hypoglossal nerve—This nerve is responsible for tongue movement; severing it leads to speech impairment and masticatory difficulties.

Lingual nerve—This is a sensory nerve; severing it causes numbness on the ipsilateral side of the tongue.

Glossopharyngeal nerve—This nerve innervates the posterior third of the tongue; damage causes difficulty swallowing and altered taste sensation on the ipsilateral side, although the contralateral side usually compensates for this.

Superficial sensory nerves—Damage to these nerves causes numbness over skin areas; sensation usually returns to large areas over time.

Facial nerve—Damage causes temporary paralysis; function usually returns to normal within 8 weeks. If the mandibular branch is sectioned, paresthesia and drooling occur on the ipsilateral side.

Spinal accessory nerve—This nerve innervates the trapezius muscle, which supports the shoulder and allows lateral abduction of the arm. The postoperative result in 50% of patients is painful shoulder droop with atrophy of the trapezius muscle; the patient can no longer raise his arm above his shoulder. He should begin an exercise program 10 to 12 days after surgery. Exercises support the shoulder while developing and strengthening the levator scapulae and rhomboid muscles of the back, aid in stretching the trapezius muscle, and also are used with patients who have had radiation therapy to the area, since radiation therapy can also decrease innervation to the trapezius muscle.

Reconstruction

Most people can adapt to the physical disfigurement of head and neck surgery; however, the changes in swallowing, articulation, and oral continence are both debilitating and crippling. Consequently the goal of reconstruction is to maintain or achieve adequate function after surgical removal of cancerous tissues.

Skin flaps help maintain remaining structures and reconstructed parts in a more normal functional position, which prevents the forces of muscle imbalance and wound contracture from shifting areas. Such procedures as intermaxillary fixation, extraoral appliances, implanted synthetic materials, or bone grafts may be used. Skin flaps can be used to cover full-thickness surface defects such as those of the floor of the nasal cavity or of the cheek; to protect and cover the carotid artery and nerves in the neck region; to line the oral mucosa or pharyngeal cavity; or to replace the mucoperiosteum overlying the alveolar ridge or hard palate. Functional support can be attained by using a flap to fill a defect that otherwise would create a gully for the entrapment and stagnation of food particles. Flaps can be used to provide surface cover and to line the oral cavity. They are particularly useful for patients who have had previous radiation therapy.

The disadvantages of skin flap reconstruction are that the skin often undergoes desquamation and, because the skin does not produce mucus, the oral cavity may be dry, causing food to stick to the flap; it also lacks sensation, and the patient may complain of a feeling of anesthesia.

The major factor in flap survival is maintaining vascular integrity. This is endangered by tension, kinking, pressure, hematoma, or infection in the flap. A healthy flap is pink or slightly reddened. Early pallor suggests a lack of capillary filling; if it persists longer than 24 hours, the flap will not survive. This is also true with early cyanosis. An edematous flap with shiny skin and blistering is likely to fail.

RADIATION THERAPY

Radiation therapy may be used as primary therapy for early lesions of the larynx, preoperatively or postoperatively, or as palliative treatment for patients with inoperable or recurrent tumors of the larynx. Given in large doses with cure as the goal (6000 to 7000 rad), radiation therapy controls the lesion while preserving the structure and function of the area treated.

Pretreatment evaluation by a dentist and fabrication of fluoride carriers may help prevent radiation-induced dental caries after treatment. The radiation port or field includes both the tumor and draining lymph nodes, since these are important sites of microscopic disease. Treatment involves two areas: a large treatment field used for part of the therapy to treat the tumor and nodes (4500 to 5000 rad) and a smaller treatment field to deliver higher doses to the tumor itself (6000 to 7000 rad). Care must be taken to block the spinal cord, since its tolerance is 4500 rad, and doses above this may result in irreversible neurologic damage. The main side effects of radiation therapy for these patients are xerostomia, mucositis, taste alterations, and throat discomfort.

Hyperthermia (e.g., superficial heating with ultrasound or microwaves) may be combined with radiation therapy to produce an enhanced effect. Catheters are inserted at the treatment site to hold temperature sensors and are left in place for the entire course of treatment. The area is heated to 41° to 45° C (105.8° to 113° F), and the temperature is maintained for 45 to 60 minutes, generally once or twice weekly during treatment. The patient may report a burning sensation and may need medication beforehand to decrease discomfort. Skin care is essential. The patient is taught to care for the catheters with aseptic technique.

LATE EFFECTS

Skin fibrosis
Bone and tissue necrosis
Trismus

If implants are used to provide radiation therapy, hollow catheters are inserted into the treatment area to hold the radioactive source, usually iridium-192 or cesium-137. The implant is left in place for 3 to 5 days to deliver a dose of 3000 to 7000 rad, depending on whether previous therapy has been given. The therapeutic goals are cure of early-stage lesions in the floor of the mouth and anterior tongue; providing a boost dose to the tumor in conjunction with external beam treatment; and treating the patient with recurrent disease within a previously treated portal.

Interstitial implants are most suitable to lesions of the lip, floor of the mouth, buccal mucosa, nasal vestibule, or skin. Pain medication may be needed; steroids and antibiotics minimize swelling and prevent infection in areas of mucositis.

Permanent implants are seeds that are inserted with an applicator. They consist of radioactive material with an inert metal. Because the source has low activity, radiation is absorbed within the tumor with little or no exposure at the skin's surface. These seeds are implanted at the time of surgery into positive margins, neck nodes, or extension of the tumor into the skull. The dose is estimated to be approximately 6000 rad in 60 days, with 12,000 rad delivered over the course of a year.

CHEMOTHERAPY

Chemotherapy has been used preoperatively for tumors classified as unresectable with the goal of reducing the size of the tumor so as to improve its response to conventional therapy. Cisplatin and 5FU are the drugs used most often. They may be given before, with, or after radiation therapy.

Adjuvant chemotherapy with methotrexate and 5FU is under study.

Patients who have refused other treatments or in whom other modalities have failed may require chemotherapy to reduce the size of the tumor and thus relieve discomfort and pain.

1 ASSESS

ASSESSMENT	OBSERVATIONS
Voice	Hoarseness
Aerodigestive function	Dysphagia; aspiration on swallowing; foreign body sensation; unilateral sore throat; earache
Respiratory	Dyspnea
Psychosocial	Fear

2 DIAGNOSE

NURSING DIAGNOSIS	SUBJECTIVE FINDINGS	OBJECTIVE FINDINGS
Impaired verbal communication related to pressure of tumor on vocal cord(s)	Complains that voice is weak, raspy	Hoarseness
Impaired swallowing related to pressure of tumor on esophagus	Reports foreign body sensation, unilateral sore throat, earache	Aspiration on swallowing

NURSING DIAGNOSIS	SUBJECTIVE FINDINGS	OBJECTIVE FINDINGS
Ineffective breathing pattern related to pressure of tumor on vocal cord(s)	Reports being short of breath	Dyspnea
Fear related to difficulty with speech, swallowing, and breathing	Expresses fear of helplessness, isolation, and possible starvation and suffocation	Depression, anger, and withdrawal

3 PLAN

Patient goals

1. The patient will be able to communicate verbally.
2. The patient will be able to swallow without difficulty.
3. The patient will be able to breathe without difficulty.
4. The patient will be less fearful about the difficulty with speech, swallowing, and breathing.

4 IMPLEMENT

NURSING DIAGNOSIS	NURSING INTERVENTIONS	RATIONALE
Impaired verbal communication related to pressure of tumor on vocal cord(s)	Teach patient to speak slowly and to articulate clearly.	To enhance effectiveness of voice.
	Provide alternate means of communication (e.g., magic slate, paper and pencil).	To conserve voice.
Impaired swallowing related to pressure of tumor on esophagus	Encourage patient to eat and drink small amounts slowly.	To avoid aspiration.
	Provide thin liquids and soft foods; offer dietary supplements.	To avoid choking and maintain nutritional balance.
	Recommend alternate methods of feeding (e.g., nasogastric tube).	To provide adequate nutrition.
Ineffective breathing pattern related to pressure of tumor on vocal cord(s)	Encourage patient to plan frequent rest periods.	To conserve energy.
	Teach patient to breathe slowly and to relax when he feels dsypneic.	To feel sense of control over breathing.
	Provide oxygen therapy as needed.	To enrich the environment.
	Position patient in semi-Fowler's position with support.	To decrease pressure on larynx.

NURSING DIAGNOSIS	NURSING INTERVENTIONS	RATIONALE
	Prepare patient for tracheostomy if deemed necessary.	To bypass obstructed airway.
Fear related to difficulty with speech, swallowing, and breathing	Assess appetite, weight loss, sleep patterns, mobility, and bowel activity.	These signs may indicate depression.
	Teach patient to use relaxation techniques, imagery, and other self-control methods.	To control anxiety related to fears.
	Listen to and accept expression of fear of helplessness, isolation, and possible starving and suffocation.	To foster expression of strong emotions.
	Involve patient in planning actions to deal with speech, swallowing, and breathing difficulties.	Gives patient sense of self-care.
Knowledge deficit	See Patient Teaching.	

5 EVALUATE

PATIENT OUTCOME	DATA INDICATING THAT OUTCOME IS REACHED
Patient's speech has improved.	Patient can speak in a normal and easily understood voice.
Patient's nutrition is adequate.	Patient can swallow without aspirating.
Patient's breathing is normal.	Patient can tolerate usual activity without dyspnea.
Patient shows progress in lessening his fears.	Patient talks about his problems in a realistic manner, with an emphasis on problem solving.

PATIENT TEACHING ▪▪▪▪▪▪▪▪▪▪▪▪▪▪▪▪▪▪▪▪▪▪▪▪▪▪▪▪▪▪▪▪▪▪▪▪

1. Teach the patient to avoid voice strain and to use alternate methods of communication when his voice needs a rest.
2. Encourage the patient to plan his diet to avoid the possibility of choking or aspirating (e.g., eat soft foods and drink liquids frequently).
3. Remind the patient to plan frequent rest periods to avoid dyspnea.
4. Encourage the patient to attend support groups in which other people discuss their fears and ways of controlling them.

Cancer of the Oral Cavity and Oropharynx

Although easily detected, oral cancers generally are discovered late; 80% to 90% are 2 cm or more in diameter at the time of diagnosis.

EPIDEMIOLOGY

Identified carcinogens in oral cancer include cigarettes, ethyl alcohol, snuff, chewing tobacco, and chemicals used in the textile and leather industries. Other factors are syphilis and vitamin deficiencies.

Although oral cavity cancers are relatively accessible to self-examination, dental evaluation, and routine physical examination, delays in diagnosis result from lack of unique symptomatology (painless lesion); confusion with traumatic, inflammatory, or infectious lesions; or patient delay due to fear and the false hope that the tumor eventually will disappear. After the larynx, the oral cavity and oropharynx are the most common sites for squamous cell carcinoma of the head and neck. These patients tend to be men in their 50s and 60s, but the number of women with this type of cancer is growing. There is also a downward trend in the age group most affected, because chewing tobacco and snuff dipping have become more common practices among women in rural areas and young boys. Use of any kind of tobacco and alcohol consumption are significant factors in the development of these cancers. Oral cancers are commonly associated with poor dentition, chronic oral infection, and local trauma of any cause. Inhalation of certain wood dusts, nickel compounds, nitrosamines, hydrocarbons, or asbestos is highly correlated with tumors of the oral cavity.

In previous years an increased incidence of oral cancer, especially of the tongue, has been observed in persons with syphilis, leading to speculation that this chronic infection may cause malignant changes in the mouth or that persons exposed to spirochetal infections are also, because of poorer socioeconomic status, more susceptible to oral cancers. Infection with *Candida albicans* is often seen in persons with leukoplakia (premalignant), as is herpes simplex virus (type 1) infection.[107]

Chronic malnutrition (particularly riboflavin deficiencies) and anemia are related to leukoplakia and mucosal changes.

Sun exposure is implicated in cancers of the exposed vermillion border of the lips, an area that also comes in contact with cigarettes, pipes, or cigars.

A relatively high incidence of Plummer-Vinson syndrome is found in persons with cancer of the oral cavity and pharynx. This syndrome is characterized by generalized nutritional deficiencies, anemia, achlorhydria, chronic dysphagia, and splenic enlargement; there may also be general signs of atrophy of the oral and pharyngeal mucous membranes. These persons often have a history of loss of teeth early in life.

PATHOPHYSIOLOGY

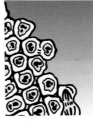

Oral cavity and oropharyngeal cancers are almost always squamous cell carcinoma. The oropharynx, which includes the lymphoid tissue of the palatal and lingual tonsils, can also be the site of lymphoma.

These lesions tend to be poorly delineated, often spread submucosally, and are not confined by the anatomic midline. Deep muscle involvement of the tongue or pterygoid musculature is an ominous finding. Invasion of bony structures (i.e., mandible, palate, maxilla, maxillary sinus, or spine) is serious in terms of both prognosis and treatment morbidity. Surgical treatment of a primary tumor that has extended across the midline is much more debilitating than for one that has remained localized.

Nodal metastases are relatively uncommon with oral cancer but are more likely when the site of the primary lesion is further into the oropharynx or when the lesion grows toward the midline. This feature, along with a higher incidence of poorly differentiated lesions, accounts to some extent for the prognosis of oropharyngeal tumors being worse than that of oral cancers.

Early lesions have a good chance for cure, whereas second primary lesions are a particular problem, especially in oral cancer. The addition of nodal disease, an advanced primary, or a recurrence after previous treatment significantly decreases survival and adds a substantial risk for distant (usually pulmonary) metastasis. The overall 5-year survival rate for oral cavity tumors is about 50%; for oropharyngeal cancers, it is about 35%. Tumors at the base of the tongue and pharyngeal walls and those that involve bone are particularly deadly.

More than 80% of those who die of oral cancer die of uncontrolled local disease rather than distant metastasis.

SIGNS AND SYMPTOMS

The most common sign is a lesion, often a white spot or sore that is slow to heal, in the oral cavity or oropharynx. Other complaints include difficulty with dentures, persistent ulcerations, and blood-tinged sputum. Complaints of difficulty with swallowing or speech indicate more extensive disease.

Fissures, ulcers, or areas of induration in patches of leukoplakia may reflect malignant changes in the mucosa. Erythroplasia or well-defined red patches with a velvety consistency among tiny areas of ulceration may be the earliest sign of malignancy.

An enlarged cervical node may be the first sign of oral cancer. Posterior tongue lesions should be suspected with hypoglossal nerve paralysis. Numbness over the chin may signal invasion of the inferior alveolar ridge and compression of the mandibular nerve.

DIAGNOSTIC STUDIES AND FINDINGS

Diagnostic test	Findings
Biopsy of areas of redness or inflammation that last >2 wk	Malignant cells
Mandible x-rays and/or bone scan	Bone involvement
Computed tomography (CT) scan	Parapharyngeal, spinal, carotid, or pterygoid muscle involvement
Endoscopy and examination under anesthesia	To evaluation the extent of the primary site and the possibility of synchronous second primaries

MEDICAL MANAGEMENT

SURGERY

Transoral, intraoral, or transcervical resection and reconstruction

Total laryngectomy

Modified or radical neck dissection

Mandibular resection and reconstruction

RADIATION THERAPY

External beam radiation

External or interstitial implant

CHEMOTHERAPY

Controversial role as adjunctive therapy

SURGERY

Surgery and radiation are equally effective in treating early-stage primary lesions of the oral cavity or oropharynx. In general, as the site of the tumor moves posteriorly, the morbidity of surgery increases. Posterior lesions are also difficult to expose to surgery. Advanced lesions generally require both surgery and radiation. Because even aggressive radical surgery for early-stage lesions of the oropharynx may not remove all gross and subclinical disease, radiation therapy is appropriate adjuvant therapy.

The transoral route may be used for anteriorly located lesions. Primary closure of the mobile tongue after partial glossectomy and also of the buccal mucosa or mouth floor often is possible. If not, split thickness or dermal skin grafting is useful. For larger or less-accessible anterior lesions and for most posterior lesions, intraoral surgery is limiting. A transcervical approach, with or without mandible or lip-splitting procedures, will be necessary. Reconstruction may require the transfer of distant tissue such as a pectoralis major myocutaneous flap, bone graft, or artificial prosthesis. The tongue base and lower pharynx are difficult areas and may require adjunctive total laryngectomy to prevent postoperative aspiration.

In the presence of known nodal disease, radical neck dissection is performed. If the spinal accessory nerve is preserved, the procedure is referred to as a modified radical neck dissection. In addition to removal of all of the nodal groups in the accessible cervical region, the internal jugular vein, sternocleidomastoid muscle, and cervical sensory nerves are also removed.

Marginal mandibulectomy is performed when the tumor is in continuity with the floor of the mouth. Because the continuity of the mandibular arch is maintained, rehabilitation is excellent. The presence of the patient's teeth allows for anchorage of a dental prosthesis. Lateral mandibulectomy involves the body and ramus of the mandible posterior to the cuspid area. Anterior facial contour is preserved but lateral facial contour is concave. Hemimandibulectomy results in greater facial disfigurement, and speech, swallowing, and salivary control are difficult. Anterior mandibulectomy creates profound functional and cosmetic deformities—that is, impaired deglutition, articulation, salivary continence, mastication, and respiration. Oral continence and facial contour are severely affected.

RADIATION THERAPY

If radiation therapy is used to treat the primary site, it can be delivered by either external beam or combined external and interstitial implant methods. Treatment of nodal disease is included in the treatment plan. Irradiation of nodes should be considered as prophylaxis for all but the smallest oral cavity tumors and for most oropharyngeal lesions.

A boost of radiation dose to the primary site can be delivered by means of interstitial implanting of radioactive material directly into the tumor.

Combined therapy may be used in the following situations: surgery first and then radiation therapy on large primary tumors; radiation therapy first and surgery second on small primary tumors; surgery plus radiation therapy with radiation therapy first if resectability is in question for a major primary tumor plus neck disease; surgery or radiation therapy for "salvage" of the primary or neck site after previous treatment failure with the other modality, adding chemotherapy or using it alone.

Cancer of the Hypopharynx

The hypopharynx is divided into the pyriform sinuses, the posterior cricoid area, and the posterior and lateral pharyngeal wall.

EPIDEMIOLOGY

The incidence of hypopharyngeal tumors is highest in men in the sixth and seventh decades of life. A history of Plummer-Vinson syndrome and alcohol and tobacco use are common risk factors.

PATHOPHYSIOLOGY

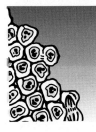

Most hypopharyngeal lesions are of squamous cell origin and are poorly differentiated. At the time of diagnosis, most patients have a large lesion and an involved node, usually large and in the midportion of the jugular chain. Local extension by mucosal spread is common. Direct extension may occur to the larynx or esophagus. Lesions of the posterior wall often extend to the posterior tonsillar pillar.

Overall survival for these patients is poor; the 5-year survival rate is 23% to 29% with treatment.

SIGNS AND SYMPTOMS

Hypopharyngeal tumors have an insidious onset. A lump in the neck may be the first sign of disease and the chief complaint. The person may have been treated previously for a persistent sore throat and may complain of a burning sensation. The most common initial symptom is odynophagia, which is sometimes unilateral. Progressive dysphagia contributes to rapid weight loss. Otalgia on the same side as the tumor indicates invasion of the superior laryngeal nerve. Hoarseness indicates invasion of the true cords or displacement of the larynx. Foul, malodorous breath may indicate a tumor that is infected and necrotic.

DIAGNOSTIC STUDIES AND FINDINGS

Diagnostic test	Findings
Mirror pharyngoscopy	Clear visualization of the tumor
Soft tissue tomograms, contrast radiograms, and direct pharyngoscopy and/or laryngoscopy with biopsy	Visualization of the tumor; malignant cells
Esophagoscopy with biopsy	Posterior invasion of the esophagus

MEDICAL MANAGEMENT

SURGERY

Resection

Total laryngectomy, pharyngectomy, and radical neck dissection

RADIATION THERAPY

External beam radiation

CHEMOTHERAPY

SURGERY

With limited laryngeal involvement, the glottic sphincter of the larynx can be preserved despite resection of a portion of the larynx and the involved pharynx. The patient may require a nasogastric tube and tracheostomy for an extended period until swallowing ability has been restored and aspiration reduced. Difficulty swallowing may be a long-term problem, because extensive postoperative scarring often results in esophageal stricture.

With involvement of the pyriform sinus, fixation of the vocal cords, and invasion of the thyroid cartilage, a total laryngectomy, pharyngectomy, and radical neck dissection are performed. The posterior pharyngeal wall is used to reconstruct a neogullet for swallowing; when it cannot be used, cervical and regional flaps are necessary to close the defect, which is done through a two- or three-stage procedure.

First, a deltopectoral flap is used to form a tube that will provide an epithelial tissue source for reconstruction of the pharyngoesophageal area. The upper end of the tube is sutured at the level of the oropharynx; the lower end is attached to the upper esophagus, with an opening on the external neck that acts as a temporary esophageal fistula. In about 3 weeks the pedicle is divided, the esophagus is anastomosed, and wound closure is completed. The patient now has a reconstructed, skin-lined conduit for saliva and food.

Surgical resections that involve the pharyngeal constrictors interfere with the normal muscular contraction that controls a bolus of food and delivers it into the esophagus during swallowing. If more than half of the middle and lower contrictors are resected and reconstructed, swallowing is impaired by scar contracture but eventually becomes adequate as scar tissue softens.

Infection is a possible complication because of the opening of the upper digestive tract, which makes surgery a contaminated procedure. Because of this, the patient receives antibiotic therapy. Meticulous wound care, adequate nutritional support, and oral hygiene are also important.

If the patient has had previous radiation therapy, wound healing is compromised and pharyngocutaneous fistula formation or infection of the anastomosis is common. This threatens the integrity of the carotid artery, and carotid rupture can be deadly.

RADIATION THERAPY

Radiation therapy and chemotherapy are alternatives available to patients with an unresectable tumor. High doses of radiation therapy to the hypopharynx and bilateral neck are necessary. The spinal cord is shielded from the radiation source after 75% of the dose has been administered.

Cancer of the Nasopharynx

The incidence of nasopharyngeal cancer is low, and the disease occurs more often in men than in women by a ratio of 3:1.

EPIDEMIOLOGY

Nasopharyngeal cancer is relatively uncommon among whites but is endemic in parts of China, where it is the most common tumor of the head and neck. The etiologic factors are believed to be environmental, particularly the Epstein-Barr virus.

PATHOPHYSIOLOGY

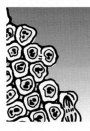 Nasopharyngeal cancers are primarily of squamous cell origin and frequently are poorly differentiated or undifferentiated. Lymphoepithelioma is the predominant malignant tumor of the Chinese.

SIGNS AND SYMPTOMS

Nasopharyngeal cancers are silent in the early stages, so many are discovered late and only after they have grown quite large. In most people unilateral lymph node metastasis, usually to the cervical chain, is the initial presenting sign.

Symptoms may include hearing impairment and tinnitus caused by obstruction of the eustachian tube and persistent otitis media. Poorly localized headache in the frontal, parietal, or temporal regions and facial pain are late symptoms, caused by bony erosion and pressure on the fifth cranial nerve. Invasion through the base of the skull results in cranial nerve compression, which is manifested in nerve-specific symptoms. For example, double vision occurs when the third, fourth, and sixth cranial nerves are affected.

Horner's syndrome indicates tumor invasion of the sympathetic nerve fibers accompanying the carotid artery as it passes intracranially. When large, the tumor causes unilateral or bilateral nasal obstruction. Epistaxis may be observed with necrosis of the tumor and vessel walls.

Cancers of the nasopharynx frequently metastasize through the bloodstream to the lungs, liver, and bone (spine, pelvis, and femur).

DIAGNOSTIC STUDIES AND FINDINGS

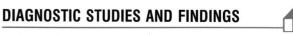

Diagnostic test	Findings
Visualization and biopsy with nasopharyngeal forceps	Observation of the tumor; malignant cells
X-rays and tomograms of the sinuses and base of the skull	Bony destruction

RADIATION THERAPY

Radiation therapy is used to irradiate all of the naso-pharynx, the retropharyngeal nodes, and all lymph nodes on both sides of the neck. Radioactive implants can be used to augment the dosage. Most tumors are relatively radiosensitive, and survival rates approach 25%.

The patient with advanced disease often has severe headaches and pain as a result of bony invasion and erosion; thus pain management is especially important. Sensory losses, visual disturbances, and palsies are common. Anorexia, severe weight loss, respiratory problems, and laryngopharyngeal edema may necessitate a tracheostomy and gastrostomy or esophagostomy.

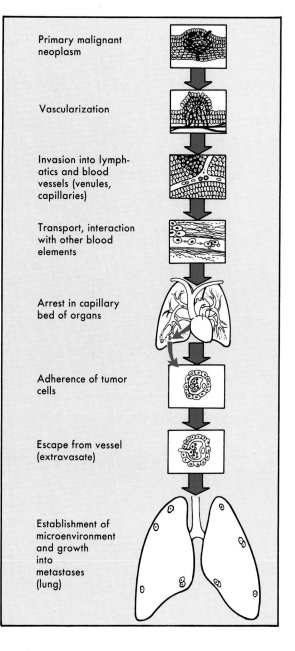

CHAPTER 12

Metastatic Disease

Metastatic disease is the major cause of death from cancer. A metastasis is a tumor that is distant from the primary tumor. The cells from the primary tumor that give rise to these metastases can be spread in many ways: for example, as a result of seeding throughout a body cavity such as the peritoneal or thoracic cavity; through mechanical transport by means of instruments or gloved hands; by lymphatic spread; or by hematogenous spread (Figure 12-1). The likelihood of one or more metastases developing is determined by several factors: how long the primary tumor has existed; a high mitotic rate; trauma, such as that caused by a biopsy of the primary tumor; heat; and the tumor's proximity to a rich lymphatic or vascular network. The following are the most common sites of metastasis:

Lungs (from such primary sites as the colorectum, breasts, renal system, testes, and bones)
Liver (from the lungs, colorectum, breasts, and renal system)
Brain (from the lungs, breasts, gastrointestinal tract, renal system, testes, uterus, and ovaries)
Spinal cord (from the lungs, breasts, prostate, renal system, and gastrointestinal tract)
Bone (from the lungs, breasts, renal system, and prostate)

In the ongoing assessment of a person with cancer, the nurse should be especially watchful for early signs and symptoms of metastatic disease. This requires a knowledge of the usual sites of spread for specific cancers, sensitivity to the patient's complaints, and attention to changes in laboratory values and alterations in function that indicate metastatic spread.

Primary malignant neoplasm

Vascularization

Invasion into lymphatics and blood vessels (venules, capillaries)

Transport, interaction with other blood elements

Arrest in capillary bed of organs

Adherence of tumor cells

Escape from vessel (extravasate)

Establishment of microenvironment and growth into metastases (lung)

FIGURE 12-1
Pathogenesis of metastasis. (From McCance and Huether.[43])

Table 12-1

LOCALIZING SIGNS AND SYMPTOMS OF BRAIN TUMORS

Location of tumor	Localizing signs and symptoms
Frontal lobe	
Anterior portion	Disturbances in mental function
Posterior portion	Motor system dysfunction, convulsions, aphasia (dominant hemisphere)
Parietal lobe	Sensory deficits (contralateral), paresthesia, hyperesthesia, astereognosis, loss of two-point discrimination, finger agnosia; convulsions; visual field defects; defects in speech and recognition (dominant hemisphere)
Temporal lobe	Psychomotor convulsions; visual field defects; auditory disturbances; Wernicke's aphasia (dominant hemisphere)
Occipital lobe	Headaches; convulsions with visual aura; visual field deficit
Cerebellar tumors	Nystagmus; ataxia; unsteady gait; dysmetria; problems with rapid alternation movements
Brainstem and cranial nerve tumors	Hemiparesis; nystagmus; extraocular nerve palsies; facial paralysis; depressed corneal reflex; hearing loss, tinnitus; problems swallowing, drooling; vertigo, dizziness; ataxia; vomiting

Table 12-2

LOCALIZING SIGNS AND SYMPTOMS OF SPINAL CORD TUMORS

Location	Signs and symptoms
Cervical tumors	
C4 and above	Sensory: vertigo
	Motor: quadriparesis, atrophy of sternocleidomastoid muscles; dysphagia; dysarthria; tongue deviation; respiratory insufficiency and/or failure
	Other: occipital headaches; nuchal rigidity; down-beat nystagmus; papilledema
C4 and below	Sensory: paresthesia; Horner's syndrome (ipsilateral pupillary constriction, ptosis, and anhidrosis)
	Motor: weakness, muscle fasciculation; muscle atrophy
	Other: shoulder and arm pain
Thoracic tumors	Sensory: hyperesthesia band immediately above level of lesion
	Motor: spastic paresis of lower extremities; positive Babinski's sign; lower motor neuron deficits
	Other: sphincter impairment
Lumbar tumors	Sensory: localized loss in legs and saddle area
	Motor: foot-drop; diminished or absent patellar and Achilles reflexes
	Other: severe low back pain with radiation down legs; perianal and bladder discomfort; decreased libido; impotence; bladder disturbances

1   ASSESS

ASSESSMENT	OBSERVATIONS
Respiratory	Cough, hemoptysis, wheezing; fever; dyspnea; chest pain; hoarseness; enlargement of neck with venous distention; clubbing of fingers
Metabolic	Nonspecific abdominal complaints (e.g., increasing distention); right upper quadrant mass; weight loss, anorexia, nausea, vomiting; signs and symptoms of cirrhosis (e.g., spider angioma and gynecomastia)

ASSESSMENT	OBSERVATIONS
Central nervous system	Headaches, nausea, vomiting; disturbances in mental, motor, and/or sensory function; focal or generalized convulsive activity; visual field, speech, or auditory defects; vertigo, dizziness, ataxia, nystagmus, depressed corneal reflex, facial paralysis (Table 12-1); pain; disturbances in sensory and/or motor function; urinary urgency, difficulty initiating urination, retention and overflow incontinence; contralateral loss of temperature and pain sensation; ipsilateral loss of motor function, touch and position sense (Table 12-2)
Communication	Difficulty with speech and hearing
Psychosocial	Expresses fear of disease progression and prognosis; anxiety, depression, anger

2 DIAGNOSE

NURSING DIAGNOSIS	SUBJECTIVE FINDINGS	OBJECTIVE FINDINGS
Altered cardiopulmonary and peripheral tissue perfusion related to pulmonary metastases	Complains of chest pain, dyspnea	Cough, hemoptysis, wheezing; fever; hoarseness; enlargement of neck with venous distention; clubbing of fingers
Altered nutrition: less than body requirements related to liver metastases	Complains of nonspecific abdominal discomfort, anorexia, nausea	Increasing abdominal distention; right upper quadrant mass; weight loss; vomiting; spider angioma; gynecomastia
Potential for injury related to central nervous system metastases	Complains of headaches, nausea, dizziness	Vomiting; disturbances in mental, motor, and/or sensory function; focal or generalized convulsive activity; visual field, speech, or auditory defects; vertigo, ataxia, nystagmus, depressed corneal reflex, facial paralysis
Pain related to bone and/or central nervous system metastases	Complains of bone pain, headache	Grimacing; holding head or guarding extremity or specific area of trunk
Impaired physical mobility related to central nervous system metastases	Complains of weakness	Disturbances in motor function, position sense
Altered patterns of urinary elimination related to central nervous system or peripheral nervous system metastases	Complains of urinary urgency and difficulty initiating urination	Urinary retention and overflow incontinence

→ › ›

NURSING DIAGNOSIS	SUBJECTIVE FINDINGS	OBJECTIVE FINDINGS
Impaired verbal communication related to central nervous system metastases	Complains of difficulty with speaking and hearing	Speech is difficult to understand; ignores comments or asks to have them repeated
Fear related to evidence of metastases	Expresses fear of disease progression and prognosis	Anxiety, depression, and anger

3 PLAN

Patient goals

1. The patient will have normal cardiopulmonary function.
2. The patient will have normal nutrition and a stable weight.
3. The patient will be ambulatory and free of injury.
4. The patient will be comfortable and without pain.
5. The patient will have normal urinary elimination.
6. The patient will be able to deal with fears in a realistic way.

4 IMPLEMENT

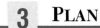

NURSING DIAGNOSIS	NURSING INTERVENTIONS	RATIONALE
Altered cardiopulmonary and peripheral tissue perfusion related to pulmonary metastases	Observe for hoarseness.	Indicates involvement of recurrent laryngeal nerve.
	Observe for signs and symptoms of pleural effusion; keep chest drainage equipment available.	Indicates involvement of viscera or parietal pleura; thoracotomy may be needed to prevent or treat pneumothorax.
	Observe for fever, hemoptysis; report to physician.	Indicates pneumonitis or abscess formation in lung.
	Administer analgesics as needed.	To relieve chest pain.
	Provide oxygen therapy as needed.	To relieve dyspnea.
	Observe for enlargement of neck with venous distention; report to physician.	Indicates compression or invasion of superior vena cava.
	Observe fingers for clubbing.	Indicates hypertrophic pulmonary osteoarthropathy.
	Position patient comfortably, with head elevated.	To promote chest expansion.
	Encourage coughing and deep breathing.	To clear and maintain patent respiratory tract.

NURSING DIAGNOSIS	NURSING INTERVENTIONS	RATIONALE
	Administer vaporized air.	To moisten secretions and to ensure adequate tissue perfusion.
	Suction airway as needed.	To relieve obstruction caused by secretions.
	Encourage adequate rest.	To decrease respiratory workload.
	Remove constrictive clothing.	To relieve pressure on chest.
	Discourage smoking.	To decrease respiratory distress.
	Observe chest for symmetric expansion; auscultate for abnormal breath sounds, voice sounds, rales, and rhonchi.	To assess respiratory status and pulmonary function.
	Monitor blood studies.	To determine adequate oxygenation.
	Be alert for complaints of cyanosis, dyspnea, wheezing, confusion, and fatigue.	Indicate increasing respiratory distress.
	Monitor pulse and respiratory rate and rhythm.	To assess for adequacy of cardiopulmonary function.
Altered nutrition: less than body requirements related to liver metastases	Offer antiemetics as prescribed.	To relieve nausea and vomiting.
	Arrange pleasant surroundings; provide appealing selection of foods; encourage family and friends to bring in food of patient's choice; provide attractive meal tray.	To enhance patient's appetite.
	Postpone feeding when patient is fatigued.	Patient is more likely to eat when rested.
	Give small, frequent feedings.	To avoid distention.
	Feed slowly, and provide rest periods.	To avoid tiring patient.
	Observe and record food intake; measure body weight daily.	To monitor nutritional status.
	Elevate patient's head.	To promote comfort.
	Encourage deep breathing; give bland food, carbonated beverages, or hot tea.	To relieve nausea.
	Observe for spider angioma, gynecomastia.	Indicates hormonal and circulatory changes caused by liver damage.

NURSING DIAGNOSIS	NURSING INTERVENTIONS	RATIONALE
Potential for injury related to central nervous system metastases	Raise and pad side rails; tape padded tongue blade or airway to head of bed.	To protect patient during convulsion.
	Maintain bed rest.	To avoid falls or other trauma.
	Provide quiet environment with subdued lighting.	To relax patient.
	Remove furniture, rugs, and other barriers.	To minimize environmental danger.
	Observe patient for abnormal body movements.	May indicate seizure activity.
	Observe for confusion, decreased pupillary response, and reduced level of consciousness.	Indicate increased intracranial pressure.
Pain related to bone and/or central nervous system metastases	Observe patient for grimacing, holding head, or guarding extremity or specific area of trunk.	To assess nonverbal signs of pain.
	Maintain body alignment.	To prevent muscular stretching.
	Position patient with support (e.g., pillows); change position slowly, and support joints.	To avoid fractures and decrease pressure.
	Apply heating pad; hot water bottle; warm, moist compress; whirlpool bath; or mentholated ointment.	To encourage relaxation and relieve pain.
	Exercise gently in range of motion.	To maintain muscle tone.
	Massage gently.	To relax muscles.
	Be alert for complaints of pain, and assess its duration and radiation.	To intervene early.
	Provide pain relief measure of patient's choice (e.g., relaxation therapy, diversion, or distraction).	To enhance effect of medication.
	Administer pain medications as ordered; evaluate pain for intensity and quality.	To control pain and determine need for further intervention.
Impaired physical mobility related to central nervous system metastases	Provide patient support when ambulating (e.g., walker, three-point cane).	To maintain mobility.
	Provide range-of-motion exercises (active and/or passive).	To avoid contractures.
	Assess patient for altered gait, position sense.	To determine need for further assistance.

NURSING DIAGNOSIS	NURSING INTERVENTIONS	RATIONALE
	Observe for signs of thrombophlebitis: calf pain, calf redness, Homans' sign, swelling, warmth; report to physician.	Indicate a common complication of immobility.
	Use antiembolic stockings.	To prevent venous stasis.
	Reposition patient q 2 h if on bed rest.	To prevent skin breakdown.
Altered patterns of urinary elimination related to central nervous system or peripheral nervous system metastases	Assess voiding pattern, palpate bladder, and monitor intake and output.	To determine need for intermittent catheterization.
	Devise schedule for intermittent catheterization.	To avoid incontinence.
	Encourage fluid intake, with even distribution during the day and decreased intake at night.	To maintain renal function while avoiding nighttime incontinence.
	Discourage use of caffeine beverages.	Caffeine has diuretic-like effect.
Impaired verbal communication related to central nervous system metastases	Listen carefully and speak clearly to patient.	To enhance ability to communicate.
	Provide paper and pencil, chalkboard, or erasable board.	To provide alternate methods of communication.
Fear related to evidence of metastases	Encourage patient to discuss fears related to disease.	To clarify specific fears and their basis in reality.
	Provide factual information as requested by patient.	To relieve anxiety.
	Encourage participation in support group or in one-to-one relationship.	To share experiences with others or with an experienced therapist.
Knowledge deficit	See Patient Teaching.	

5 EVALUATE

PATIENT OUTCOME	DATA INDICATED THAT OUTCOME IS REACHED
Patient maintains optimal cardiopulmonary and peripheral tissue perfusion.	Skin, nails, lips, and earlobes are warm, moist, and of natural color; respirations, pulse, blood pressure, and temperature are within normal limits.
Patient maintains optimal nutrition.	Diet is balanced and adequate, and fluid intake equals output; weight is maintained within normal limits.

PATIENT OUTCOME	DATA INDICATED THAT OUTCOME IS REACHED
Patient is free of injury.	Patient observes appropriate safety precautions.
Patient is comfortable.	Patient does not complain of pain, and facial expression and body are relaxed.
Patient ambulates frequently.	Patient uses assistive devices as needed.
Patient has normal urinary elimination.	Patient voids without difficulty, and intake equals output.
Patient can communicate.	Patient speaks without difficulty or uses assistive devices effectively; can hear those speaking.
Patient is able to deal with her fears.	Patient discusses fears openly and uses appropriate problem-solving techniques to deal with disease progression and prognosis.

PATIENT TEACHING

1. Teach the patient and family to avoid stress, exposure to environmental pollution, and others' infections.
2. Instruct the patient to plan for periods of activity balanced with rest.
3. Teach the patient and family to change the home (e.g., furniture) as necessary to enhance the patient's safety.
4. Teach the patient the importance of eating a varied and balanced diet.
5. Teach the patient how to manage pain without using drugs (e.g., through guided imagery, relaxation, and distraction).
6. Encourage the patient to walk, using assistive devices as needed.
7. Encourage the patient to communicate with others, using assistive devices as needed.
8. Teach the patient bladder training strategies as needed to avoid incontinence.
9. Encourage the patient to continue discussing fears and to use problem-solving techniques to deal with them in a realistic manner.

CHAPTER 13

Oncologic Emergencies

As many as 20% of persons with cancer develop at least one oncologic emergency in the course of the disease. As patients survive longer with cancer, the incidence of these emergencies increases. Among the oncologic emergencies are hypercalcemia, obstruction of the superior vena cava, cardiac tamponade, disseminated intravascular coagulation, carotid rupture, spinal cord compression, syndrome of inappropriate antidiuretic hormone, sepsis, and tumor lysis syndrome.

A number of factors must be considered before treatment of an oncologic emergency is begun; these include the current signs and symptoms, the natural history of the primary tumor, the efficacy of available treatment, and the treatment goals (see box). Aggressive treatment is indicated if a histologic diagnosis of cancer has not been established; if the patient has a good prognosis with therapy or a chance for cure or prolonged palliation; or if there is a likelihood of restoring functional status. The approach to oncologic emergencies is to treat the underlying malignancy and to start treatment promptly to prevent complications and permanent disability. For the terminally ill, withholding treatment and focusing on symptom management is believed to be more appropriate.

MANAGEMENT FACTORS IN THE EVALUATION AND TREATMENT OF AN ONCOLOGIC EMERGENCY

Symptoms and signs

1. Are the symptoms and signs caused by the tumor or by complications of treatment?
2. How quickly are the symptoms of the oncologic emergency progressing?

Natural history of the primary tumor

1. Is there a previous diagnosis of malignancy?
2. What is the disease-free interval between the diagnosis of the primary tumor and the onset of the emergency?
3. Has the emergency developed in the setting of terminal disease?

Efficacy of available treatment

1. Has there been extensive previous treatment, or any previous treatment?
2. Should treatment be directed at the underlying malignancy, the urgent complication, or both?
3. Will the patient's general medical condition influence the ability to administer effective treatment?

Treatment and goals

1. What is the potential for cure?
2. Is prompt palliation required to prevent further debilitation?
3. What is the risk-benefit ratio of treatment?
4. Should treatment be withheld if the patient is terminally ill with minimal chance of response to available antitumor therapies?

From Holleb et al.[33]

Hypercalcemia

Hypercalcemia is a condition that exists when the serum calcium is above 11 mg/dl (normal range, 8.5 to 10.5 mg/dl). It occurs when the bones release more calcium into the extracellular fluid than can be filtered by the kidneys and excreted in the urine.

EPIDEMIOLOGY

Hypercalcemia is observed most often in patients with multiple myeloma or cancers of the breast, lung, kidney, head and neck, esophagus, and thyroid. In addition, some tumors produce parathyroid hormone or a substance with the same physiologic effects, which causes increased resorption of calcium from the bone, increased intestinal absorption of calcium, and reduced renal excretion. The most common cause of hypercalcemia is thought to be destruction of bone by invasive metastases. Other causes are tumor production of vitamin D−like substances and osteoclast-activating factors, dehydration, and immobilization.

PATHOPHYSIOLOGY

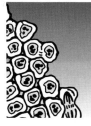 Approximately 40% to 50% of women with metastatic breast cancer develop hypercalcemia. This is caused not only by destruction of the bone by disease but also by hormonal therapy. Estrogen and anti-estrogens stimulate breast cancer cells to produce osteolytic prostaglandins and to increase bone resorption; the resultant hypercalcemia must be treated before the medication is reinstituted.

Twenty percent of the solid tumors associated with hypercalcemia show no evidence of bony involvement; it has been shown that humoral substances such as parathyroid hormone−like substances or osteolytic prostaglandins are secreted by tumor cells. Patients with multiple myeloma have osteoclast activating factor (OAF) produced by the abnormal plasma cells. However, patients with elevated OAF levels do not develop hypercalcemia unless renal function is inadequate. Patients with lymphoma caused by the human T-cell lymphotrophic virus (HTLV) have severe hypercalcemia related to ectopic production of OAF, colony-stimulating factor, interferon gamma, and an active vitamin D metabolite.

SIGNS AND SYMPTOMS

Hypercalcemia affects a variety of body systems, including the gastrointestinal tract, renal system, musculoskeletal system, central nervous system, and cardiopulmonary system. The presenting signs and symptoms vary with the serum calcium level and include the following:

Gastrointestinal symptoms: anorexia, nausea and vomiting, weight loss, constipation, vague abdominal pain
Fluid and electrolyte imbalance: polyuria (early sign), polydipsia, dehydration, renal calculi, pruritus
Altered musculoskeletal status: hypotonia, fatigue, muscle weakness, hyporeflexia of deep tendon reflexes, bone pain
Central nervous system excitability: confusion and disorientation, drowsiness and lethargy, reduced memory span, shortened attention span, inappropriate behavior, headache, and stupor and coma (late signs)
Altered cardiopulmonary function: chest pain, irregular pulse, bradycardia

DIAGNOSTIC STUDIES AND FINDINGS

Diagnostic test	Findings
Ionized serum calcium	Elevated
Alkaline phosphatase	Elevated
Serum phosphate	Decreased
Serum potassium	Decreased
Immunoreactive parathyroid hormone	Elevated with hypophosphatemia (suggests ectopic hormone production)
Electrocardiogram	Shortening of QT interval, widening of T wave, and PR prolongation

MEDICAL MANAGEMENT

Intravenous fluids
Drug therapy
  Furosemide (Lasix)
  Plicamycin (Mithracin)
  Corticosteroids (usually prednisone)
  Calcitonin
  Phosphates
  Gallium nitrate (Ganite)

INTRAVENOUS FLUIDS AND MEDICATIONS

Acute hypercalcemia is treated initially with intravenous normal saline, which increases urinary calcium excretion. Aggressive hydration (250 to 300 ml/h) and intravenous furosemide are used when hypercalcemia is life threatening.

Most patients are treated effectively with hydration, mobilization, effective antitumor therapy, and gradually tapering doses of plicamycin, calcitonin, or corticosteroids. If effective cancer chemotherapy is not available, the patient must be maintained on hypocalcemic therapy indefinitely, and the serum calcium level should be monitored at least twice a week.

Many patients are treated with plicamycin, a chemotherapeutic drug that decreases bone reabsorption by reducing the number and activity of osteoclasts. The drug is effective in patients with hypercalcemia caused either by bone metastasis or by bone reabsorption from ectopic humoral substances; it must be given as a bolus through a freshly started intravenous line. The dosage usually is one or two injections at 15 to 20 µg/kg/wk, with initial response expected within 6 to 48 hours. A second dose is given if there is no response within the first 2 days. Since only low doses of plicamycin are needed to control hypercalcemia, most patients do not develop side effects. When the drug is used chronically, the interval between injections generally can be lengthened.

Corticosteroids block bone reabsorption caused by osteoclast activating factor and may also have hypocalcemic effects by increasing urinary calcium excretion, inhibiting vitamin D metabolism, decreasing calcium absorption, and producing negative calcium balance in bone (after long-term use). High doses usually are required for several days; most patients require 40 to 100 mg of prednisone daily. This can be gradually tapered to the lowest effective therapeutic dosage.

Calcitonin inhibits bone reabsorption, causing the serum calcium level to fall within hours. However, tachyphylaxis develops unless a glucocorticoid is given with calcitonin. Calcitonin is given in daily doses intravenously or twice daily in intramuscular or subcutaneous injection (100 to 400 MRC units/kg). The injection interval can be gradually increased from 12 to 24 hours.

Intravenous phosphate may rapidly decrease serum calcium, but it is rarely used because of the high incidence of severe complications such as hypotension, hypocalcemia, and renal failure. A 50 mmol infusion of monobasic or dibasic anhydrous potassium phosphate may be administered over 6 to 8 hours to treat hypercalcemia associated with cardiac dysrhythmias and coma. Oral phosphates (1 to 3 g of sodium acid phosphate daily) are effective and relatively safe in controlling mild hypercalcemia.

Gallium nitrate (Ganite) exerts a hypocalcemic effect by inhibiting calcium resorption from bone, possibly by reducing increased bone turnover. It is essential to establish adequate hydration before initiating therapy. The usual recommended dosage is 200 mg/ml daily as a continuous 24-hour infusion for 5 consecutive days or until the calcium level returns to normal, whichever occurs first.

Patients should be mobilized to prevent osteolysis, and constipation should be corrected. Reducing the patient's oral calcium intake may be of some value. Medications such as thiazide diuretics and vitamins A and D (which elevate the calcium level) should not be used. The patient and family should be taught the signs and symptoms of hypercalcemia so that it can be detected early and treatment can be started before serious problems such as renal failure and coma develop.

Superior Vena Cava Syndrome

When the superior vena cava (SVC) is obstructed by an adjacent, expanding mass, venous blockage produces pleural effusion and facial, arm, and tracheal edema. Severe obstruction may result in brain edema and impaired cardiac filling.

EPIDEMIOLOGY

Most cases of superior vena cava syndrome are caused by mediastinal cancers. More than 75% of these obstructions are secondary to small cell or squamous cell lung cancers; 10% to 15% are secondary to mediastinal lymphomas, most often of the diffuse large cell subtypes. Other causes of this syndrome are breast cancer and gastrointestinal tract metastases. The most common nonmalignant cause of obstruction of the superior vena cava is thrombus in a central venous catheter. Most patients with superior vena cava syndrome do not present with a histologic diagnosis of cancer; thus the least invasive technique is used to establish the diagnosis (i.e., biopsy or cytologic tests).

SIGNS AND SYMPTOMS

Signs and symptoms depend on the extent and rapidity of compression of the superior vena cava. If the superior vena cava is compressed gradually and collateral circulation develops, signs and symptoms may be indolent and more subtle.

In order of frequency, the common signs and symptoms of superior vena cava syndrome are thoracic vein distention, neck vein distention, edema of the face, tachypnea, plethora of the face, cyanosis, edema of the upper extremities, paralyzed true vocal cord, and/or Horner's syndrome. The patient may also complain of headache and visual disturbances. Brain edema and impaired cardiac filling may cause altered consciousness and focal neurologic signs. Pedal edema may occur with inferior vena cava obstruction.

DIAGNOSTIC STUDIES AND FINDINGS

Diagnostic test	Findings
Venography	Compression of superior vena cava
Radionuclide scans	Compression of superior vena cava
Chest computed tomography (CT) with intravenous contrast or magnetic resonance imaging (MRI)	Anatomic detail and definition of radiation portals
Biopsy or cytologic tests	To establish diagnosis of cancer
Superior vena cavagram, radionuclide vena cavagrams, or angiography	Complete obstruction of superior or inferior vena cava

MEDICAL MANAGEMENT

Radiation therapy
  External beam radiation
Chemotherapy
  Cyclophosphamide (Cytoxan)

RADIATION THERAPY

Radiation therapy is quite effective for most cases of superior vena cava syndrome caused by cancer. Radiation therapy is initially given in high daily fractions; the dose depends on the tumor's size and radioresponsiveness and the probability of achieving a response with systemic therapy.

Patients with locally advanced non–small cell lung cancer without distant metastases should have irradiation of the mediastinal, hilar, and supraclavicular lymph nodes and any adjacent parenchymal lesions. Radiation therapy is palliative for superior vena cava syndrome in 70% of patients with lung cancer and in more than 95% with lymphoma. Corticosteroids decrease the edema associated with inflammatory reactions following radiation-induced tumor necrosis. Steroids are administered for 3 to 7 days.

If superior vena cava syndrome is caused by a thrombus around a central venous catheter, the patient may be treated with antifibrinolytics or anticoagulants. The catheter may require surgical removal.

If the signs and symptoms are not relieved by radiation therapy, persistence of the tumor outside the treatment portals must be suspected. If this occurs, invasive diagnostic procedures (e.g., contrast venography) should be used to determine the cause of treatment failure and to modify treatment to achieve a more extensive response.

CHEMOTHERAPY

Chemotherapy may be the treatment of choice in patients with disseminated disease if a prompt response is anticipated (e.g., with small cell anaplastic carcinoma or lymphoma).

■ ■ ■

During the acute episode, the patient should be kept in Fowler's position. Diuretics may be helpful; however, the obstruction must be relieved to prevent cerebral anoxia, hemorrhage, or strangulation.

Cardiac Tamponade

Cardiac tamponade is caused by the formation of pericardial fluid, which compresses the heart and causes life-threatening changes in cardiac function.

EPIDEMIOLOGY

At autopsy, as many as 20% of cancer patients are found to have cardiac or pericardial metastases. Cancers of the lung or esophagus grow by direct extension into the pericardium, whereas distant primary cancers metastasize to the pericardium via the bloodstream.

PATHOPHYSIOLOGY

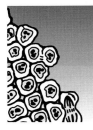

Cardiac tamponade occurs as the result of the formation and accumulation of excessive amounts of fluid in the pericardial sac, although encasement of the heart by tumor or post-irradiation pericarditis can mimic it. The severity of tamponade depends on the rate of fluid formation and the volume accumulated. Slow pericardial fluid accumulation may stretch the pericardium, so that cardiac contractility is not impaired. The normal diastolic filling is impaired by elevated pericardial pressures, and stroke volume is reduced. As stroke volume falls, hypotension, compensatory tachycardia, and equalization and elevation of the mean left atrial, pulmonary arterial and venous, right atrial, and vena caval pressures occur. Tachycardia and peripheral vasoconstriction develop in an attempt to maintain arterial pressure, increase blood volume, and improve venous return. If the tamponade goes untreated, circulatory collapse occurs.

SIGNS AND SYMPTOMS

Signs and symptoms depend on how quickly the fluid accumulates in the pericardial sac. Frequent signs of tamponade include rapid, weak pulse; distended neck veins during inspiration (Kussmaul's sign); pulsus paradoxus (inspiratory decrease in arterial blood pressure of more than 10 mm Hg from baseline); ankle or sacral edema; pleural effusion; ascites; hepatosplenomegaly; lethargy; and altered level of consciousness. The patient may complain of dyspnea, cough, and retrosternal pain that is relieved by leaning forward.

Occasionally a patient with a large effusion develops hoarseness, hiccups, nausea, vomiting, and epigastric pain.

DIAGNOSTIC STUDIES AND FINDINGS

Diagnostic test	Findings
Chest x-ray	Cardiac enlargement, mediastinal widening, or hilar adenopathy
Electrocardiogram	Nonspecific abnormalities; low QRS voltage in limb leads, sinus tachycardia, ST elevations, and T-wave changes in pericarditis
Echocardiogram	Two distinct echoes, one from effusion and the other from the posterior heart border; space between these echoes indicates the size of the effusion or thickness of the pericardium
Right heart catheterization	Pericardial tamponade or constriction
Pericardiocentesis	Positive cytologic test results in patient with metastatic cancer; inconclusive with lymphoma and mesothelioma
Pericardial biopsy	Malignant cells

MEDICAL MANAGEMENT

Pericardiocentesis
Sclerosis
Pleural-pericardial windows
Radiation therapy
Pericardiectomy
Chemotherapy

PERICARDIOCENTESIS

Emergency pericardiocentesis is performed when the patient develops one of the following: cyanosis, dyspnea, shock or impaired consciousness; a pulsus paradoxus greater than 50% of the pulse pressure; a decrease of more than 20 mm Hg in pulse pressure; or peripheral venous pressure above 13 mm Hg. Oxygen should be administered. Before pericardiocentesis, isoproterenol and volume expansion can be used to improve cardiac contractility and filling.

Tamponade will recur in 24 to 48 hours unless treatment is started promptly to prevent pericardial fluid reaccumulation. The therapeutic options depend on the sensitivity of the primary tumor to systemic chemotherapy, hormonal therapy, or local radiation therapy; previous treatment; and the patient's life expectancy. The duration of response to various treatments and of survival are influenced by the extent of metastatic disease and the chance of response to concurrent systemic hormonal therapy or chemotherapy.

SCLEROSIS

Tamponade can be controlled by inserting an indwelling pericardial catheter until pericardial drainage stops; then tetracycline (500 to 1000 mg) is instilled through the cannula and flushed with normal saline. The procedure is repeated every 2 to 3 days until there has been no fluid drainage in the preceding 24 hours. The inflammatory response and fibrosis caused by the intrapericardial tetracycline obliterates the space between the parietal and visceral pericardium, thus preventing fluid formation.

A single instillation of bleomycin (30 mg or 60 mg) has also been shown to be an effective sclerosing agent. Bleomycin is instilled after all pericardial fluid has been evacuated for 24 hours; the catheter is then clamped for 10 minutes, after which the drug is withdrawn. Bleomycin may have fewer side effects than tetracycline (especially less pain for the patient).

PLEURAL-PERICARDIAL WINDOWS

Performed under local anesthesia, inferior pericardiotomy provides immediate relief of cardiac compression, as well as tissue for histologic diagnosis. Symptoms recur in fewer than 5% of patients.

RADIATION THERAPY

The sensitivity of the tumor determines the response to radiation therapy and the duration of palliation. Radiation therapy has been reported to control more than 50% of malignant pericardial effusions.

PERICARDIECTOMY

Pericardiectomy is needed if radiation-induced pericardial disease cannot be controlled with conservative medical management. Because surgical morbidity and mortality rates are high, this procedure should not be performed if an extensive pericardial tumor is present.

CHEMOTHERAPY

After the patient is clinically stable, systemic chemotherapy should be administered, if effective treatment is available (e.g., as in lymphoma and small cell lung cancer). Chemotherapy may also be effective in leukemia and breast cancer patients with pericardial effusion.

Disseminated Intravascular Coagulation

Disseminated intravascular coagulation (DIC) is a syndrome characterized by indiscriminate formation of fibrin in small blood vessels throughout the circulation, with a consumption of fibrinogen and other procoagulant factors that results in paradoxic bleeding.

EPIDEMIOLOGY

Sepsis, malignancy, and shock syndromes are the most common disorders predisposing to the development of disseminated intravascular coagulation. Malignant tumors arising from the pancreas, stomach, or colon may produce mucin; the sialic acid component of this mucin may directly activate clotting factor X, triggering systemic thrombin generation and acute disseminated intravascular coagulation. Adenocarcinomas of the prostate are rich in procoagulant factors; prostatic tissue is also rich in plasminogen activator, which can independently lead to the formation of potent enzymes that fragment both fibrinogen and fibrin, as well as other proteins. Acute promyelocytic leukemia cells contain granules replete with both procoagulant and fibrinolytic activators, inducing disseminated intravascular coagulation and a fibrinolytic state.

PATHOPHYSIOLOGY

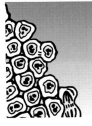 Disseminated intravascular coagulation is initiated by the introduction or release of procoagulant substances into the circulation, triggering intravascular clotting and followed by secondary fibrin dissolution. An uncontrollable triggering of the internal or external pathway of the clotting cascade occurs, resulting in accelerated coagulation and the formation of excessive thrombin. As long as coagulation occurs, the fibrinolytic system is activated, so that clotting and bleeding continue at a life-threatening pace.

SIGNS AND SYMPTOMS

Signs and symptoms of disseminated intravascular coagulation include systemic bleeding, ranging from petechiae to hematuria to acute gastrointestinal hemorrhage; organ dysfunction (e.g., pulmonary emboli, thromboemboli in the extremities, and renal failure); decreased blood pressure and pulse; cool, clammy skin; anemia; pallor; and shortness of breath. Hemorrhagic signs of disseminated intravascular coagulation include persistent oozing from venipuncture sites; bleeding around intranasal, endotracheal, and urethral catheters; hemoptysis; hematemesis; hematuria; and melena.

DIAGNOSTIC STUDIES AND FINDINGS

Diagnostic test	Findings
Thrombin time, prothrombin time, partial thromboplastin time	Prolonged
Platelets	Decreased
Fibrinogen	Decreased
Fibrin-split products	Elevated
Erythrocytes	Fragmented (indicating partial occlusion of small vessels by fibrin thrombi)

MEDICAL MANAGEMENT

Medications
  Antibiotics, chemotherapy, heparin
Blood component therapy

MEDICATIONS

Disseminated intravascular coagulation rapidly resolves when infections are controlled by appropriate antibiotic therapy, when tumors can be eradicated or brought into remission, or when thrombosis is controlled with small amounts of an anticoagulant such as heparin (e.g., as with migratory thrombophlebitis in a patient with prostatic malignancy).

BLOOD COMPONENT THERAPY

Administration of platelets may prevent intracranial bleeding in patients with acute promyelocytic leukemia; a continuous infusion of fresh-frozen plasma may control bleeding in patients with gastrointestinal bleeding secondary to tumor-induced disseminated intravascular coagulation.

The nurse should continuously monitor sites and amount of bleeding, as well as laboratory values; assess the adequacy of tissue perfusion; and prevent or minimize further bleeding.

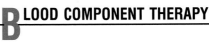

Carotid Rupture

Carotid rupture or blowout is the loss of large amounts of blood via a damaged artery, with resultant life-threatening bleeding.

EPIDEMIOLOGY

Patients with an invasive tumor in the head and neck area, as well as those who have undergone head and neck surgery for the removal of cancer, are at risk for carotid rupture.

PATHOPHYSIOLOGY

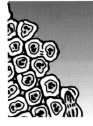 A carotid artery weakened by tumor invasion or surgical manipulation is likely to rupture. Related causes of vessel weakness include simultaneous infection or skin flap necrosis.

SIGNS AND SYMPTOMS

The first sign of carotid blowout usually is a small trickle of blood from the neck area. The rupture may be sudden, with forceful expulsion of large volumes of blood from the artery.

MEDICAL MANAGEMENT

Digital pressure
Surgery

DIGITAL PRESSURE

If carotid blowout occurs, a saline-soaked cotton dressing is wrapped around the two middle fingers and constant digital pressure is applied directly to the area over the artery. The nurse must not check to see whether the bleeding has stopped nor attempt to apply a hemostat because of the likelihood of further blood loss. A clot of blood is drawn and sent to the blood bank for typing and cross-matching, and an intravenous line is started. Only after the patient is in the operating room and the operative area has been prepared can the pressure be released.

SURGERY

The treatment of choice is ligation of the damaged vessel. Hemiparesis remains a strong possibility as a post-operative complication, but preventing shock and replacing fluid for adequate perfusion of the brain via the opposite internal carotid artery help decrease this risk.

Spinal Cord Compression

Spinal cord compression, which is always an emergency, may result in permanent neurologic dysfunction if not diagnosed and treated promptly.

EPIDEMIOLOGY

The tumors most commonly associated with spinal cord compression are carcinomas of the breast, lung, and prostate; multiple myeloma; and lymphoma. At autopsy, more than 5% of patients with metastatic disease have been found to have epidural tumors, which usually arise within the vertebral body and grow along the epidural space anterior to the spinal cord. Patients with paraspinal tumors may develop epidural metastases when the tumor grows through the intervertebral foramina from adjacent lymph nodes.

PATHOPHYSIOLOGY

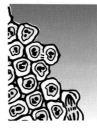 In addition to compression caused by metastatic disease, both spinal cord and nerve root compression can occur secondary to an epidural tumor or to vertebral collapse from destructive bony metastases. Permanent neurologic damage may also occur if vascular compromise produces prolonged ischemia or hemorrhage.

SIGNS AND SYMPTOMS

More than 95% of patients with spinal cord compression complain of progressive central or radicular back pain, which often is aggravated by lying down, weight bearing, coughing, sneezing, or the Valsalva maneuver and is relieved by sitting. The earliest neurologic symptoms are sensory changes such as numbness, paresthesia, and coldness. Although bladder and bowel dysfunction are rarely the first signs of cord compression, metastases to the cauda equina often produce impaired urethral, vaginal, and rectal sensations; bladder dysfunction; saddle anesthesia; and decreased sensation in the lumbosacral dermatomes.

The level of cord compression can be identified by pain elicited by straight leg raising, neck flexion, or vertebral percussion. The upper limit of the sensory level often is one or two vertebral bodies below the site of compression. Decreased rectal tone and perineal sensation often are noted with autonomic dysfunction. Deep tendon reflexes may be brisk with cord compression and diminished with nerve root compression.

DIAGNOSTIC STUDIES AND FINDINGS

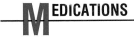

Diagnostic test	Findings
Myelogram or computed tomography (CT) scan	Spinal tumor
Magnetic resonance imaging (procedure of choice)	Complete or partial block of spinal cord with epidural deposits at other level
Cerebrospinal fluid	Malignant cells

MEDICAL MANAGEMENT

Radiation therapy
Surgery
    Laminectomy
Medications
    Corticosteroids, chemotherapy, hormonal therapy

RADIATION THERAPY

The decision to use radiation therapy is based on the tumor's radiosensitivity, the surgeon's clinical expertise with surgical decompression, the level of cord compression, the rate of neurologic deterioration, and previous radiotherapy. Radiation therapy is the primary therapy for most patients with epidural metastases and should be initiated as soon as the diagnosis of cord compression has been confirmed. Radiation portals include the entire area of blockage and two vertebral bodies above and below it. More than half of patients with rapid neu-

rologic deterioration improve with radiation therapy; however, the prognosis for patients with autonomic dysfunction or paraplegia is poor despite surgery or radiation therapy.

SURGERY

Posterior laminectomy achieves immediate decompression of the spinal cord and nerve roots; however, it is difficult to remove the tumor, since most metastases arise in the vertebral bodies anterior to the spinal cord. Because of this, postoperative radiation therapy is given to decrease residual tumor, relieve pain, and improve functional status. Surgery usually is contraindicated if there are several areas of cord compression or a collapsed vertebral body. Laminectomy may be used for both diagnosis and treatment if there is no previous histologic diagnosis of cancer or if infection or epidural hematoma must be ruled out.

If surgery is not possible for high cervical cord compression, the patient's neck should be stabilized in halo traction to prevent death from respiratory paralysis. If neurologic signs progress for 48 to 72 hours despite high doses of steroids and radiation therapy, emergency decompression should be attempted.

MEDICATIONS

Corticosteroids may quickly reduce peritumoral edema and improve neurologic function. Dexamethasone is administered before emergency diagnostic procedures to patients with neurologic symptoms. Dexamethasone (4 to 10 mg q 6 h) usually is continued during radiation therapy and then tapered. Although steroids initially improve neurologic function, it is not clear whether they affect the final outcome.

Chemotherapy rarely has a major role, but if the tumor is sensitive, the drug regimen can be administered concurrently with or soon after completion of radiation therapy or surgery. Chemotherapy may play a role in patients with multiple myeloma who have had previous radiation therapy. Systemic hormonal therapy or chemotherapy may be useful with certain types of tumors; for example, patients with lymphoma have been observed to experience neurologic recovery with single-agent chemotherapy; paraplegia caused by prostate cancer has been found to respond to hormonal therapy without radiation therapy.

Pain management should include administering appropriate analgesics, bed rest, and supporting the patient for transfer and position changes.

Syndrome of Inappropriate Antidiuretic Hormone

The abnormal production or stimulation of antidiuretic hormone results in excessive water retention and hyponatremia.

EPIDEMIOLOGY

The causes of the syndrome of inappropriate antidiuretic hormone (SIADH) include tumor secretion (e.g., as is seen in patients with small cell lung cancer, lymphoma, and pancreatic and prostate cancers); stimulation by drugs such as vincristine and cyclophosphamide; viral or bacterial pneumonia; or neurologic trauma.

PATHOPHYSIOLOGY

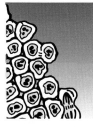 Antidiuretic hormone, which normally is released from the posterior pituitary in response to increased plasma osmolarity or decreased plasma volume, may be abnormally produced or stimulated. The results of this alteration are excessive water retention and hyponatremia.

SIGNS AND SYMPTOMS

Signs and symptoms of the syndrome of inappropriate antidiuretic hormone include confusion, irritability, weakness, lethargy, headache, hyporeflexia, nausea, vomiting, anorexia, diarrhea, and weight gain without edema.

DIAGNOSTIC STUDIES AND FINDINGS

Diagnostic test	Findings
Serum sodium level	<130 mEq/L
Serum osmolarity	<280 mOsm/kg H_2O
Urine sodium level	>20 mEq/L

MEDICAL MANAGEMENT

Medications
  Antineoplastic agents, antibiotics, diuretics, demeclocycline
Intravenous fluids
  Hypertonic saline

MEDICATIONS

Chemotherapy, antibiotics, diuretics, and demeclocycline may be used to eradicate the cause of the syndrome or to control symptoms. If a chemotherapeutic agent is identified as causing the disorder, it should be discontinued.

INTRAVENOUS FLUIDS

Hypertonic saline (3% to 5% sodium chloride) is the fluid of choice.

The nurse should maintain an accurate record of intake and output, restrict fluids as necessary, monitor laboratory reports of fluid and electrolyte balance, and provide safety measures for weak and confused patients.

Sepsis

Bacterial invasion of the circulatory system results in inadequate tissue perfusion.

EPIDEMIOLOGY

This oncologic emergency is most often seen in neutropenic patients whose immunologic response is weakened by the decreased number of functional neutrophils. The most common causative agents are gram-negative bacteria.

PATHOPHYSIOLOGY

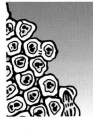

Sepsis results from the release of an endotoxin from the cell walls of gram-negative bacteria, which causes increased capillary permeability and leakage. This in turn causes stagnation of the blood, lactic acidosis, a decrease in the circulating blood volume, and decreased cardiac output.

Sepsis is the most common cause of death in immunocompromised patients.

SIGNS AND SYMPTOMS

Signs and symptoms of sepsis include fever; chills; restlessness; confusion; tachycardia; hypotension; decreased pulses; cool, clammy skin; decreased urinary output; and bleeding from one or more sites (which may be caused by disseminated intravascular coagulation).

DIAGNOSTIC STUDIES AND FINDINGS

Diagnostic test	Findings
Blood cultures	Positive for gram-negative bacteria
Chest x-ray	Infiltrates
White blood cell count	Decreased or elevated
Arterial blood gas analysis	Metabolic acidosis
Prothrombin time and partial thromboplastin time	Prolonged

MEDICAL MANAGEMENT

Medications
  Antibiotics
Supportive care
  Interventions include administering antibiotics as prescribed; reducing the temperature with antipyretics, ice packs, a hypothermia blanket, and other techniques; fluid volume replacement; monitoring of vital signs, arterial blood gas values, and hemodynamic stability; and performing blood cultures as needed.

Tumor Lysis Syndrome

Tumor lysis syndrome is a metabolic imbalance caused by rapid cancer cell death; it results in uric acid nephropathy.

EPIDEMIOLOGY

A patient's risk of developing tumor lysis syndrome increases with the presence of bulky tumors that have a high growth fraction. The syndrome usually begins 1 to 5 days after initiation of chemotherapy for non-Hodgkin's lymphoma or leukemia. There have also been reports of tumor lysis syndrome in patients with chronic myeloproliferative syndromes, multiple myeloma, and squamous cell carcinoma of the head and neck.

PATHOPHYSIOLOGY

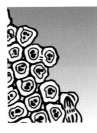

Rapid cell death increases the production of uric acid and results in hyperuricemia and deposition of uric acid crystals throughout the urinary tract. Most episodes are associated with effective cytotoxic chemotherapy or radiation therapy, but spontaneous nephropathy has occasionally been reported.

The incidence and severity of tumor lysis syndrome have decreased with the use of allopurinol, aggressive hydration, and urine alkalinization. With current therapy most patients regain normal renal function in a few days.

SIGNS AND SYMPTOMS

Signs and symptoms of tumor lysis syndrome include oliguria, anuria, urine crystals, flank pain, hematuria, nausea, vomiting, cardiac dysrhythmia, muscular cramps, tetany, lethargy, and confusion.

DIAGNOSTIC STUDIES AND FINDINGS

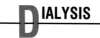

Diagnostic test	Findings
Serum uric acid	Elevated
Blood urea nitrogen, creatinine	Elevated
Serum phosphate	Elevated
Serum calcium	Decreased
Urinary uric acid-to-creatinine ratio	>1
Renal ultrasound	To exclude ureteral obstruction

MEDICAL MANAGEMENT

Medications
  Allopurinol, calcium supplements
Intravenous fluids
Dialysis

MEDICATIONS

The goal of treatment should be to prevent tumor lysis syndrome. Patients at risk should receive allopurinol, aggressive hydration, and urinary alkalinization for at least 48 hours before chemotherapy. Drugs that block tubular reabsorption of uric acid should be avoided (e.g., aspirin, radiographic contrast, probenecid, and thiazide diuretics). Before chemotherapy, the serum uric acid level should be within normal limits and the urine pH above 7.

Serum potassium and magnesium levels should be monitored closely and allopurinol administered in dosages ranging from 300 to 800 mg/day. Allopurinol decreases uric acid production by inhibiting xanthine oxidase.

INTRAVENOUS FLUIDS

Intravenous hydration should be given to ensure a urine volume of more than 3 L per day. To alkalinize the urine, intravenous sodium bicarbonate (100 mEq/m^2) should be given daily.

If oliguria or anuria develops, ureteral obstruction must be excluded. Once this is ascertained, mannitol or high-dose furosemide should be given in an attempt to restore urine flow.

A Foley catheter should be inserted so that the nurse can measure urine output accurately.

DIALYSIS

If diuresis does not occur within a few hours, hemodialysis is necessary. Within 6 hours of initiating treatment, uric acid levels usually fall by 50%. Most patients require 6 days of dialysis before the hyperuricemia resolves and renal function returns to normal. A low-calcium dialysate is used to prevent calcium phosphate precipitation. Aluminum hydroxide antacids may help decrease gastrointestinal phosphate absorption.

If peritoneal dialysis is used, albumin added to the dialysate increases uric acid protein binding and removal.

Cancer Therapies

Surgery

Surgery historically has been the treatment of choice for most cancers. A decision to use surgery as primary therapy is based on analysis of a variety of data, including a thorough history and physical examination; laboratory, radiologic, and other specialized diagnostic procedures; and histologic evidence of malignancy.

A radical surgical approach to operable tumors is no longer routinely used, because a greater variety of surgical procedures, more sophisticated staging techniques, and multimodality options (e.g., preoperative, intraoperative, or postoperative radiation therapy) are available. The more conservative surgical management of breast cancer is an excellent example of this trend.

The preferred surgical approach is excision of the primary tumor and enough surrounding tissue and lymph nodes to offer maximum protection against local recurrence; these are called curative resections. Palliative resections may be done when the cancer has spread to distant, previously undetected sites, with the goal of relieving symptoms of obstruction, pressure, and infection. A primary tumor is considered inoperable if it is large or in a difficult-to-reach location or if there is evidence of extensive local invasion or metastasis.

Staging operations, such as a laparotomy, may be performed to determine the appropriate therapy. Secondary operations may be done for local recurrence. "Second look" operations may be performed without clinical evidence of recurrent disease, but the overall effectiveness of this procedure for finding recurrent disease is questionable.

Distant metastases, such as pulmonary or hepatic cancers, may respond to direct surgical resection. In the past, indirect ablative procedures such as adrenalectomy and hypophysectomy were believed to be useful in the palliation of hormonally sensitive cancers of the breast or prostate; however, advances in hormonal therapy have resulted in less frequent use of these procedures. Other indirect palliative procedures include cordotomy for relief of intractable pain and ostomy to relieve gastrointestinal obstruction.

Reconstructive surgery of the head and neck, breast, and extremities has become an important aspect of cancer rehabilitation in recent years. For example, the development of maxillofacial prosthodontics has enabled individuals treated with radical neck dissection to regain an acceptable cosmetic appearance and to eat and drink in a more natural manner. Breast reconstruction is an option for women whose disease and treatment enable the surgeon to implant a prosthesis or to transplant tissue from other areas of the body to create a more natural breast.

Whatever the surgical procedure, the patient's nutritional status, both before and after surgery, has been found to be a significant factor in the amount of surgery that can be tolerated, the rate of recovery from the surgery, and the adequacy of wound healing.

Photodynamic Therapy

Photodynamic therapy (PDT) involves injecting the patient with intravenous dihematoporphyrin ether (DHE) or some other photosensitizing agent, waiting 48 to 72 hours for the drug to clear healthy tissues and concentrate in malignant cells, and then exposing the cancerous area to laser light delivered through a scope (e.g., cystoscope or bronchoscope).

Photodynamic therapy is used as a possible cure for early stages of skin and bladder cancers and for palliation of advanced lung, esophageal, and pelvic cancers. Patients selected for this therapy may have had previous treatment, may be undergoing conventional therapy, or may be newly diagnosed.

Although all cells absorb the photosensitizing agent, retention is higher in malignant tissue, the liver, spleen, kidneys, and skin. The laser emits powerful red light that penetrates tissue and activates the photosensitizer in the malignant cells. A superoxide, which is produced by the chemical reaction between the laser beam and the photosensitizer, changes the cell membrane, destroying the malignant cells.

The procedure is painless, since no tissue is burned or cut. However, because the photosensitizer causes profound photosensitivity, patients must stay out of sunlight for up to 6 weeks after the treatment. Like the laser, sunlight contains red light that easily penetrates the skin; thus exposure to sunlight could cause severe swelling and redness.

If photodynamic therapy is used to treat bladder cancer, the patient may complain after the procedure of severe urinary frequency and urgency caused by edema and hemorrhage. Bladder capacity may be decreased as a result of edema, the high-energy source, or overdistention of the bladder during the procedure. Bladder capacity usually returns to normal within 3 months after treatment. Oral analgesics, antispasmodics, and prophylactic antibiotics may be prescribed.

Photodynamic therapy can also alleviate symptoms caused by obstructive primary or secondary cancer. Debulking of the tumor can relieve bleeding, infection, pain, and symptoms of obstruction.

Bone Marrow Transplantation

Bone marrow transplantation (BMT) is a treatment for certain cancers that involves intravenous infusion of bone marrow into the patient to replace the defective host hematopoietic system with healthy stem cells. As these undifferentiated cells (from which all other cell lines arise) engraft, both the cellular and humoral elements of immunity are replaced. Most bone marrow transplantations are performed to treat cancer, including a variety of leukemias, non-Hodgkin's lymphoma, Burkitt's lymphoma, multiple myeloma, osteosarcoma, and breast cancer.

There are three types of transplantations: autologous, syngeneic, and allogeneic. An autologous transplantation involves harvesting the patient's marrow after treatment with cytoreductive therapy. The marrow may be further treated with chemotherapy to remove any remaining tumor cells and is then frozen until the patient needs it.

Syngeneic transplant involves using an identical twin as donor, which ensures that donor cells are matched with those of the recipient at all genetic loci. Allogeneic transplant usually involves a sibling as donor, but the donor may be any relative or an unrelated donor with compatible human leukocyte antigens (HLA) and mixed lymphocyte culture (MLC). The advantages and disadvantages of each type are given in Table 14-1.

The steps involved in bone marrow transplantation are donor selection, bone marrow harvest, preparative regimen, infusion of bone marrow, aplasia, engraftment, and discharge from inpatient to outpatient setting. The type of transplantation to be performed is based on the disease or disorder, the availability of histocompatible donors, and the health status of potential donors. The allogeneic transplant is used most frequently and is preferred in the treatment of hematologic malignancies.

Once a compatible donor has been selected, the marrow usually is harvested from the posterior iliac crest of the donor, but it may be taken from the ante-

Table 14-1

TYPES OF BONE MARROW TRANSPLANTS

Type	Advantages	Disadvantages
Autologous	Low risk of graft versus host disease Availability of donor Fewer treatment-related side effects and complications	Greater risk of relapse
Syngeneic	Low risk of graft versus host disease Fewer treatment-related side effects and complications	Greater risk of relapse Few donors available
Allogeneic	Less risk of relapse Greater availability of donors (compared with syngeneic type)	Greater risk of graft versus host disease Increased number and severity of treatments, related side effects, and complications

From Freedman et al.[22]

rior iliac crest or the sternum (see Patient Teaching Guide). This is a relatively safe procedure that rarely causes problems for the donor. The marrow is filtered through a screen to remove fat particles and bone chips and then is placed in a heparinized saline solution. T cells or red blood cells may be removed before the marrow is infused into the recipient.

Preparation of the recipient involves either high-dose chemotherapeutic agents or high-dose chemotherapy and total body irradiation (TBI). It may take as long as 10 days to prepare the patient for the transplant. The purposes of the preparative phase are to eliminate residual tumor, create space for donor marrow, and provide immunosuppression to decrease the risk of rejection.

Side effects of the high-dose chemotherapy and/or total body irradiation include common side effects (e.g., nausea, vomiting, anorexia, mucositis, parotitis, xerostomia or excessive salivation, diarrhea, low-grade fever, alopecia, electrolyte imbalances, and aplasia) and life-threatening side effects (e.g., severe thrombocytopenia, syndrome of inappropriate antidiuretic hormone, renal failure, sepsis, venous occlusive disease, and capillary leak syndrome).

Before the marrow infusion, the recipient is hydrated with a bicarbonate solution to force a brisk alkaline urine flow, which prevents the renal complication of red blood cell hemolysis. Emergency drugs for treating an anaphylactic reaction are kept at the bedside. (The patient who is to receive an allogeneic transplant is premedicated with diphenhydramine hydrochloride, hydrocortisone sodium succinate, and mannitol to lessen the chance of adverse reactions and to ensure a brisk urine flow.) Bone marrow then is infused via a central line without a filter over a period of 1 to 4 hours.

After the bone marrow transplant, the recipient progresses through stages of severe, prolonged aplasia; lingering side effects of the preparatory therapy; and then engraftment of the donor marrow. If there are no complications, the patient remains in the hospital for 1½ to 2 months and is closely followed as an outpatient for at least 1 year.

Acute complications may occur simultaneously and may cause or exacerbate other complications. Acute complications include mucositis, viral infection, bacterial and fungal sepsis, renal failure, interstitial pneumonias, veno-occlusive disease, and graft versus host disease.

For at least 2 to 4 weeks after the transplant, the patient is at high risk for fungal and bacterial sepsis; the most common causative organisms are gram-negative pathogens (*Pseudomonas* sp., *Klebsiella* sp., and *Escherichia coli*), gram-positive pathogens (*Staphylococcus* and *Streptococcus* organisms), and fungal pathogens (*Aspergillus* and *Candida* spp.). Both primary viral infections and reactivation of latent viruses are a perplexing problem during the first months after the transplant. Viral pathogens include varicella zoster, herpes simplex virus, and cytomegalovirus. As many as 60% of patients' interstitial pneumonias, a major cause of mortality, are associated with cytomegalovirus infection.

Efforts to prevent infections in these patients include protective isolation or laminar air flow rooms; prophylactic systemic antibiotics and antiviral agents (primarily acyclovir); and routine cultures of the blood, urine, throat, and stool. Despite these and other interventions, the patient can become septic in a matter of hours, with multisystem failure.

Another serious complication is veno-occlusive disease, which has a mortality rate of about 50%. It is caused by the accumulation of fibrous material in the small venules of the liver after high-dose chemotherapy and total body irradiation. The fibrous material eventually creates a plug and occludes hepatic and renal blood flow.

A unique complication of bone marrow transplantation is graft versus host disease (GVHD), which occurs in as many as 60% of allogeneic recipients and up to 10% of autologous and syngeneic recipients. The new bone marrow produces immunocompetent cells, which recognize their environment as foreign and try to destroy their new host body. In acute graft versus host disease, which usually appears within 2 weeks to 3 months after transplantation, these donor-derived T cells mount a cytotoxic response that may cause erythema, a maculopapular rash, blistering and desquamation, liver failure, diarrhea, abdominal pain, and denuding of the gastrointestinal tract. Mild cases usually are self-limiting. Severe cases require such agents as high-dose steroids, antithymocyte globulin (ATG), and the monoclonal antibody OKT-3.

Chronic graft versus host disease occurs 3 months to 1 year after transplantation. It is caused by autoreactive T cells and autoantigens and is manifested as scleroderma-like changes in the skin, gastrointestinal tract, and liver; immune deficiency; marrow suppression; and changes in respiratory and musculoskeletal function. It

is treated with prednisone and azathioprine. Agents such as cyclosporin A, methotrexate, and steroids may be used alone or in combination for prophylaxis of graft versus host disease.

Survival after bone marrow transplantation depends on the patient's age, remission status, and clinical status at the time of transplantation. Long-term problems are related to the preparatory regimen before transplantation, the sequelae of the transplant, relapse, and secondary malignancies. Potential long-term problems include neurologic damage, cataract formation, endocrine problems, and changes in the skin, eyes, mouth, and gastrointestinal tract.

The psychosocial impact of bone marrow transplantation on patients and their families requires further study, in light of the increasing disease-free survival. The "cured" patient may be chronically ill and experiencing an altered quality of life. Fear of death and dying may yield to feelings of guilt, depression, and anxiety among survivors. Changes in life priorities and perspective may not be shared by the patient's loved ones, leaving the patient feeling isolated. The nurse, whose care during each stage of the transplantation is vital to the patient's survival, must also help the patient deal with the challenges of survival.

Radiation Therapy

Radiation therapy is a major modality in the treatment of cancer. It involves using high-energy ionizing radiation to treat malignancies. It is estimated that 60% of individuals with cancer receive radiation at some point during the course of their disease. Radiation is used at all phases of the cancer trajectory. As a primary therapy, radiation is used with curative intent in early-stage Hodgkin's disease, skin cancers, and head and neck and gynecologic malignancies. Radiation is used as an adjuvant treatment in small cell lung cancer and head and neck cancer; after definitive chemotherapy in small cell cancer; and after surgery with head and neck malignancies. In the palliative phase of treatment, radiation alleviates pain from bony metastases, controls bleeding from extensive gynecologic malignancies, and relieves obstruction and compression from advanced lung cancer and brain and spinal cord lesions.

Radiation is one of the oldest treatments for cancer.

From the discovery of x-rays by Roentgen in 1895, radioactivity by Becquerel in 1896, and radium by the Curies in 1898, attempts have been made to use radiation to treat cancer. Early efforts were hampered by lack of equipment and an inadequate understanding of radiobiology. Treatment units could deliver significant radiation doses to the skin but lacked the energy to treat tumors below the skin's surface without causing unacceptable side effects. Skin cancers and other superficial lesions could be treated, but it was not until high-energy cobalt and linear accelerators (Figure 14-1) were developed in the 1950s that tumors well below the skin's surface could be treated. Linear accelerators deliver the maximum radiation below the skin's surface and are known as skin sparing.

Along with the development of sophisticated equipment, the sciences of radiation biology and physics emerged. Understanding the effect of radiation on nor-

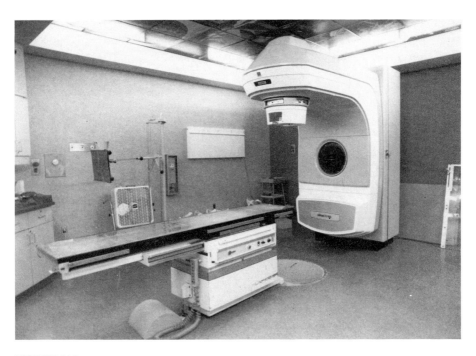

FIGURE 14-1
Linear accelerator. Used for the treatment of patients with a
wide variety of cancers.

mal and tumor cells and the properties of ionizing radiation was essential to the safe, effective use of radiation in individuals with cancer.

The types of radiation commonly used in treatment include electromagnetic radiation with x-rays and gamma rays. X-rays are photons generated within a machine; gamma rays are photons emitted from a radioactive source. Particulate radiation uses electrons, protons, and, less commonly, neutrons and pi mesons produced within a machine. Radiation is measured in units known as the rad (radiation absorbed dose) or the Gray, which is equal to 100 rad.

The target organ in the cell for radiation damage is the DNA. Cellular death from radiation is mitotically linked in that the cell can function but cannot survive division. The rate at which normal and cancer cells react to radiation is determined by their mitotic rate. Normal cells with high mitotic rates (e.g., hair follicles, gastrointestinal mucosa, and bone marrow cells) and cancers such as lymphomas, leukemias, and seminomas respond quickly to treatment. These are radiosensitive tumors. Cells with slower rates (e.g., muscles, nerves, and vessels) and tumors such as rhabdomyosarcomas are radioresistant, requiring a higher radiation dose and a longer response time.

The cellular response to radiation occurs in several phases (see box).

**CELLULAR RESPONSE
TO RADIATION**

Physical: Phase of excitation and ionization; the energy imparted by the radiation disrupts molecules by ejecting electrons from orbit

Physicochemical: Powerful oxidizing and reducing agents are formed within the cells

Chemical: Chemical reactions occur within the cell, producing changes in DNA

Biologic: Cellular death occurs as cells divide; single- and double-stranded breaks in chromosomes occur, rendering cells incapable of proliferation

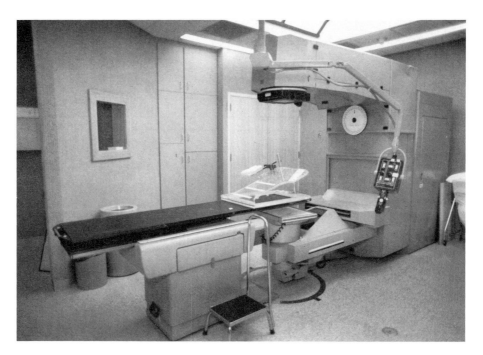

FIGURE 14-2
Simulator. Used to take treatment planning films and to set up treatment fields.

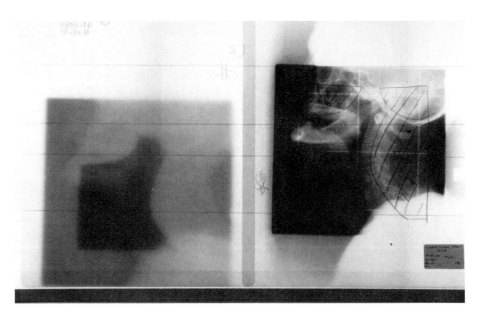

FIGURE 14-3
Treatment planning for radiation therapy. The film on the left is a port film of a patient with head and neck cancer. The film on the right is a simulation film showing the treatment field with blocks.

Normal cells are better able to recover from the damage caused by radiation than are cancer cells. Because malignant cells lack the capacity for repair, more cancer cells than normal cells are damaged by radiation. However, normal cells do have a maximum dose of radiation that they can tolerate before irreversible damage occurs. Simulation and treatment planning are designed to minimize the radiation dose to normal structures (Figures 14-2 and 14-3). Radiation tolerance varies widely, from sensitive organs (e.g., the gonads and small intestine) to tolerant tissue (e.g., the uterus and bladder). Spinal cord tolerance, at 4,500 rad, is a dose-limiting factor, since overdose to the spinal cord causes cord necrosis and results in functional loss. Meticulous planning and recording of spinal cord dose are essential.

RADIATION DELIVERY SYSTEMS

Radiation may be delivered in several ways. Most commonly individuals are treated with external beam radiation or teletherapy (treatment at a distance). The individual lies on a table at a distance from the source and is exposed to a prescribed dose of radiation on a daily basis (Monday through Friday). The area encompassed in the radiation field generally includes the tumor and draining lymphatics.

Implant therapy, or brachytherapy (close therapy), is a method of implanting sealed sources directly into the tumor or a cavity surrounding the tumor. The sources used for brachytherapy (cesium, iridium) are nonpenetrating and deposit most of the dose in a small area, with rapid fall-off in normal tissue. The goal of brachytherapy is to deliver a high dose to a small volume of tissue. It is used in clinical situations (e.g., head and neck and gynecologic tumors) where high local doses are needed that would not be well tolerated by the surrounding normal structures. Precautions are necessary when caring for these individuals, who are radioactive for the period of time the source is in place (usually 3 to 5 days). Since the sources are sealed, there is no contamination of body fluids.

The nurse who is caring for patients receiving internal radiation should observe the principles of radiation safety. These are time (planning care to minimize time in the room), distance (standing as far as possible from the source), using shielding as available, and performing care from behind the shield whenever possible.

Radiopharmaceutical, or isotope, therapy is the use of unsealed sources to treat cancers. The sources used have a short half-life, and because they are unsealed, body fluids do become contaminated. The most commonly used radioisotope is iodine-131 (^{131}I) for thyroid cancer. Iodine-131 has a half-life of 8 days. Individuals

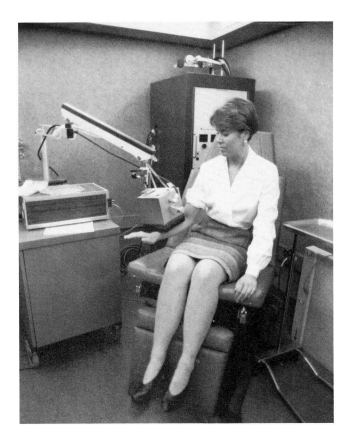

FIGURE 14-4
Hyperthermia system.

are hospitalized for the period of time the isotope is most active and then discharged.

Combining heat (hyperthermia) with radiation appears to result in thermal potentiation of the effects of radiation, which may be the result of (1) excess thermal sensitivity of hypoxic-acidotic tumor cells; (2) the differential effects of heat and radiation on various phases of the cell cycle; and (3) the impaired ability of tumor cells to repair sublethal or potentially lethal radiation damage. The goals of interstitial thermoradiotherapy are to improve disease-free and long-term survival and to promote comfort and control in cases of recurrent tumor growth. This treatment (Figure 14-4) has achieved high response rates and local tumor control for a variety of advanced or recurrent cancers of the pelvis, head and neck, breast, and other sites (e.g., skin, colorectum, and oral cavity). Hyperthermia can be delivered locally, regionally, or systemically (whole body) by electromagnetic, radiofrequency, or ultrasound techniques. Research is under way to allow more precise temperature monitoring throughout the treatment volume, to identify prognostic factors that influence response, and to determine the optimum fractionation and sequencing for heat in combination with radiation.

EFFECTS OF RADIATION

Radiation effects may be categorized as acute (during treatment to 6 months), subacute (after 6 months), and chronic (with variable time to expression). The effects are seen sooner in cell lines with a high mitotic index (the skin, mucous membranes, and hair follicles) and later in cell lines that divide more slowly (the vascular system and muscles). Early side effects are believed to be reparable, whereas late effects are more often permanent.

Radiation produces most of its effects in the area being treated; however, general effects such as fatigue and anorexia do occur. Fatigue is a commonly reported problem that has been shown to increase during the course of treatment. Research suggests a weekly pattern to the fatigue, with patients feeling better on some days than others. Fatigue is expected to occur by the third or fourth week of treatment. The patient should be encouraged to chart a pattern of fatigue and to plan activities accordingly, with rest planned before activities.

Megavoltage radiation therapy with skin-sparing techniques has resulted in less severe skin reactions than in the past. However, patients continue to express a fear of being burned. Transient erythema may appear as early as the first treatment, but it is usually during the second or third week of therapy that a lasting reaction appears. A dry desquamation may develop, with peeling of the skin. The cells may become darker before they peel off because of radiation effects on melanocytes. Patients complain of dryness and itching. Areas of wet desquamation may occur in areas subjected to higher doses or pressure (e.g., skin folds, perineum, axilla, collar area, and areas under the breast). This is a result of the destruction of all cells of the basal layer, exposing the dermis, which creates small but painful oozing areas. Permanent skin changes may result from dermal fibrosis and atrophy. The skin may feel hard, look shiny, and become darker than surrounding tissue. Telangiectasia (a dilation of capillaries related to late vascular effects and increased pressure of blood flowing through superficial vessels) results in spidery purple-red vessels visible in the treated area. This area may always react differently to sun exposure and should be protected (see Patient Teaching Guide).

Acute pulmonary effects of chest radiation therapy include increased cough, which may become more productive with the release of material that has been trapped in blocked alveoli as a result of lung cancer. As the mucosa dries during treatment, the cough becomes nonproductive and may require cough suppressant

therapy if it becomes persistent and debilitating. Patients also report dyspnea, which is difficult to manage and heightens the patient's anxiety. The primary acute effect is pneumonitis, with symptoms such as dyspnea, cough, fever, and night sweats appearing within 3 to 6 weeks after radiation therapy is begun, although pneumonitis often may be asymptomatic. The late effect is fibrosis in the treated area. This usually is asymptomatic, although extensive fibrosis with very high doses of radiation therapy may cause infection, fever, chills, dyspnea, clubbing, and abscesses.

Gastrointestinal effects reflect the area being irradiated. Irradiation of the small and large intestine causes vomiting, anorexia, diarrhea, and gastric distention. Gastric emptying is delayed, returning to normal 1 to 2 weeks after treatment ends. Patients receiving radiation therapy to the gastrointestinal tract may complain of nausea, vomiting, and diarrhea.

Radiosensitive cells, those most likely to be adversely affected by radiation, include relatively undifferentiated and rapidly dividing cells such as those of the gonads, the mucosa of the gastrointestinal tract, and lymphoid tissue. The most radioresistant cells are those originating from the connective tissue. At the cellular level the degree of sensitivity is related to the degree of cellular differentiation, rate of mitosis, and mitotic potential. The degrees of vascularity and oxygenation are also important in determining tissue responsiveness.

The toxic effects of radiation therapy depend on the site of irradiation, the volume of tissue irradiated, the total dosage delivered, and the time frame within which it is administered. Although newer technology has allowed tumors to be treated more precisely, surrounding or underlying healthy tissue will still be damaged.

The dose of radiation that can be delivered to any tumor is limited by the radiation tolerance of the adjacent normal tissues. A method of allowing for recovery of normal tissue is the fractionation of treatment, or dividing the total dosage of radiation into several equal daily doses (five days a week). This allows the following processes to occur: repair of sublethal tissue damage, repopulation of clonogenic cells, reassortment of cells in the cell cycle, and reoxygenation of hypoxic cells. The best results are achieved with predetermined doses given five times a week for 4 to 6 weeks (depending on the type of tumor).

Before initiating therapy, the radiation oncologist localizes the treatment field with a simulator, which reproduces the geometric factors of actual therapy. Computed tomography (CT) scanning that defines both the tumor-bearing volume and critical normal structures is also used. The information obtained is used, with computer assistance, to devise an individualized treatment plan (see photographs).

Using chemotherapy with radiation requires careful monitoring of peripheral blood counts and observation for combined modality disorders such as dysuria (cyclophosphamide) and enhanced mucositis (methotrexate, bleomycin). Actinomycin D and doxorubicin produce a recall phenomenon in which skin reactions appear in previously irradiated tissues when the drug is given as late as 1 year after the patient's radiation therapy. When radiation therapy is combined with other treatment modalities, acute and chronic reactions may be exacerbated. The nurse caring for these individuals must coordinate assessments and interventions to provide continuity of care.

PATIENT TEACHING

Teaching patients receiving radiation involves explaining the complex treatment in terms they can understand, predicting anticipated acute and long-term effects, and providing information about symptom management. With these tools, patients can undergo treatment with minimal disruption of their activities. Symptom management is a critical aspect of the care of the individual receiving radiation therapy.

1 ASSESS

ASSESSMENT	OBSERVATIONS
Gastrointestinal tract	Nausea and vomiting, anorexia, taste changes, esophagitis, sore throat, xerostomia, mucositis, tooth decay, diarrhea, perianal irritation
Genitourinary	Bladder irritation, vaginal discharge, amenorrhea, impotence, sterility
Dermatologic	Hair loss, dry desquamation, moist desquamation
Central nervous system	Headache, irritability, confusion, restlessness
Neuromuscular system	Fatigue, transient myelitis
Cardiopulmonary	Pneumonitis, pericarditis, myocarditis
Hematologic	Leukopenia, thrombocytopenia

2 DIAGNOSE

NURSING DIAGNOSIS	SUBJECTIVE FINDINGS	OBJECTIVE FINDINGS
Fluid volume deficit related to nausea and vomiting	Complains of nausea	Vomiting

➜ ❯ ❯

NURSING DIAGNOSIS	SUBJECTIVE FINDINGS	OBJECTIVE FINDINGS
Altered nutrition: less than body requirements related to gastrointestinal irritation and increased body requirements	Complains of anorexia, taste changes, sore throat	Esophagitis, xerostomia, mucositis
Diarrhea related to gastrointestinal irritation	Complains of urgency to defecate, perianal irritation	Frequent loose, liquid, or semiliquid stools
Altered oral mucous membranes related to treatment-induced irritation	Complains of sore throat, dry mouth	Mucositis, xerostomia
Altered patterns of urinary elimination related to bladder irritation	Complains of urgency, burning during urination	Frequency, hematuria
Sexual dysfunction related to treatment-induced changes in hormonal status and local effects of radiation	Complains of impotence; discomfort during sexual activity	Vaginal discharge, amenorrhea, sterility, vaginal dryness
Impaired skin integrity related to treatment-induced changes	Complains of dry, itchy feeling	Hair loss, dry desquamation (reddened area, dry in appearance), moist desquamation (blistering, sloughing)
Pain (headache) related to increased intracranial pressure	Complains of headache	Grimacing, holding head in hands, pupillary changes, increased blood pressure
Impaired physical mobility related to fatigue and myelitis	Complains of fatigue, painful sensations	Weakness, guarding of extremities, Lhermitte's sign
Altered cardiopulmonary tissue perfusion related to pneumonitis, pericarditis, myocarditis, anemia, and bleeding	Complains of chest pain	Cough, dyspnea, friction rub, electrocardiogram (ECG) changes, dysrhythmias, anemia, thrombocytopenia

3 PLAN

Patient goals

1. The patient will maintain adequate hydration and nutrition.
2. The patient will maintain normal fecal and urinary elimination patterns.
3. Sexual function will be normal.
4. The patient will have healthy skin.
5. The patient will have no pain.
6. The patient will ambulate without difficulty.
7. The patient will have adequate oxygenation, as evidenced by normal cardiopulmonary function.

4 IMPLEMENT

NURSING DIAGNOSIS	NURSING INTERVENTIONS	RATIONALE
Fluid volume deficit related to nausea and vomiting	Administer antiemetic as needed before treatment of areas known to cause nausea and vomiting.	To control incidence of nausea and vomiting.
	Plan rest periods before and after meals.	To enhance patient's appetite.
	Provide small, bland feedings and increased fluids.	To maintain nutrition and hydration.
	Offer frequent mouth care.	To promote comfort and appetite.
	Provide clean environment with fresh air and no odors.	To decrease noxious stimuli.
	Administer intravenous therapy as ordered.	To maintain hydration.
	Monitor intake and output, daily weight, and electrolytes.	To determine need for further intervention.
Altered nutrition: less than body requirements related to gastrointestinal irritation and increased body requirements	Encourage patient to eat high-calorie, high-protein diet.	For maximum nutrition.
	Offer small, frequent feedings.	To increase intake.
	Do not rush meals.	To increase intake.
	Keep room free of odors and clutter.	To reduce noxious stimuli.
	Provide meticulous mouth care.	To increase comfort and appetite.
	Use enteral feeding tube or total parenteral nutrition if necessary.	To maintain nutritional balance.
	Monitor weight daily.	To detect nutritional imbalance.
	Encourage clear liquids, low-residue diet, and antacids.	To increase comfort.

NURSING DIAGNOSIS	NURSING INTERVENTIONS	RATIONALE
Diarrhea related to gastrointestinal irritation	Offer antidiarrheal agents per physician's order.	To control intestinal irritability.
	Maintain good perineal care.	To prevent pain, infection, and fear of eating caused by painful bowel movement.
	Test stools for occult blood.	To identify intestinal bleeding.
	Record number and consistency of stools.	To monitor effect of therapy.
	Observe for dehydration and electrolyte imbalances.	To determine need for further intervention.
Altered oral mucous membranes related to treatment-induced irritation	Encourage good oral hygiene with use of dental floss or Water Pik unless thrombocytopenia is present.	To prevent infection and assist in healing.
	Discourage foods that are spicy, hot, dry, or thick.	They increase discomfort.
	Offer topical relief of pain—viscous lidocaine.	To promote comfort and nutrition.
	Apply water-soluble lubricant (K-Y Jelly) to lips.	To maintain moisture.
	Offer sugar-free popsicles.	To increase comfort and hydration.
	Offer artificial saliva.	To moisten mucosa.
	Encourage increased fluid intake with meals.	To maintain hydration.
	Use mouth irrigations (e.g., salt and bicarbonate with water).	For oral hygiene.
	Encourage use of sugarless lemon drops or mints.	To promote feeling of freshness and to stimulate saliva.
	Discourage smoking, alcohol, or ginger ale.	They irritate mucosa.
	Assess mouth for dryness, lesions, bleeding, discharge, and tooth decay.	To determine need for specific interventions.
	Consult dentist before treatment for dental problems, including fluoride therapy.	To prevent further irritation and infection and to prevent radiation caries.
Altered patterns of urinary elimination related to bladder irritation	Force fluids.	To maintain renal and bladder hydration.
	Encourage patient to empty bladder completely.	To avoid distention.

NURSING DIAGNOSIS	NURSING INTERVENTIONS	RATIONALE
	Administer urinary antiseptics as prescribed.	To reduce inflammation.
	Observe for signs of infection (e.g., burning, cloudy urine, hematuria, and fever).	To determine the need for antibiotics and other interventions.
Sexual dysfunction related to treatment-induced changes in hormonal status	*For sterility:* Help patient explore alternatives (e.g., sperm banking) if an option and hormonal therapy.	To counteract sterility.
	Refer patient to sexual counselor as necessary.	To treat impotence.
	For vaginal discharge: Encourage patient to douche as needed and to perform thorough perineal care.	To maintain hygiene.
	Observe for redness, tenderness, discharge, or drainage.	These may indicate need for further intervention.
	For vaginal dryness: Observe for skin integrity and lubrication of mucosa; offer lubricants and vaginal dilator.	To maintain integrity of mucosa, facilitate comfort during intercourse, and prevent vaginal fibrosis.
Impaired skin integrity related to treatment-induced changes	*For alopecia:* Help patient plan for wig with soft underside to minimize skin irritation; use only for special occasions.	To avoid scalp damage.
	Have patient wear scarf or turban.	For daily protection of scalp.
	Have patient gently wash and comb hair.	To avoid further hair loss.
	Tell patient that hair loss secondary to whole brain radiation for primary brain tumors is permanent.	To avoid false hope about regrowth.
	For dermatitis: Observe irradiated area daily.	To monitor for inflammation or other reactions.
	Apply baby oil or ointment as prescribed: lanolin or Aquaphor.	To maintain moisture.
	Keep reddened area dry and aerated.	To avoid infection.
	Use cornstarch, A & D ointment, hydrocortisone ointment, aloe vera.	To relieve dryness and itching.
	For moist desquamation: Provide saline soaks, moisture-permeable dressings, topical vitamins, steroids, or antibiotic ointments; expose area to air.	To enhance healing.
	Do not use adhesive tape.	It irritates the skin.

➡ ❯ ❯

NURSING DIAGNOSIS	NURSING INTERVENTIONS	RATIONALE
	Help patient with bathing.	To maintain markings.
	Have patient avoid excessive heat, sunlight, soap, and tight, restrictive clothing.	They further irritate damaged skin.
	Provide special skin care to tissue folds (e.g., buttocks, perineum, groin, and axilla).	They are subject to increased pressure and damage.
	Do not apply deodorant or aftershave lotion to treated area.	They may irritate the skin.
Pain (headache) related to increased intracranial pressure	Assess presence and characteristics of headache.	To monitor need for intervention.
	Administer medications (e.g., steroids, analgesics) as prescribed.	To relieve pain.
	Offer patient other pain relief measures if desired.	To encourage patient involvement in pain management.
	Monitor pupillary response and changes in vital signs, irritability, confusion, and restlessness.	These indicate increasing intracranial pressure.
Impaired physical mobility related to fatigue and myelitis	Plan frequent rest periods.	To avoid fatigue.
	Assist patient with ambulation and remove environmental barriers.	To avoid injury.
	Assess reflexes, tactile sensation, and movement in extremities; report abnormal findings.	To detect complications.
	Observe for Lhermitte's sign (sensation of electric shock running down back and over extremities).	This indicates transient myelitis.
Altered cardiopulmonary tissue perfusion related to pneumonitis, pericarditis, myocarditis, anemia, and bleeding	Auscultate lungs, and report signs of pleural rub.	To detect respiratory problems early.
	Observe for cough, dyspnea, and pain on inspiration.	These indicate respiratory dysfunction.
	Treat with antibiotics and steroids as prescribed.	To reduce irritation and prevent infection.
	Auscultate heart, and report signs of friction rub, dysrhythmia, or hypertension.	To detect complications.
	Observe for chest pain and weakness.	These indicate cardiac dysfunction.
	Monitor ECG reports.	To monitor cardiac function.

NURSING DIAGNOSIS	NURSING INTERVENTIONS	RATIONALE
	Administer drugs as prescribed.	To counteract dysrhythmias.
	Encourage adequate rest; alternate rest and activity periods.	To avoid stress on respiratory system.
	Observe patient for dyspnea and increased weakness.	These are signs of further anemia.
	Administer oxygen therapy as needed.	To increase oxygenation of tissues.
	Monitor hemoglobin and hematocrit.	To determine effect of therapy on bone marrow.
	Administer transfusions as ordered.	To increase circulating red blood cells.
Knowledge deficit	See Patient Teaching.	

5 EVALUATE

PATIENT OUTCOME	DATA INDICATING THAT OUTCOME IS REACHED
Patient has adequate hydration. 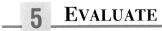	Patient has no nausea or vomiting, intake and output are balanced, and electrolytes are within normal limits.
Patient's nutrition is adequate.	Patient has no complaints of anorexia or unusual taste sensations and can eat and swallow without pain; weight is normal.
Patient has normal bowel elimination.	Patient has no diarrhea.
Patient's oral mucous membranes are healthy.	Mucous membranes, lips, tongue, and gingiva are moist and normal in color; the teeth are clean and saliva is adequate; patient can swallow and has a normal voice.
Patient has normal urinary elimination.	Patient has no complaints of urinary distress, and intake and output are balanced.
Patient's sexual function is normal.	Patient has a satisfactory libido and has made plans for dealing with possible sterility; there is no vaginal discharge (women) or erectile ability has been maintained (men).
Patient's skin is healthy and intact.	Patient has no complaints of itching, and there is no evidence of rash, blistering, or redness.
Patient has no pain.	Patient has no complaint of headache.
Patient has normal physical mobility.	Patient can ambulate without assistance.
Patient has adequate cardiopulmonary tissue perfusion.	Patient has no complaints of chest pain, cough, or dyspnea, and CBC is within normal limits.

➜ ❯ ❯

PATIENT TEACHING

1. Discuss the need for skin care such as maintenance of dye markings, avoiding soap and other ointments, and avoiding sunbathing or heat applications (see Patient Teaching Guide).
2. Emphasize the need to avoid injury to the skin (see Patient Teaching Guide).
3. Explain the maintenance of adequate nutrition and hydration (see Patient Teaching Guide).
4. Explain the patient's "radioactive state," if present, and precautions to be taken.
5. Discuss how to manage fatigue and maintain mobility.

Chemotherapy

Chemotherapy is still considered a relatively new form of cancer treatment, the first patient having been treated with nitrogen mustard in 1942. Chemical agents are especially important in the treatment of systemic disease. Researchers strive to discover drugs that kill cancer cells without extensively damaging normal tissues. In addition, combinations of chemotherapeutic agents, as well as chemotherapy combined with other treatments, have increased the number of cures, remissions, and palliative outcomes.

The following are some general principles that guide the use of cancer chemotherapeutic agents:

1. Combination chemotherapy, when carefully designed, has been consistently superior to single-agent therapy.
2. Complete remission is the minimum requirement to achieve cure and even significantly prolonged survival.
3. The best chance for a significant response is with the first attempt; thus the type of treatment should be the approach with maximum effectiveness.
4. Drugs should be used in the highest possible doses to attain maximum tumor-cell kill.
5. Drug dosage reduction to minimize toxicity is itself the most toxic side effect of chemotherapy.
6. Adjuvant chemotherapy is now well established in the treatment of breast cancer and holds promise for other types of cancer.
7. The development of analogs of existing drugs has made it possible to at least partly modify those drugs' toxicity while preserving their antitumor activity (e.g., carboplatin and iproplatin are second-generation platinum compounds that are less nephrotoxic than cisplatin).
8. Various therapeutic maneuvers are used to lessen toxicity (e.g., doxorubicin is much less toxic when given by 96-hour infusion than when given as a bolus).
9. "Neoadjuvant," or induction, chemotherapy is the initial use of drugs to reduce a tumor's bulk and lower its stage, making it amenable to cure with local therapy (e.g., as in osteogenic sarcoma).
10. Chemoprevention of cancer is becoming a reality (e.g., 13-cis-retinoic acid has been shown to produce marked regression of leukoplakia, a premalignant lesion in the oral cavity).

Chemotherapeutic agents are highly toxic, attacking all rapidly dividing cells, both normal and malignant. Thus the contraindications for and precautions in the use of the various agents reflect the patient's pretreatment condition, stage of disease, response to therapy, and allergies or sensitivities. The nurse involved in administering the drugs and monitoring the patient's responses must have a comprehensive baseline assessment for evaluating the patient's condition and ability to tolerate the therapy. Many health care providers monitor the patient's functional status in a systematic manner, using such instruments as the Karnofsky Performance Scale (Table 14-2). Preset values guide the health care provider in determining the patient's tolerance of the therapy, as well as the need to delay or discontinue treatment.

Table 14-2

KARNOFSKY PERFORMANCE SCALE

Activity status	Point	Description
Normal activity	10	Normal, with no complaints or evidence of disease
	9	Able to carry on normal activity but with minor signs or symptoms of disease present
	8	Normal activity but requiring effort; signs and symptoms of disease more prominent
Self-care	7	Able to care for self but unable to work or carry on other normal activities
	6	Able to care for most needs but requires occasional assistance
	5	Considerable assistance required, along with frequent medical care; some self-care still possible
Incapacitated	4	Disabled and requiring special care and assistance
	3	Severely disabled; hospitalization required but death from disease not imminent
	2	Extremely ill; supportive treatment, hospitalized care required
	1	Imminent death
	0	Dead

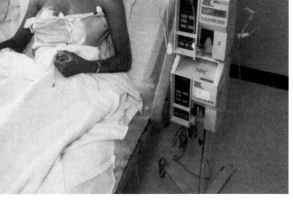

FIGURE 14-5
Hickman-Broviac catheter. This patient has a Hickman-Broviac catheter for venous access. Note the catheter's lift over the right breast, with a protective dressing and tape to prevent dislodgment. The patient is receiving multiple intravenous infusions via the catheter.

ROUTES OF ADMINISTRATION

Depending on the drug's pharmacodynamics, chemotherapy may be administered by a variety of routes: oral, intravenous, central venous catheter, venous access via an implantable access device, intraarterial, intraperitoneal, intrapleural, or intrathecal via the Ommaya reservoir. The intramuscular and subcutaneous routes are used less frequently than other routes.

In recent years venous access has become increasingly important because of the ease of access to the venous system for drug delivery, increased patient comfort, and the addition of external or internal pump systems for more continuous infusion of drugs (Figure 14-5) (see Patient Teaching Guide). Although most central venous lines have similarities, the nurse should become familiar with the variations; for example, a Broviac line has a smaller inner lumen than a Hickman catheter. Injection caps, repair kits, and surgical insertion techniques also vary with the brand, as do the materials the catheters are made of. Most central venous lines (ex-

cept the Groshong catheter) should be flushed with 2 to 5 ml of normal saline before medication is administered. After the medication has been instilled, the nurse or patient should flush again with saline and then a heparin solution. When not in use, the catheter should be flushed regularly with a heparin solution to maintain patency. There is increasing evidence that the catheter does not have to be flushed daily; nursing research continues in this area. Unlike other central lines, the Groshong catheter has a rounded tip and a valve that prevents venous blood from entering the catheter and also blocks out air if the line is left uncapped. This catheter should be flushed with normal saline after use; no heparinization is required. The Groshong is a more transparent and flexible catheter and should not be clamped when uncapped. When caring for a patient who has a central line, the nurse should don a mask and sterile gloves, hold the catheter away from the patient's body, and clean the site and 3

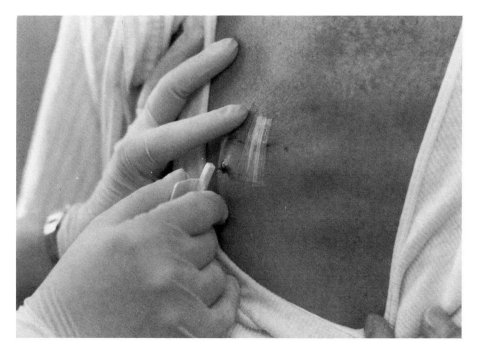

FIGURE 14-6
Implanted pump. The nurse is accessing the patient's implanted pump for the purpose of infusing a chemotherapeutic
agent. The needle is taped to the skin surface for the duration
of the infusion and then removed.

inches up the catheter with povidone-iodine. It is also
important to observe the site for redness, tenderness,
drainage, or swelling, each of which requires further assessment and intervention.

Unlike central venous lines, which provide external
access, the implanted venous infusion device remains
completely under the patient's skin, which serves as a
defense against infection. Vascular access ports (Figure
14-6) such as the Infuse-A-Port and the Port-A-Cath
consist of a resealable silicone rubber septum, a hous-
ing or body of molded plastic and silicone rubber or
stainless steel, and an attached silicone rubber catheter
or a separate catheter and locking ring. The port is implanted subcutaneously with the indwelling catheter
positioned in a vein, artery, peritoneum, pericardial
cavity, or pleural cavity. The advantages of the port include repeated access to blood vessels or a body cavity
with minimal trauma and distress for the patient; the
ability to inject bolus or continuous infusions of drugs,
blood, nutritional products, or other fluids; access to
blood samples; and promotion of the patient's normal
body image and ability to conduct activities of daily living. The system is flushed weekly or monthly, depending on whether the catheter is in an artery or a vein.

The implantable pump provides a refillable reservoir; a permanent, nonreplaceable power source; few
moving parts; a variable infusion rate; and a double
septum for continuous and bolus drug delivery. The
pump is approved for use with floxuridine (FUDR),
methotrexate, heparin, morphine, and some aminoglycosides.

The Ommaya reservoir (Figure 14-7) is a mush-
room-shaped device made of silicone rubber and connected to a catheter in the lateral ventricle. The hollow
dome, a reservoir with an internal volume of 1.25 ml, is
made of specially thickened self-sealing silicone rubber
which allows for at least 200 separate needle punctures.
The dome also functions as a pump when compressed
through the skin with a fingertip. The Ommaya reservoir is used to deliver drugs directly into the cerebrospinal fluid (CSF), to obtain CSF specimens, and to
measure CSF pressure, thus eliminating the need for
repeated lumbar punctures. In addition, drug distribution is better when the drug is delivered into the ven-
tricles.

Intraperitoneal chemotherapy is used to treat minimal residual disease, with the goal of enhancing local
tumor control while decreasing systemic exposure to

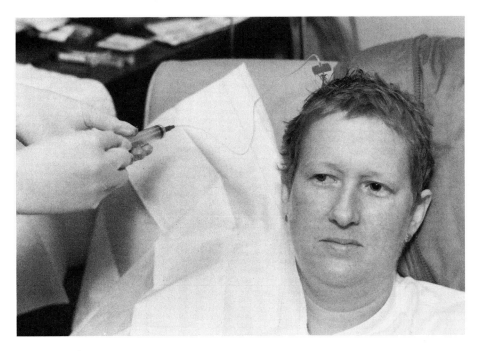

FIGURE 14-7
Ommaya reservoir. This patient is receiving chemotherapy via the Ommaya reservoir, which is implanted within the scalp. The drug is delivered directly into the cerebrospinal fluid.

drug toxicity (see Patient Teaching Guide). The peritoneal cavity acts as a tumor refuge, since it is separated from the bloodstream by a cellular enclosure similar to the blood-brain barrier. Direct administration of chemotherapeutic drugs ensures greater exposure of malignant cells to the drugs. The slower peritoneal clearance or absorption leads to greater pharmacologic advantage. In addition, the drug is partly detoxified and metabolized by the liver before entering the systemic circulation, thus reducing the number and severity of systemic toxicities. Cisplatin currently is the drug of choice for intraperitoneal infusion, although interferon-alpha, methotrexate, fluorouracil (5FU), doxorubicin, and other agents are being studied.

The Tenckhoff peritoneal dialysis catheter most often is used for intraperitoneal chemotherapy, with the intraperitoneal end surgically placed in the abdominal cavity. The distal end of the catheter and the abdominal exit site are cared for meticulously to prevent infection. The nurse must help the patient in the management of abdominal fullness or pressure, which results from drastic fluid changes in the abdominal cavity. Effective interventions include having the patient wear loose-fitting clothing and change position every 15 minutes,

and maintaining the bed in semi-Fowler's position during the infusion. If the patient experiences severe dyspnea during the procedure, the nurse may need to withdraw the fluid early. If leakage occurs around the catheter site, the placement of the catheter should be checked. Complications include bacterial peritonitis and infection at the exit site.

CLINICAL TRIALS

A comprehensive description of cancer chemotherapeutic agents is given in Chapter 16. Many other agents currently are under study. Patients often are asked to participate in clinical trials of single agents or combinations of drugs. It is important for the nurse to understand the phases of drug testing to teach the patient about clinical trials and to ensure the patient's informed consent if he or she agrees to participate (see Patient Teaching Guide).

OTHER ISSUES RELATED TO CHEMOTHERAPY

Although chemotherapy often is of great value to the patient with cancer, it may also create chemotherapy-related malignancies. The class of drugs most commonly associated with long-term damage to normal cells is the alkylating agents, which include busulfan (Myleran), chlorambucil (Leukeran), cyclophosphamide (Cytoxan), and melphalan (Alkeran). The most frequently reported second cancer is acute nonlymphocytic leukemia (ANL), which has a short latency period (2 to 5 years after treatment). Most patients die within 6 months of diagnosis. Patients at greatest risk for second malignancies are those treated for Hodgkin's lymphoma, non-Hodgkin's lymphoma, multiple myeloma, ovarian cancer, breast cancer, gastrointestinal cancers, lung cancer, and testicular cancer.

Another interesting phenomenon is multidrug resistance, which is seen in cancers that are (1) highly responsive to chemotherapy and frequently curable but that show a drug-resistant relapse (e.g., diffuse lymphomas and testicular cancers); (2) initially highly responsive to cytoreductive therapy but eventually relapse or progress (e.g., disseminated breast cancer, ovarian cancer, and small cell lung cancer); or (3) refractory at initial diagnosis; that is, de novo resistance (e.g., colon cancer and disseminated malignant melanoma). If satisfactory tumor-cell kill is achieved only at the cost of unacceptable patient toxicity, then for all practical purposes the tumor is resistant.

The nurse who administers cancer chemotherapeutic drugs must be concerned about and careful with not only the patient but also herself. It has been proved that unsafe handling of these drugs may heighten the nurse's reproductive risks as well as endanger the environment. The Occupational Safety and Health Administration (OSHA) offers recommendations for safe handling of antineoplastic drugs, which can be obtained from the U.S. Department of Labor. Nurses preparing and administering chemotherapy must be familiar with these guidelines and see that they are implemented for the protection of all who come into contact with these drugs. The guidelines address avoiding exposure via inhalation, absorption through the skin, and ingestion. There are also recommendations for protective equipment, safe disposal, and monitoring of biologic safety cabinets and personnel health.

1 ASSESS

ASSESSMENT	OBSERVATIONS
Gastrointestinal	Nausea and vomiting, diarrhea, constipation, stomatitis, esophagitis, anorexia
Dermatologic	Alopecia, dermatitis, changes in skin color, hyperpigmentation of nail beds, rash, jaundice, pruritus, extravasation
Hematologic	Fatigue and dyspnea (anemia), petechiae, ecchymoses, frank bleeding (thrombocytopenia), fever, chills, hypotension (leukopenia)
Reproductive	Sterility, amenorrhea, decreased libido
Urinary	Hemorrhagic cystitis, as evidenced by hematuria, burning during urination, and backache; nephrotoxicity, as evidenced by renal failure or decrease or absence of urinary output
Neurologic	Ototoxicity, as evidenced by vertigo, tinnitus, and loss of hearing; peripheral neuropathies, as evidenced by muscular weakness, paresthesia, absence of deep tendon reflexes
Musculoskeletal	Myalgia, muscle weakness, osteoporosis, gout
Respiratory	Pulmonary fibrosis, as evidenced by dyspnea, chest pain, or cyanosis

ASSESSMENT	OBSERVATIONS
Cardiac	Congestive heart failure, as evidenced by exertional dyspnea, cough, rales, and ECG changes
Psychosocial	Fear, depression, anger, anxiety

2 DIAGNOSE

NURSING DIAGNOSIS	SUBJECTIVE FINDINGS	OBJECTIVE FINDINGS
Fluid volume deficit related to nausea and vomiting	Complains of nausea	Vomiting
Constipation related to impaired intestinal motility	Complains of fullness, inability to defecate	Absence of bowel movements
Diarrhea related to intestinal irritation	Complains of urgency to defecate	Frequent loose, liquid, or semiliquid stools
Altered oral mucous membranes related to poor oral hygiene, preexisting dental disorders, or drug-induced irritation	Complains of pain in mouth, difficulty swallowing, unusual taste sensations	Redness, ulcers or lesions, dry or cracked lips, coated tongue, thick saliva, edematous gums, plaque or debris around teeth, deep, raspy voice
Altered nutrition: less than body requirements related to gastrointestinal irritation and increased body requirements	Complains of anorexia, unusual taste sensations	Stomatitis, esophagitis
Impaired skin integrity related to drug-induced changes, extravasation	Complains of itching	Alopecia, dermatitis/rash, changes in skin color (e.g., jaundice), hyperpigmentation of skin and nail beds
Impaired gas exchange related to anemia, pulmonary fibrosis, cardiotoxicity	Complains of fatigue, chest pain	Pallor, exertional dyspnea, cough, fever, ECG changes
Altered peripheral tissue perfusion related to bleeding	Complains of weakness	Tachycardia, hyperpnea, hypotension, petechiae, ecchymoses, melena, hematuria, frank bleeding

NURSING DIAGNOSIS	SUBJECTIVE FINDINGS	OBJECTIVE FINDINGS
Potential for infection related to leukopenia, bone marrow suppression	Complains of fever	Chills; hypotension; damp, warm, red skin; odor; leukocytosis or leukopenia
Sexual dysfunction related to drug-induced changes in hormonal status	Complains of decreased libido	Sterility, amenorrhea
Altered patterns of urinary elimination related to drug-induced nephrotoxicity	Complains of burning during urination, urgency, backache	Frequency, decreased urination, hematuria
Sensory/perceptual alterations (auditory, tactile) related to drug-induced neurotoxicity	Complains of vertigo, dizziness, loss of hearing, numbness and tingling, weakness	Appears not to hear speaker; asks speaker to repeat words; muscle weakness; loss of deep tendon reflexes
Impaired physical mobility related to drug-induced gout, osteoporosis, myelotoxicity	Complains of weakness, muscle pain	Muscle weakness, difficulty ambulating
Altered cardiopulmonary tissue perfusion related to drug-induced cardiac damage	Complains of chest pain	Exertional dyspnea, cough, rales, ECG changes
Ineffective individual coping related to stress of dealing with chemotherapy	Expresses fear, anger, sadness	Appears afraid, angry, anxious, withdrawn

3 PLAN

Patient goals

1. The patient will maintain adequate hydration and nutrition.
2. The patient will maintain normal fecal and urinary elimination patterns.
3. The patient will have healthy oral mucous membranes and skin.
4. The patient will have adequate oxygenation, as evidenced by normal cardiopulmonary function and warm, pink skin.
5. The patient will have no evidence of infection.
6. Sexual function will be normal.
7. The patient will demonstrate normal sensory/perceptual function with regard to hearing, touch, and sensation.
8. The patient will ambulate without difficulty.
9. The patient will be able to cope with the stress of chemotherapy.

4   IMPLEMENT

NURSING DIAGNOSIS	NURSING INTERVENTIONS	RATIONALE
Fluid volume deficit related to nausea and vomiting	Administer antiemetic (prochlorperazine, thiethylperazine, trimethobenzamide, mito-clopramide, intravenous dexamethasone, or tetrahydrocannabinol [THC]) prophylactically before chemotherapy and on regular schedule after therapy per physician order.	To decrease incidence of nausea and vomiting.
	Withhold food and fluids for 4 to 6 hours before treatment.	To decrease gastric irritation.
	Provide small feedings and increase fluids.	To maintain nutrition and hydration.
	Provide frequent mouth care.	To promote patient's comfort.
	Provide clean environment with fresh air and no odors.	To reduce noxious stimuli.
	Monitor intake and output, weight, and electrolytes.	To avoid dehydration.
	Administer intravenous therapy as ordered.	To maintain fluid and electrolyte balance.
	Use relaxation techniques, guided imagery, self-hypnosis, and distraction as indicated.	To reduce nausea.
Constipation related to impaired intestinal motility	Offer fluids and foods high in fiber and bulk; offer stool softeners or laxatives.	To stimulate motility.
	Avoid enemas.	They may traumatize the intestinal mucosa.
	Use warmth, such as a heating pad.	To relieve discomfort caused by abdominal distention.
Diarrhea related to intestinal irritation	Offer clear liquids.	To prevent dehydration.
	Offer antidiarrheal agent, such as Kaopectate or diphenoxylate (Lomotil), per physician's order.	To control amount and frequency of diarrhea.
	Maintain good perineal care.	To avoid irritation and discomfort.
	Test stools for occult blood.	To identify evidence of blood.
	Record number and consistency of stools.	To monitor need for further intervention.
	Observe for dehydration and electrolyte imbalance.	To detect complications early.

➔ 〉 〉

NURSING DIAGNOSIS	NURSING INTERVENTIONS	RATIONALE
Altered oral mucous membranes related to poor oral hygiene, preexisting dental disorders, or drug-induced irritation	Avoid alcohol and tobacco.	They irritate mucous membranes.
	Encourage good oral hygiene.	To promote comfort and prevent infection.
	Discourage spicy and hot foods.	To avoid irritation or pain.
	Offer topical agents for relief of pain (lidocaine or dyclonine) per physician's order.	To soothe irritated mucous membranes.
	Apply water-soluble lubricant (K-Y Jelly) to lips.	To maintain moisture.
	Offer popsicles.	For hydration and comfort.
	Use oral assessment guide to monitor changes in voice and ability to swallow, as well as condition of lips, tongue, mucous membranes, gingiva, teeth, and saliva.	To evaluate response to interventions.
	Avoid foods that are difficult to chew, such as apples, and highly acidic beverages such as citrus juices.	To avoid irritation.
	Administer nystatin oral suspension or suppository or clotrimazole (Mycelex) troche per physician's order.	To combat infection.
	Have patient postpone dental work if possible; have patient brush teeth gently and use toothettes.	To avoid further trauma.
Altered nutrition: less than body requirements related to gastrointestinal irritation and increased body requirements	Offer bland or pureed foods.	To facilitate swallowing.
	Have patient avoid spicy foods, alcohol, and tobacco.	To decrease irritation.
	Offer antacids.	To counteract gastric acid.
	Identify food preferences.	To increase patient's interest in eating.
	Offer small, frequent feedings.	To avoid distention.
	Do not rush meals.	So patient will increase intake.
	Keep room free of odors and clutter.	To reduce noxious stimuli.
	Provide meticulous mouth care.	To enhance appetite.
	Use enteral feeding tube or total parenteral nutrition if necessary.	To maintain nutritional balance.
	Weigh daily.	To monitor nutritional status.

NURSING DIAGNOSIS	NURSING INTERVENTIONS	RATIONALE
Impaired skin integrity related to drug-induced changes, extravasation	*For alopecia:* Help patient plan for wig, scarf, or hat before hair loss.	To enhance patient's self-image.
	Offer tourniquet or ice cap preventive therapy based on policy and diagnosis.	To decrease hair loss.
	Have patient wash and comb remaining hair gently.	To decrease hair loss.
	Reassure patient that hair will grow back after therapy.	To lessen patient's anxiety regarding hair loss.
	For dermatitis: Use cornstarch, Alpha Keri, calamine lotion, or other agent.	To relieve itching.
	Warn against overexposure to sun.	To avoid further irritation.
	Keep skin clean and dry.	To avoid infection.
	For changes in color of skin or nail beds: Assure patient that discoloration will fade with time.	To lessen patient's anxiety regarding discoloration.
	Use nail polish according to patient's wishes.	To mask discoloration.
	For jaundice: Monitor hepatic enzymes.	To determine liver function.
	Assess skin and sclera daily.	For evidence of increase or decrease in discoloration.
	For extravasation: Observe for early signs, which include pain or burning sensation at or above IV site, blanching, redness, swelling, slowing of infusion, absence of blood return.	To detect problem before tissue damage occurs.
	Stop infusion; aspirate remaining drug from needle, inject antidote, and apply topical ointment, heat, or cold as dictated by protocol.	To prevent tissue damage.
Impaired gas exchange related to anemia, pulmonary fibrosis, cardiotoxicity	Monitor respiratory function with pulmonary function tests.	To detect changes in status.
	Note limitation of lifetime dosage of bleomycin.	To prevent irreversible toxicity.
	Help with pulmonary function studies.	To detect changes in status.

➜ ➤ ❯

NURSING DIAGNOSIS	NURSING INTERVENTIONS	RATIONALE
	Provide oxygen therapy, sedative, cough suppressants, and steroids as prescribed.	For symptom management.
	Have patient change position slowly, and encourage adequate rest.	To conserve energy.
	Observe patient for dyspnea and increased weakness.	As evidence of further dysfunction.
	Monitor hemoglobin and hematocrit.	To determine effect of therapy.
	Administer transfusions as ordered.	To increase red blood cell count.
	Monitor heart rate, blood pressure, and ECG.	To detect cardiac dysfunction.
Altered peripheral tissue perfusion related to bleeding	Protect patient from injury (e.g., use precautions when shaving with razor blade, do not permit cluttered environment, and do not administer rectal suppositories).	To avoid trauma.
	Have patient avoid using aspirin and aspirin products.	They increase clotting time.
	Avoid giving injections; if they are necessary, apply pressure at site for 3 to 5 minutes afterward.	To prevent bleeding.
	Use toothettes for oral care.	To avoid trauma to mucosa.
	Monitor skin (petechiae, ecchymoses), urine, and platelet count.	For evidence of bleeding.
	Evaluate neurologic status.	To identify intracranial bleeding.
	Have nasal packing available.	In case bleeding occurs.
	Administer platelet transfusions as necessary.	To control bleeding.
	Monitor vital signs.	To detect bleeding early.
	Support patient in ambulation.	To prevent injury related to weakness.
Potential for infection related to leukopenia, bone marrow suppression	Warn patient to avoid crowds and people with colds, flu, or cold sores.	To prevent exposure to infection.
	Use sterile technique whenever needed.	To prevent infection.
	Initiate reverse isolation as indicated.	To protect patient from pathogens.

NURSING DIAGNOSIS	NURSING INTERVENTIONS	RATIONALE
	Monitor temperature and leukocyte count; observe skin temperature, color, and odor.	To detect signs of infection.
	Encourage careful hygiene.	To prevent infection.
	Discourage fresh-cut flowers.	They may carry microorganisms.
	Avoid using indwelling catheters or performing rectal procedures or examinations.	To prevent infection.
	Administer antibiotics as prescribed.	To treat infection.
	Provide analgesics as ordered.	To reduce fever.
	Encourage fluids.	To prevent dehydration.
Sexual dysfunction related to drug-induced changes in hormonal status	Help patient explore alternatives for sterility (e.g., sperm banking, hormonal therapy during treatment, and postponement of conception and childbearing). Refer to sexual counselor as needed.	To provide support regarding possible changes in sexuality.
Altered patterns of urinary elimination related to drug-induced nephrotoxicity	Force fluids.	To maintain renal blood flow.
	Monitor blood urea nitrogen, serum creatinine, creatinine clearance, and electrolytes.	They indicate renal function.
	Monitor intake and output; check for edema.	To detect renal dysfunction.
	Administer diuretics as ordered.	To enhance renal excretion.
	Encourage foods high in potassium.	To prevent diuretic-related hypokalemia.
	Administer normal saline and mannitol before cisplatin therapy per physician's order.	To maintain fluid and electrolyte balance.
	Administer allopurinol as prescribed with high fluid intake.	To prevent uric acid accumulation in kidneys.
	Encourage patient to empty bladder frequently, especially at night.	To avoid stasis, inflammation, and infection.
	Provide adequate hydration.	To maintain renal function.

→ 〉 〉

NURSING DIAGNOSIS	NURSING INTERVENTIONS	RATIONALE
Sensory/perceptual alterations (auditory, tactile) related to drug-induced neurotoxicity	Monitor hearing with baseline and periodic audiograms.	To detect hearing loss early.
	Speak clearly and in normal tone of voice.	To enhance communication.
	Assess patient for numbness and tingling in extremities.	To detect development of paresthesias.
	Prohibit smoking and have patient observe placement of feet and hands.	To encourage safety.
Impaired physical mobility related to drug-induced gout, osteoporosis, myelotoxicity	Monitor calcium level.	To determine bone status.
	Provide safety measures.	To prevent injury.
	Be alert for complaint of pain over bony area; if patient has such a complaint, maintain bed rest until x-rays are taken for fracture.	To detect bone disease.
	Use assistive devices for ambulation.	To enhance tolerance of activity.
	Encourage range-of-motion exercises.	To maintain mobility.
	Position patient in proper anatomic alignment.	To avoid stretching, pressure, or fracture.
Altered cardiopulmonary tissue perfusion related to pneumonitis, pericarditis, myocarditis, anemia, and bleeding	Auscultate lungs, and report signs of pleural rub.	To detect respiratory problems early.
	Observe for cough, dyspnea, and pain on inspiration.	These indicate respiratory dysfunction.
	Treat with antibiotics and steroids as prescribed.	To reduce irritation and prevent infection.
	Auscultate heart, and report signs of friction rub, dysrhythmia, or hypertension.	To detect complications.
	Observe for chest pain and weakness.	These indicate cardiac dysfunction.
	Monitor ECG reports.	To monitor cardiac function.
	Administer drugs as prescribed.	To counteract dysrhythmias.
	Encourage adequate rest; alternate rest and activity periods.	To avoid stress on respiratory system.
	Observe patient for dyspnea and increased weakness.	These are signs of further anemia.

NURSING DIAGNOSIS	NURSING INTERVENTIONS	RATIONALE
	Administer oxygen therapy as needed.	To increase oxygenation of tissues.
	Monitor hemoglobin and hematocrit.	To determine effectiveness of therapy.
	Administer transfusions as ordered.	To increase circulating red blood cells.
Ineffective individual coping related to stress of dealing with chemotherapy	Assess patient's coping behavior, and determine its effectiveness.	To detect need for new coping strategies.
	Reassure patient that mood changes are temporary and dose related.	To reduce anxiety regarding mood changes.
	Allow independence in self-care.	To maintain patient's self-esteem and promote effective coping.
	Maintain supportive, nonjudgmental attitude.	To foster patient coping.
	Encourage use of resources, such as support groups.	To assist patient in coping.
	Encourage patient to express fears.	To identify problem-solving strategies.
Knowledge deficit	See Patient Teaching.	

5 EVALUATE

PATIENT OUTCOME	DATA INDICATING THAT OUTCOME IS REACHED
Patient has adequate hydration.	Patient has no nausea or vomiting, intake and output are balanced, patient's weight is normal, and electrolytes are within normal limits.
Patient has normal bowel elimination.	Patient has no constipation, diarrhea, or distention.
Patient's oral mucous membranes are healthy.	Mucous membranes, lips, tongue, and gingiva are moist and normal in color; patient's teeth are clean, and saliva is adequate; patient can swallow and speaks in a normal voice.
Patient's nutrition is adequate.	Patient has no complaints of anorexia or unusual taste sensations; patient can eat and swallow without pain, and weight is normal.
Patient has healthy, intact skin.	Patient has no complaints of itching, and there is no evidence of rash or changes in pigmentation; patient has hair on head.
Patient has adequate gas exchange and peripheral tissue perfusion.	Patient has no complaints of fatigue or weakness, and skin is warm and pink; respirations, pulse, blood pressure, and ECG are normal; there are no signs or symptoms of bleeding or cardiac dysfunction.

➤ ➤ ➤

PATIENT OUTCOME	DATA INDICATING THAT OUTCOME IS REACHED
Patient has no infection.	Patient's temperature and WBC are normal; skin is cool and dry.
Patient has normal sexual function.	Patient has satisfactory libido and has made plans for dealing with possible sterility.
Patient has normal urinary elimination.	Patient has no complaints of urinary distress, and intake and output are balanced.
Patient has normal hearing and sense of touch.	Patient can hear speaker and is aware of sensations on body.
Patient has normal physical mobility.	Patient can ambulate without assistance.
Patient can cope with stress of therapy.	Patient discusses fears, anger, and sadness but focuses on problem solving.

PATIENT TEACHING

1. Encourage the patient to maintain adequate nutrition and hydration.
2. Emphasize the need for self-care to control nausea, vomiting, constipation, diarrhea, urinary distress, oral irritation, and itching, which may include appropriate use of medications (see Patient Teaching Guide).
3. Discuss the warning signs of bleeding that should be reported to the physician, as well as safety measures (see Patient Teaching Guide).
4. Emphasize the need to take temperature, use good hand-washing techniques, identify and report signs of infection, and avoid exposure to infected individuals (see Patient Teaching Guide).

Biologic Response Modifiers

Biologic response modifiers is the term used to describe therapy with immunologic agents as well as other substances derived from biologic sources. Immunotherapies can be classified as active or passive. Active immunotherapies attempt to induce in the patient a state of immune responsiveness to a tumor. This responsiveness may be specific or nonspecific. Passive immunotherapies transfer directly to the patient immunologically active agents that mediate an antitumor response themselves. This responsiveness may also be specific or nonspecific (Table 14-3).

The rationale for using biologic response modifiers to treat cancer is based on animal studies and clinical observations such as the following:

1. After surgery patients often are found to have malignant cells in circulating blood and in operative wound washings but may never be diagnosed as having cancer.
2. Among transplant patients who receive immunosuppressant therapy, cancer occurs at a rate at least 80 times that of the general population.

Table 14-3 _____

IMMUNOLOGIC TREATMENT OF CANCER

Active immunotherapy
Specific
Inactivated tumor vaccines (autologous, allogeneic)
Human tumor hybrids (with xenogeneic antigen bearing fusion partners)
Monoclonal tumor antiidiotypic antibodies

Nonspecific
Chemical immunostimulants—levamisole, picabanyl, cimetidine, lysosomes containing macrophage-activating substances
Biological immunostimulants—BCG, MER, cyclophosphamide, *C. parvum*, OK432, etc.
Cytokines—interferon, IL-2, tumor necrosis factor
Chemotherapy—cyclophosphamide, melphalan, cisplatin, doxorubicin, vinca alkaloids

Passive (adoptive) immunotherapy
Specific
Heterologous antiserum—from immunized human
Monoclonal antibodies—murine, human, chimeric
    Biologic—via opsonization, complement fixation, or antibody-dependent cellular cytotoxic mechanisms (direct or antibody heteroconjugates)
    Radiotherapeutic—coupled to alpha- or gamma-emitting radionuclides
    Chemotherapeutic—adriamycin, methotrexate, diphtheria or ricin conjugates
T lymphocytes—autologous, allogeneic, xenogeneic
    From in vitro sensitization
    From tumor-draining lymph nodes
    From TILs
Monoclonal lymphocytes—from any of the sources listed above under T lymphocytes
Allogeneic bone marrow transplants with ablative chemotherapy or radiation therapy (graft versus tumor)

Nonspecific
LAK cells—generated by IL-2, IL-4 (?)
Activated macrophages—interferon, phorbol esters
Cytostatic or cytotoxic cytokines—interferons alpha, beta, and gamma; TNF

From Lotze and Rosenberg.[41]
Key: BCG, bacillus Calmette-Guérin; MER, methanol extracted residue of BCG; IL-4, interleukin-4; TILs, tumor-infiltrating lymphocytes; LAK, lymphokine-activated killer; IL-2, interleukin-2; TNF, tumor necrosis factor.

3. Rapidly progressive, recurrent cancer sometimes appears 10 to 20 years after an apparent cure.
4. Patients with congenital or acquired immunologic deficiencies have a greater incidence of cancer than does the general population.
5. Individuals with faulty immune systems cannot be sensitized to certain chemicals and thus are classified as anergic; an anergic patient usually has a rapidly growing tumor and a poor prognosis.

NONSPECIFIC ACTIVE IMMUNOTHERAPY

One group of nonspecific, active immunologic agents is the cytokines, which include interferon, interleukin-2 (IL-2), and tumor necrosis factor. Interferon is subdivided into three major species—alpha (derived from leukocytes), beta (derived from fibroblasts), and gamma (immune- or lymphocyte-derived). Interferons have been observed to inhibit viral replication and may have a direct antiproliferative effect on the tumor. This effect may be augmentation or induction of host-effector mechanisms such as natural killer cell activity or induction of membrane antigens on tumor cells, which produces immune recognition. The tumors most responsive to interferon are hematologic, including non-Hodgkin's lymphomas, cutaneous T-cell lymphoma, and chronic myelogenous and hairy cell leukemias.

Lymphokines such as interleukin-1 (IL-1) and interleukin-2 (IL-2) cause T-cell proliferation, activation of the lytic mechanisms of lymphokine-activated killer (LAK) cells, emigration of lymphoid cells from the peripheral blood, and the release of other lymphokines such as tumor necrosis factor (TNF), and interferon-gamma, and other hormones, such as adrenocorticotropic hormone (ACTH), cortisol, and growth hormone. Toxicity is a major deterrent to the use of interleukin-2; the patient may experience chills and fever, nausea and vomiting, diarrhea, cutaneous erythema, weight gain, anemia, hypotension, tachycardia, and hepatic and renal dysfunction. Interleukin-2 has demonstrated responses in renal cell cancer and malignant melanoma.

NONSPECIFIC PASSIVE IMMUNOTHERAPY

The nonspecific, passive immunologic agents include the cytokines and lymphokine-activated killer (LAK) cells. LAK cells—for example, natural killer cells—lyse the tumor.

SPECIFIC ACTIVE IMMUNOTHERAPY

Many attempts have been made since the early 1960s to immunize patients with their own tumors or with similar ones from other persons. Most of the studies that have been reported were empirical, with little evidence of a specific immune response. Because researchers have not been able to induce a response to specific agents, apparently because of the host's inability to respond to his own tumor, the focus has more recently been on increasing the immunogenicity of human tumors—that is, nonspecific active immunotherapy.

SPECIFIC PASSIVE IMMUNOTHERAPY

Monoclonal antibodies are the result of the genetic fusing of cancer cells with leukocytes to produce specific antibodies, which provide passive immunity and serve as carriers of cytotoxic agents to malignant cells. For example, they are being labeled with such isotopes as iodine-131 (^{131}I) to seek occult tumor deposits throughout the body. Monoclonal antibodies may also activate complement, a stage in the immune response that eventually leads to cell death.

Supportive Care

BLOOD TRANSFUSIONS

Infusion of blood may be lifesaving for the patient with cancer, whose blood loss may be caused by the disease, surgical intervention, bone marrow suppression during chemotherapy or radiation therapy, or an oncologic emergency, such as disseminated intravascular clotting. The transfusion immediately increases the body's ability to receive oxygen and transmit it to the cells, thereby avoiding severe and sometimes irreversible tissue damage. Contraindications and cautions for the use of blood are as follows:

1. Blood to be transfused must be checked by at least two care providers to prevent infusion of mismatched blood, which causes a severe hemolytic reaction characterized by chills and fever, tachycardia, nausea and vomiting, hematuria or oliguria, headache, backache, dyspnea, cyanosis, and chest pain. If such a reaction occurs, the transfusion should be discontinued immediately, the remaining blood and a sample of the patient's blood sent to the laboratory for repeat type and cross-match, and intravenous fluids, oxygen, and such drugs as vasopressor agents, epinephrine, sedatives, and mannitol administered.

2. Contaminated blood can cause a bacterial reaction; thus the nurse must observe the patient for fever, chills, lumbar pain, headache, malaise, bloody vomitus, diarrhea, or red shock (skin warm, dry, and pink); if these occur, the transfusion should be discontinued immediately, the remaining blood and a sample of the patient's blood sent to the laboratory for repeat type and cross-match, and intravenous fluids, cooling measures, and medications such as vasopressors, steroids, broad-spectrum antibiotics, analgesics, and antiemetics administered.

3. Allergic reactions can occur, although their cause is unknown; the signs and symptoms vary from mild edema and hives to bronchial wheezing or anaphylaxis; if a mild reaction occurs, the nurse should slow the rate of transfusion; if the reaction is severe, the nurse should stop the transfusion, administer intravenous fluids, give medications such as a bronchodilator or epinephrine, and provide oxygen therapy.

4. Too rapid an infusion or too great a quantity of blood can result in circulatory overload, particu-

larly if the patient has concurrent renal or cardiac disease. The signs and symptoms include cough; dyspnea; tachycardia; hemoptysis; frothy, pink-tinged sputum; and distended neck veins. If these occur, the nurse should slow the rate of transfusion, notify the physician, give digitalis as ordered to enhance cardiac output, prepare for venisection or rotating tourniquets, and monitor vital signs.

Blood component therapy, which is the transfusion of a specific part of the blood rather than whole blood, conserves precious resources, allows for treatment of specific problems such as thrombocytopenia and anemia, and is the best method for patients who require numerous transfusions of a specific blood component. The most frequently used blood components in individuals with cancer are packed red blood cells to treat anemia and platelets to prevent hemorrhage. The use of granulocyte concentrates is controversial and expensive and carries the possibility of numerous recipient complications. However, this therapy may be of value to the neutropenic patient with a diagnosed infection that is unresponsive to antibiotic management. Plasma products are used to treat such coagulopathies as disseminated intravascular clotting (DIC) or liver failure.

The nurse must have a sound knowledge of modern transfusion principles, since it is the nurse who administers and monitors the procedure, identifies adverse reactions, and provides immediate intervention.

COLONY-STIMULATING FACTORS

One of the most exciting and promising developments of recent years in the area of supportive care has been the identification and use of hematopoietic colony-stimulating factors (CSFs). It is believed that colony-stimulating factors could ameliorate or even eliminate the major hazards of treatment, including neutropenia and thrombocytopenia. Colony-stimulating factors are involved in all aspects of hematopoiesis, including proliferation, differentiation, maturation, and functional activation. They may be categorized by the number of blood cell lines affected (e.g., multilineage, such as interleukin-3 and hemopoietin-1, or single lineage, such as erythropoietin) or by biologic function.

The major endogenous human colony-stimulating factors are produced in the hematopoietic microenvironment of the bone marrow by T lymphocytes, monocytes/macrophages, endothelial cells, and fibroblasts. Each colony-stimulating factor binds to and activates its unique, high-affinity protein receptor on the surface membrane of target cells. Receptors for G-CSF are found predominantly on the mature elements of the neutrophil line; receptors for GM-CSF are found pre-

dominantly among early cells. M-CSF receptors predominate on the more mature cells of the monocyte/macrophage series.

Both G-CSF and GM-CSF sustain the viability and potentiate the functions of neutrophils. GM-CSF also stimulates production of such cytokines as tumor necrosis factor and interleukin-1. M-CSF enhances monocyte production of colony-stimulating activity, interferon, and tumor necrosis factor. Interleukin-3 may regulate the functions of mature eosinophils and monocytes.

Colony-stimulating factors have been studied in leukopenic individuals with acquired immunodeficiency syndrome (AIDS), cancer patients receiving chemotherapy, and bone marrow transplant patients. Side effects of CSF therapy include fatigue, fever, myalgias, loss of appetite, transient bone pain, rash, edema, and weight gain.

Nursing management of patients receiving CSF therapy includes pretreatment assessment, patient and family education, monitoring for side effects and toxicities, and implementing specific instructions that depend on the treatment protocol.

NUTRITIONAL SUPPORT

Patients with cancer must deal not only with the metabolic effects of the disease on their nutritional status but also with the effects of treatment. In addition, being unable to eat or having difficulty eating may affect the patient psychologically, since eating is not only a basic human need but often a source of social interaction. Patients with cancer who have anorexia, nausea and vomiting, stomatitis, changes in taste, and difficulty swallowing face the challenge of eating when they least want or are able to do so, yet have the greatest need for good nutrition. Numerous research studies have shown that poor nutritional status adversely affects the patient's ability to tolerate both cancer and its treatment.

The body of an individual with cancer responds to the increased demand for glucose, which is required by both normal and cancer cells, by increasing the rate of gluconeogenesis. This is the synthesis of glucose by the liver and renal cortex from noncarbohydrate sources such as lactate and amino acids. When protein is broken down to provide amino acids for gluconeogenesis, muscle wasting is the result. Progressive muscle wasting, called cachexia, gives the patient a characteristic appearance of emaciation.

Fat metabolization is also adversely affected in individuals with cancer. Fat stored in the form of fatty acids is mobilized from adipose tissue and released into the bloodstream for use as fuel. This process, which is controlled by the inhibitory effects of insulin, is compromised in people with cancer, so that body stores of fat are depleted as the disease progresses.

People with cancer also have deficiencies in such vitamins as A, thiamine, and C. Iron deficiency may also occur. Fluid and electrolyte imbalances include hypercalcemia, hyperuricemia, hyperphosphatemia, and hyperkalemia. These alterations result from either the direct or indirect effects of tumors, such as paraneoplastic syndromes (see Chapter 4).

Poor nutrition also adversely affects immunocompetence, by decreasing the size of the lymphoid tissues, including the spleen, lymph nodes, and thymus. The resulting decreased function of B- and T-cell lymphocytes, directly correlated with the degree of malnutrition, produces delayed hypersensitivity response.

Local effects of cancer, such as tumors that adversely affect chewing, swallowing, and peristalsis, can alter the patient's nutritional status. Obstruction, pain, and distention affect the patient's ability to digest and metabolize food.

As discussed earlier, the treatment modalities (surgery, chemotherapy, radiation therapy, and the biologic response modifiers) also compromise the patient's nutritional status. Thus the nurse must assess the patient's nutritional status frequently to obtain a baseline measure and to identify the need for aggressive intervention. Clinical observation, including identification of concurrent health problems (diabetes, hypertension, malabsorption), psychosocial factors (home environment, methods of food preparation, the patient's body image), and physical assessment provide the data needed to monitor the patient's nutritional status. Examining the hair, teeth, gums, and general muscle tone can facilitate detection of early signs of nutritional deficiencies.

Dietary evaluation is also useful and includes a 24-hour food diary, a complete dietary history with food allergies and preferences, direct observation of dietary intake, and evaluation of nutrient composition. Biochemical measurements include such laboratory values as serum albumin, serum transferrin, total lymphocyte count, and urine urea nitrogen. Anthropometric measurements include the patient's midarm muscle circumference (MAMC), triceps skin fold thickness (SFT), subscapular skin fold thickness (SST), and weight for height.

Nutritional interventions for the person with cancer have been shown to decrease the morbidity and mortality of cancer by preventing weight loss, increasing response to therapy, minimizing the side effects of treatment, and improving the quality of life. The type of nutritional support the patient requires is based on functional abilities and limitations, severity of the nutritional deficiency, potential for complications, duration of therapy, cost, and psychologic effect.

Nutritional support may include oral, enteral, and parenteral nutritional management. The oral route is preferred, because it is more natural and least invasive. Oral nutritional support may range from adding sauces and gravies to foods to more complex interventions such as dietary supplements. The patient with anorexia may benefit from frequent small meals and snacks. Foods high in protein and calories are recommended, such as cheese, fish, poultry, milkshakes, peanut butter on crackers, and prepackaged puddings.

If the patient has stomatitis or taste alterations, a high-calorie bland diet may be helpful. The patient should avoid seasoning and liquids with high acidity such as orange and lemon juices. Measures such as using a topical analgesic, good mouth care, and avoiding commercial mouthwashes reduce oral discomfort. Cold foods such as popsicles and ice cream have a numbing effect, which patients tolerate better than warm or hot foods.

Psychosocial support is also critical. Both the patient and family should be encouraged to try a variety of strategies and to be supportive of one another, since this is a difficult and challenging problem. Sometimes eating at the table with family and friends in an attractive sociable environment can enhance the patient's appetite. Using small plates, eating more often, and decreasing exposure to strong food odors may also be helpful. Antiemetics and artificial saliva can be used to control the symptoms of gastrointestinal irritation.

High-calorie, high-protein supplements such as Isocal, Polycose, and Vivonex may be helpful to the patient; however, they are not well tolerated by patients with lactose intolerance.

The enteral route via a feeding tube may be needed by patients who are anorectic, hypermetabolic, or unconscious, as well as those who have a mechanical impairment. Parenteral feeding is indicated only for patients with totally nonfunctioning gastrointestinal tracts, who require bowel rest, or who cannot tolerate enteral nutritional support.

Patients with functioning gastrointestinal tracts who cannot ingest adequate nutrients to meet their metabolic demands should be considered for enteral feeding. These include patients with anorexia; cachexia; cancers of the head or neck, esophagus, and stomach; central nervous system disease that impairs swallowing; and intractable diarrhea.

Tube feedings may be administered by the nasogastric, nasoduodenal, nasojejunal, esophagostomy, gastrostomy, and jejunostomy routes (Figure 14-8). The most common routes involve passage of a small, flexible feeding tube through the nose into the stomach or intestine. Feeding ostomies, such as the gastrostomy, usually require surgical percutaneous insertion and are preferred for long-term nutritional support. The cervical esophagostomy is a surgically created, skin-lined ca-

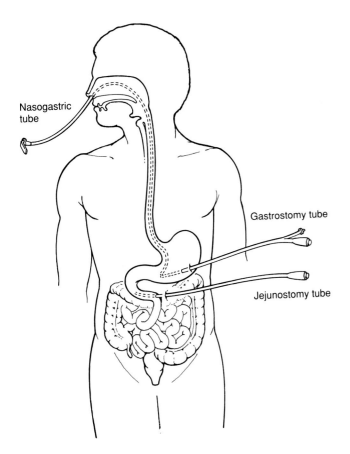

Nasogastric tube

Gastrostomy tube

Jejunostomy tube

FIGURE 14-8
Three routes for tube feeding. (From Otto.[48])

nal extending from the border of the neck to the area below the cervical esophagus; the feeding tube is passed through this opening to the stomach for each feeding and then removed.

Aspiration may occur more often with gastric feedings, because only the gastroesophageal sphincter is functioning to prevent gastric reflux, whereas the intestinal feedings use both the gastroesophageal and pyloric sphincters to prevent reflux. When feedings are improperly selected or administered, nausea, diarrhea, and cramps can occur.

The volume and concentration of the nutriment provided by tube feeding should meet the needs of the individual and should be compatible with the size and location of the tube and the patient's tolerance of formula strength and rate of administration. Feedings may be delivered by bolus or gravity, as well as by enteral pump. The position of the tube and gastric residual should be checked frequently. The patient should be monitored for the development of dumping syndrome, aspiration, weight loss, or diarrhea, each of which re-

quires evaluation of the formula and infusion rate for changes.

The patient may also complain of thirst, taste deprivation, and inability to satisfy the appetite, as well as a sense of altered body image. The patient may be permitted to chew gum or suck on hard candies, drink fluids, and eat soft, bland foods. Referral to a support group may help the patient accept the changes in the social and aesthetic aspects of eating.

Complications of tube feedings may be mechanical (nasal irritation and erosion, esophagitis or pharyngitis, tube dislocation or occlusion), gastrointestinal (abdominal distention, nausea and vomiting, constipation, or diarrhea), respiratory (aspiration pneumonia), or metabolic (hyperglycemia, hypokalemia, hyperkalemia, hypernatremia, and dehydration). The nurse and patient should monitor the feedings to identify problems early and intervene before serious alterations occur. Since many patients now receive enteral feedings in the home, a caregiver and the patient should be taught general care of the patient and the tube to ensure safe and effective therapy.

Parenteral nutrition, also called hyperalimentation, supplies all of the essential nutrients by intravenous infusion. Total parenteral nutrition (TPN) supplies all of the daily requirements for protein and calories directly into the patient's bloodstream; it is indicated for patients with cancer of the gastrointestinal tract, other obstructions, radiation enteritis, and intractable diarrhea, to name but a few conditions.

Total parenteral nutrition is delivered via peripheral veins, most often those of the arm or the external jugular vein. Limitations of peripheral infusion include provision of limited calories, vein irritation, and limited usefulness for long-term therapy. Use of a central line into a major vein such as the superior vena cava provides for a large amount of calories and protein, high dextrose and amino acid concentrations, and usefulness for long-term therapy. Central lines used for total parenteral nutrition include ports, triple lumen catheters, and Broviac, Hickman, and Groshong catheters. When central infusion is used, the solution must be tapered by rate and concentration to discontinue therapy without inducing profound hypoglycemia.

Total parenteral nutrition contains glucose, amino acids, and fats to provide both immediate and long-term energy. Patients receiving total parenteral nutrition usually have a multilumen central venous catheter inserted to serve as access for administering medications and drawing blood.

Total parenteral nutrition may be given continuously or by cycling; cycling at night is used most often for patients receiving TPN at home. Cycling enables the patient to be mobile during the day but does require the ability to tolerate a high-volume load. Programmable pumps are used to prevent or minimize hypoglycemia and hyperglycemia. Ambulatory patients benefit from using the portable pump, which is worn in a backpack-type carrying bag.

The nurse should assess the patient's life-style, home environment, family and support systems, body image, and perceptions about total parenteral nutrition to plan for optimum acceptance of and adaptation to the therapy. Daily monitoring of vital signs, weight, and laboratory values enables the nurse to determine the need for adjusting the formula or rate of administration before the patient's discharge. Follow-up visits in the home are important and ensure the patient's compliance with and tolerance of TPN.

The nurse's role in nutritional support is a critical one that involves comprehensive assessment, monitoring, and patient education to maintain the individual with cancer in optimum nutritional status.

PAIN MANAGEMENT

Patients with cancer may have pain at any point during the course of their disease and its treatment. In fact, of the 4 million people throughout the world who die from cancer each year, 70% experience pain as a primary symptom. Unfortunately, many people believe that pain is an early symptom of cancer and do not seek diagnosis until pain occurs. Pain is almost without exception a late symptom of cancer and indicates tumor obstruction, pressure on nerves, invasion of bone, phantom sensation, peripheral neuropathy, postherpetic neuralgia, mucositis, and/or incisional irritation.

It is estimated that 85% of patients with cancer pain can be managed effectively with appropriate therapy. The American Cancer Society, the American Pain Society, the World Health Organization, and the Oncology Nursing Society, as well as many other organizations, consider pain control to be a major issue in the management of a person with cancer. If not relieved, pain contributes to nausea, vomiting, anorexia, and insomnia. Anxiety, fear, and depression contribute to this pain and interfere with the patient's ability to cope with it.

One of many challenges facing the nurse who cares for the patient with pain is the assessment of the pain. The nurse must accept the definition of pain as whatever the person experiencing the pain says it is, existing wherever the person says it does.[42] This is frustrating to many nurses and physicians, who may doubt the presence and nature of the patient's pain when there are no physiologic parameters by which to measure it. Because there are no direct measures of pain, the nurse must gather data from the patient for use in diagnosing the pain, describing its characteristics, and deciding on the appropriate interventions.

A pain history gathered from the patient should include the following data:

Onset of the pain (when it started)
Precipitating factors (what triggers the pain)
Alleviating factors (what lessens the pain)
Location of the pain
Associated signs and symptoms
Medications taken by the patient and the extent to which they provide relief
Quality and intensity of the pain
Patient's view of the pain
Actions that have helped or not helped to relieve the pain

In addition, the nurse should use observational skills to assess the patient's appearance, motor behavior, affective behavior, verbal behavior, brainstem automatic responses (e.g., increase in heart rate, respirations, and blood pressure), spinal cord reflex responses, and nonverbal pain clues. The psychosocial dimensions of the pain must also be explored. These include personality factors, cultural factors, religious factors, the patient's interpretation of pain, the patient's prior experience with pain, and the physical environment in which the patient is experiencing the pain.

General guidelines for the use of pain relief measures are:

1. Use a variety of pain relief measures.
2. Use pain relief measures before the patient's pain becomes severe.
3. Include pain relief measures that the patient believes will be helpful.
4. Determine the patient's ability or willingness to participate actively in the use of pain relief measures.
5. Rely on patient behavior that indicates pain severity rather than relying on known physical stimuli.
6. Encourage the patient to try a pain relief measure at least two times before abandoning it as ineffective.
7. Have an open mind as to what may relieve the patient's pain, including nonpharmacologic measures.
8. Keep trying to relieve the pain; do not become discouraged and stop working with the patient.

Chemical means of pain management include the use of narcotics and nonnarcotics. Nonnarcotic analgesics of value in the treatment of cancer pain are acetaminophen, aspirin, and nonsteroidal antiinflammatory drugs such as ibuprofen, indomethacin, and naproxen. One potential drawback of aspirin is its antiplatelet effect, which can create problems in the myelosuppressed patient. Acetaminophen may be a problem in patients with impaired liver function. Both aspirin and the nonsteroidal antiinflammatory drugs are generally well tolerated but have the potential to cause gastrointestinal ulceration, renal toxic effects, and inhibition of platelet aggregation. If a nonnarcotic does not have a therapeutic effect initially, then the dosage should be increased before another type of drug is tried. When a ceiling is reached with a nonnarcotic, a moderately potent narcotic such as oxycodone or codeine can be added. Some individuals with cancer require such a combination from the start of treatment.

Narcotics (opioids) used in the management of cancer pain include morphine (the prototype), hydromorphone, and methadone. Sustained-release morphine in an oral form, such as MS Contin or Roxanol SR, has been found to be of particular value in the management of the terminally ill person with pain. Administering narcotics via intravenous drips, intrathecally, and epidurally enhances the analgesic effect of the opioids. Avoiding the peaks and valleys of pain relief with bolus injections has provided a more constant analgesic effect for patients with cancer pain. The need for around-the-clock dosage has been noted, so that fixed dosage schedules with adequate doses for pain relief provide more constant blood levels and predictable pain relief. Some patients have breakthrough pain that requires additional doses, but the fixed dosage schedule should be maintained. Side effects of the narcotics that require monitoring and intervention by the nurse include constipation, vomiting, and respiratory and central nervous system depression.

Another category of drugs that may be used for pain management is the narcotic agonist/antagonists such as nalbuphine (Nubain), butorphanol (Stadol), pentazocine (Talwin), and buprenorphine (Buprenex). Analgesic potentiators include the phenothiazine derivatives such as promethazine (Phenergan), prochlorperazine (Compazine), and chlorpromazine (Thorazine); hydroxyzine (Vistaril); diazepam (Valium), lorazepam (Ativan); and diphenhydramine (Benadryl). Also used are stimulants such as cocaine, methylphenidate (Ritalin), dextroamphetamine, and caffeine; tricyclic antidepressants such as amitriptyline (Elavil), imipramine (Tofranil), and doxepin (Sinequan); and butyrophenones such as droperidol (Inapsine) and haloperidol (Haldol).

Patient self-control methods include distraction, massage, relaxation, biofeedback, hypnosis, and imagery (see Patient Teaching Guide). Many patients respond positively to the opportunity for self-care in the management of their pain and perceive that such self-control measures enhance the effectiveness of other prescribed pain interventions.

Pain technology includes using the following:

1. External pumps for the intravenous, epidural, and intrathecal administration of narcotic analgesics
2. Implantable pumps for the intravenous, epidural, and intrathecal administration of narcotic analgesics
3. Patient-controlled analgesia, particularly for the management of acute pain such as postoperative pain
4. Transcutaneous electrical nerve stimulation (TENS)
5. Continuous subcutaneous infusion (CSCI) with an ambulatory infusion pump

In each instance the nurse must develop the technical skill needed to initiate and monitor the therapy and to teach the patient and family how to use and maintain the system. Each of these technologies has expanded the options for the patient with pain and increased the degree of self-control.

Other interventions for pain include (1) anesthetic procedures such as nerve blocks, trigger point injections, and the use of nitrous oxide; (2) neuroaugmentive therapies such as counterirritation, rubbing, TENS, and percutaneous nerve stimulation; (3) neuroablative procedures such as cordotomy; and (4) physiatric supportive measures such as using a prosthesis, physical therapy, and occupational therapy.

The nurse's unique contributions to pain management are acting as key link between the patient and the health care team, the amount of time spent with the patient, the ability to assess the patient's response to the pain and its management, and the role of patient and family educator. In addition, the nurse has the ability to articulate a concise pain assessment, use equianalgesic charts for dosage guidelines, and anticipate and address patient, family, and health care provider misconceptions about pain management. For example, many patients and their families have opioid phobia, the irrational and undocumented fear that even appropriate use of narcotics causes addiction. This fear of addiction among both health care providers and the public seems to be a major reason for the undertreatment of pain. The nurse must understand and be able to articulate the differences between addiction, tolerance, and physical dependence in order to use pain management strategies appropriately and to enable patients and their families to accept the therapeutic value of drugs such as the narcotics.

CHAPTER 15

Patient Teaching Guides

Patient education has always been an important part of the nursing process. In today's hospitals, teaching patients about their disease and its treatment poses a great challenge as diagnostic and treatment methods become increasingly complex. Hospitalized patients often are confronted by an array of threatening-looking equipment, and many procedures are based on technology that is unfamiliar to the general public. Compounding these problems is the shortened hospital stay for most patients.

Written materials can help patients understand their treatments and what they must do to manage at home. This chapter provides handouts that can be photocopied and given to patients or their caregivers to take home and use for self-care. Specific materials that explain intraperitoneal chemotherapy or skin care during external radiation are used by nurses who care for these special patients. Some of the guides list step-by-step instructions for certain procedures.

More than one guide may be needed for a particular patient. For example, a patient undergoing chemotherapy will need to know how to deal with loss of appetite, how to prevent infection and bleeding, and how to manage pain without drugs. Guides that explain preventive measures are also included.

Mosby's
Clinical Nursin
Series

Prevention, Screening, and Early Detection

The number of people who develop cancer is on the rise—it is estimated that one in three Americans will have some type of cancer. Some of these cancers can be cured in the early stages, but not when the disease is too advanced. Early detection and treatment are the keys to curing cancer; preventing cancer in the first place is even better.

General prevention guidelines

There is much you can do to help prevent cancer. Smoking has been scientifically proven to cause cancer, so if you smoke, stop. What you eat can also have an effect on whether you develop cancer. The following are dietary recommendations for preventing cancer:

Reduce the amount of fat in your diet to 30% of your total daily calorie intake.

Limit the amount of alcohol you drink to one or two drinks a day.

Limit the amount of charbroiled, smoked, and salted foods you eat.

Maintain your ideal weight.

Eat foods high in:

Vitamin A—apricots, peaches, carrots, spinach, asparagus, squash, and sweet potatoes

Vitamin C—oranges, lemons, grapefruit, strawberries, tomatoes, cabbage, and walnuts

Vitamin E—lettuce, alfalfa, and vegetable oils

Fiber—fresh vegetables and fruits, whole grain breads and cereals, nuts, beans, and peas

Prevention, screening, and early detection guidelines for common cancers

Breast Cancer. Reduce the amount of fat in your diet. Any one or a combination of these signs may be a warning signal for cancer: a lump in the breast; dimpling of the skin; a sinking in of the nipple, or discharge from the nipple; swelling in the breast; or a change in the size or shape of the breast. Early detection includes breast self-examination once a month (see pages 238-239); a yearly breast examination by a health care provider; a baseline mammogram between the ages of 35 and 39; and a yearly mammogram after age 40. If you have a family history of breast cancer, you should start having mammograms at age 30.

Cervical Cancer. Avoid sex at an early age (especially before age 18), and don't have numerous partners. Use condoms, and practice good perineal hygiene. Cancer warning signs include abnormal vaginal bleeding and spotting after having sex. Early detection involves an annual Pap smear for women over age 18. After at least three normal examinations, the test can be done less often.

Colon/Rectal Cancer. Follow the dietary guidelines listed above. Have colorectal polyps removed. Cancer warning signs include rectal bleeding, a change in stools, pain in the abdomen, and pressure on the rectum. Early detection includes an annual digital rectal examination starting at age 40; an annual stool blood test starting at age 50; and an annual inspection of the colon with a special instrument (sigmoidoscopy) starting at age 50.

Endometrial Cancer. Follow the dietary guidelines listed above. Discuss with your doctor the benefits and risks of estrogen therapy if you are past menopause. Cancer warning signs include abnormal vaginal bleeding and pain or a mass in the abdomen. Early detection includes pelvic examinations and endometrial biopsy at menopause and in high-risk women.

Head and Neck Cancer. Follow the dietary guidelines listed above. Avoid tobacco in all forms. Practice good oral hygiene. Cancer warning signs include difficulty chewing; a persistent sore throat; hoarseness; a color change in the mouth; earache; a lump in the neck; loss of sense of smell; and difficulty breathing. Early detection includes monthly oral self-examination and an annual physical exam.

Lung Cancer. Do not smoke. Follow guidelines at work to reduce exposure to cancer-causing substances. Warning signs include a persistent cough or cold; pain in the chest; wheezing; difficulty breathing; and a change in the volume or odor of phlegm. No tests exist for early detection.

Prostate Cancer. There are no prevention guidelines for prostate cancer. Warning signs include difficulty urinating, painful and frequent urination, and blood in the urine. Early detection includes an annual digital rectal exam starting at age 40.

Skin Cancer. Use a sunscreen with a sun protection factor (SPF) of at least 15 (the SPF is shown on the bottle), and wear protective clothing when in the sun. Avoid tanning booths. Cancer warning signs include a change in a wart or mole, and a sore that does not heal. Early detection includes an annual physical examination, monthly self-examination of the skin, and paying particular attention to moles, warts, and birthmarks.

Testicular Cancer. No prevention guidelines exist for testicular cancer. Cancer warning signs include swelling, a lump, or a heavy feeling in the testicle. Early detection includes an annual physical exam and monthly testicular self-exam.

Breast Self-Examination

Performing breast self-examination once a month could save your life. Many breast cancers are discovered by patients who had regularly done self-exam and thus were able to distinguish a change from what is normal in their breasts. If you are still menstruating, examine your breasts right after your period ends. If you have reached menopause, pick a day of the month that is easy to remember.

How to do breast self-examination

1. Undress and stand in front of a mirror with your arms at your sides. Look for any changes in the shape or size of your breasts or anything unusual, such as discharge from the nipples or puckering or dimpling of the skin (Figure 1).
2. Raise your arms above and behind your head, and press your hands together. Look for the same things as in step 1 (Figure 2).
3. Place the palms of your hands firmly on your hips; look again for any changes (Figure 3).
4. Raise your left arm over your head. Examine your left breast by firmly pressing the fingers of your right hand down and around in a circular motion until you have examined every part of the breast. You may use the wedge section, circular, or vertical strip examination method (page 239). Be sure to include the area between your breast and armpit and the armpit itself. You are feeling for any lump or mass under the skin. If you find a lump, notify your doctor (Figure 4).
5. Gently squeeze the nipple, and look for any discharge. If there is any, see your doctor (Figure 5).
6. Repeat steps 4 and 5 on your right breast. (You may also perform steps 4 and 5 in the shower.)
7. Now, lie down on your back with a pillow under your right shoulder. Put your right arm over your head. This position flattens the breast and makes it easier to examine. Examine your right breast just as you did in steps 4 and 5. Repeat on your left breast (Figure 6).

Don't panic if you notice anything unusual. This doesn't necessarily mean you have cancer. Notify your doctor and let him or her examine you. *Remember: Breast self-examination is important, but it is not a substitute for a doctor's examination and regular mammograms for women over age 35.*

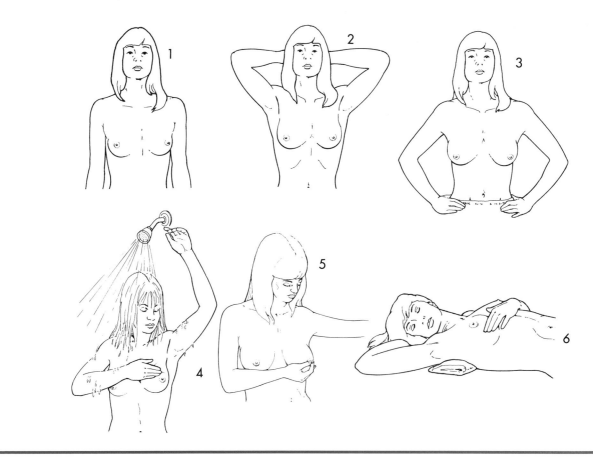

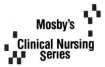
Different Methods for Breast Self-Examination

One important aspect of breast self-examination is the method you use to examine your breasts. Three methods have been developed—the circular method, the wedge method, and the vertical strip method—that are believed to be equally effective, as long as every part of the breast is checked. You may want to try each of them and then choose the one you find easiest and most comfortable.

Wedge method

Place the flat surface of the middle three fingers against the outer edge of the breast. Press gently from the outer edge in a straight line toward the nipple. Move your fingers in parallel lines around the breast until each area is covered. Then squeeze the nipple.

Circular method

Place the flat surface of your middle three fingers against the outer edge of the breast. Press gently in small, circular motions around the breast. Move your fingers in smaller circles around the breast until you reach the nipple (try not to lift your fingers off the breast as you move from one point to another). Then squeeze the nipple.

Vertical strip method

Place the flat surface of the middle three fingers against the top outer edge of the breast. Press gently from the top outer edge down to the bottom edge. Continue up and down until you reach the inner aspect of the breast. Then squeeze the nipple.

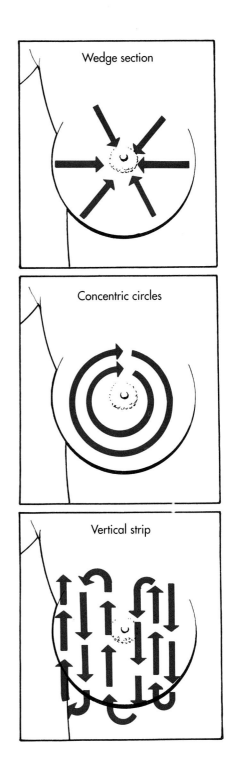

Wedge section

Concentric circles

Vertical strip

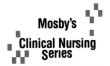

Mosby's
Clinical Nursing
Series

Testicular Self-Examination

Testicular cancer is a curable disease if discovered and treated early. Performing testicular self-examination (TSE) once a month greatly increases the chances that you will discover a cancerous lump or mass early enough for effective treatment.

When you do TSE you should be looking for hard nodules or lumps in the testes. Testes that are enlarged may also indicate a cancerous condition, and any enlargement or swelling that doesn't respond to antibiotics should be investigated further.

How to do testicular self-examination

It is best to do TSE after a warm bath or shower, when the scrotal skin is loose and relaxed. Use both hands during the examination.

1. Lift your penis with your left hand. With the right hand, locate the epididymis, the cordlike structure at the back of your right testicle.

Feel along it with your thumb and first two fingers. The epididymis extends upward into the spermatic cord. Squeeze along the length of this cord, feeling for lumps and masses as you progress upward.

2. To examine the right testicle, place your right thumb on the front of the testicle and your first two fingers behind it. Gently press your fingers and thumb together until they meet. Check the entire testicle in this manner.

3. Repeat steps 1 and 2 with the left testicle, using the left hand.

Normal testicles should feel firm to the touch, but you should be able to move them. They should feel smooth and rubbery and should be free of lumps. If you notice any lumps or masses or anything unusual, call your doctor.

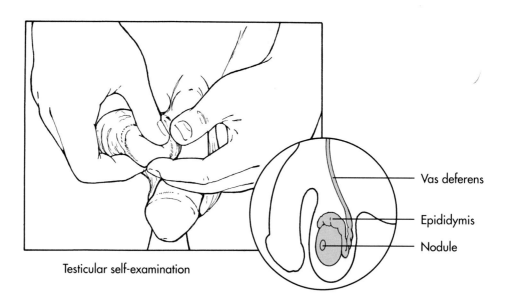

Testicular self-examination

Vas deferens

Epididymis

Nodule

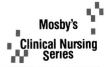
Skin Self-Examination

The number of cases of skin cancer is on the rise. Steps for preventing skin cancer include wearing a sunscreen with a high sun protection factor (SPF 15 or higher); staying out of the midday sun, if possible; and performing a monthly skin self-examination.

Examining your skin once a month can help you detect any moles, blemishes, or birthmarks that have changed in size, shape, or color, or a sore that doesn't heal. If you find any of these signs, see your doctor at once.

How to do skin self-examination

You will need a hand mirror and a full-length mirror to examine yourself.

1. Using a full-length mirror, examine the front and back of your body. Then raise your arms and examine the sides of your body (Figure 1).
2. Check the skin under your forearms and upper arms and on the palms of your hands.
3. Sit down and look at the backs of your legs. Examine your feet, including the soles and between your toes (Figure 2).
4. Examine the back of your neck and your scalp with a hand mirror (Figure 3).

Examining your skin once a month will help you familiarize yourself with the normal appearance of your skin. It is also a good idea to visit a dermatologist once a year for a thorough skin examination.

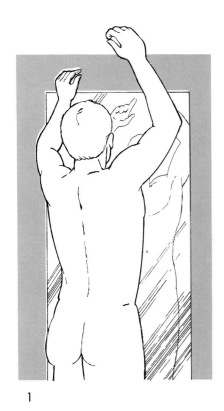

1

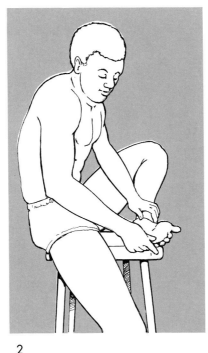

2

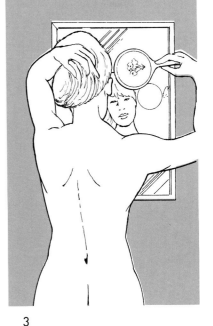

3

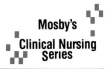
Vulvar Self-Examination

Cancer of the vulva is still a rare disease, but it is occurring more frequently. Women over age 50 are most susceptible to this cancer, but it can occur at any age. Examining your vulvar area once a month can help you discover the first symptoms of vulvar cancer, which can be cured if treated early. The vulvar area includes all the female external genital organs: the pubic mound, clitoris, urinary opening, vaginal opening, and anus (Figure 1).

How to do vulvar self-examination

Use a flashlight and a hand mirror to make viewing easier. You may do the examination while sitting on the edge of the toilet seat, your bed, or the bathtub. Sit with your legs spread apart, and check the entire vulvar region (Figure 2).

Examine both sides of the labia (the opening folds of the vulva), and see if they are similar.

With your fingers, separate the inner lips of the vulva, and check the clitoris, the urinary opening, the vagina, and the skin between the vagina and anus (Figure 3).

Press down on all areas of the vulva, feeling for any lumps or masses (Figure 4).

Gently squeeze the vaginal opening between your thumb and forefinger. It should feel soft and moist (not be tender or sore) (Figure 5).

If you see any of the following, see your doctor:

Lumps, masses, or growths

Any change in skin color

Moles or birthmarks on the vulva that change color, bleed, or enlarge

Burning in the vulva during urination

Persistent itching

Soreness or tenderness that doesn't go away

Usually these signs don't indicate cancer, but check with your doctor to make sure.

What causes vulvar cancer, and what can I do to prevent it?

It is unclear what causes cancer in the vulvar area, but certain conditions are thought to lead to the disease. These include poor hygiene, certain types of sexually transmitted diseases, cancer of other reproductive organs, and a condition called dystrophy, in which the skin of the vulva may thin or thicken, and red or white patches and sores may appear. You can help prevent some of these problems by seeing your gynecologist at least once a year, reporting any changes you find during your vulvar self-examination, and practicing good hygiene. Good hygiene of the vulva includes the following:

Wiping from front to back after urination or a bowel movement

Avoiding scented and perfumed products such as tampons, sanitary pads, feminine hygiene products, and scented soaps

Using unscented, white toilet paper

Wearing all-cotton underwear

Avoiding tight clothing such as girdles, pantyhose, and form-fitting jeans

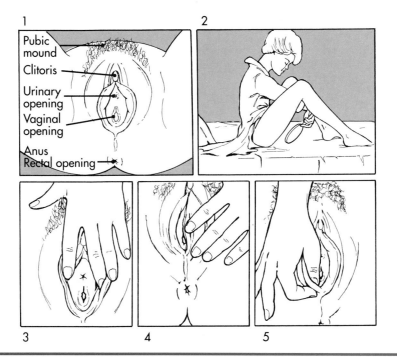

1
Pubic mound
Clitoris
Urinary opening
Vaginal opening
Anus
Rectal opening

2

3   4   5

Care of the Hickman-Broviac External Venous Catheter

An external venous catheter is a convenient way to deliver medications, including drugs for chemotherapy, and to take the many blood samples needed without having to insert a needle into your vein. The catheter is a soft, plastic tube that is implanted in your chest. One end of the tube is placed in a large vein close to your heart; the other end stays outside your body. The catheter has a cap that can be removed when blood samples are needed or drugs for chemotherapy must be given.

You will need to follow three procedures to care for your external venous catheter: changing the dressing, changing the cap, and flushing the catheter. Follow the procedures carefully to prevent infection and clotting of the tube.

Changing the dressing

You must change the dressing on your catheter frequently (at least every other day) until the wound site has healed. (After the site has healed, your doctor may allow you to clean around the wound site with soap and water while you shower; then dry the area and apply a small gauze pad or adhesive bandage to the exit site.)

Assemble the following equipment:
Hydrogen peroxide
Small container to pour hydrogen peroxide in
Alcohol wipes
Antibiotic ointment
Dressing
Tape
Cotton-tipped ear swabs

1. Wash your hands.
2. Remove old dressing and wash hands again.
3. Pour the hydrogen peroxide into the container, and dip a cotton swab into the hydrogen peroxide. Starting at the wound site and using a circular motion, clean the skin around the wound site, working your way out. Use a new cotton swab whenever you need more hydrogen peroxide.
4. Clean the length of the catheter with an alcohol wipe.
5. Apply antibiotic ointment to the wound site with a cotton swab.
6. Tape a new dressing over the wound site.

Changing the catheter cap

Catheter caps should be changed every 7 days.
Assemble the following equipment:
Catheter cap
Catheter clamp
Alcohol wipes

1. Wash your hands.

2. Clamp the catheter.
3. Unscrew the old cap. Wipe around the end of the catheter with alcohol wipes. Screw on a new cap. Unclamp the catheter.

Flushing the catheter

You need to flush your catheter as directed by the nurse (as often as once a day) to prevent blood clots from forming inside it.

Assemble the following equipment:
Vial of heparin-saline solution
Disposable syringe and needle
Alcohol wipes

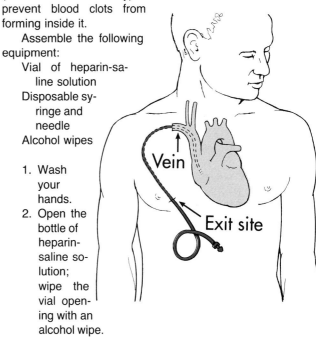

Vein

Exit site

1. Wash your hands.
2. Open the bottle of heparin-saline solution; wipe the vial opening with an alcohol wipe.
3. Remove the needle guard from the syringe, and pull back the plunger. Insert the needle into the vial, turn the vial upside down, and pull back on the syringe to fill it (tap on the side of the syringe to remove air bubbles).
4. Clean the catheter cap with an alcohol wipe. Insert the needle into the cap, and push down on the plunger to inject the solution into the catheter.
5. Remove the needle and carefully discard it and the syringe.

Catheter maintenance

Be sure to buy a catheter repair kit to use when a leak occurs. If the catheter continues to leak despite your repairs, call your physician or nurse.

Call your doctor or nurse if:

Pain, redness, or puffiness develops around the catheter site.
You notice drainage from the catheter site.
Your temperature is above 100° F.
The catheter slips.
There is blood in the catheter.
You are unable to flush the catheter.

Mosby's
**Clinical Nursing
Series**

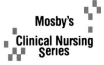

Care of the Implanted Port

An implanted port is a convenient way to deliver medications, including drugs for chemotherapy, and to take the many blood samples needed without damaging your veins. The implanted port consists of a soft, plastic catheter that is placed in a large vein close to your heart and a port with a metal base and rubber top through which medications will be administered and blood will be drawn. The implanted port is surgically placed in your chest or abdomen, and there are no external parts.

Because an implanted port is completely under the skin, it doesn't require a lot of care. You must watch for signs of infection, protect the needle during ambulatory infusion pump treatments, and prevent the skin over the port from becoming irritated.

Watching for signs of infection

Call your doctor if:

Redness, pain, or puffiness develops around the port.

You notice drainage from the incision site.

Your temperature is above 100° F.

You become short of breath.

You have chest pain.

Protecting the needle during infusion

Sometimes you may need to receive treatments over an extended period. For these occasions, a bent needle (Huber needle) is inserted into the port and connected to an ambulatory infusion pump. The needle is left in the port until the treatment is finished, sometimes for several days. The pump is attached to your body by a belt or pouch and is worn for the duration of the treatment.

During this time you will need to prevent the needle from becoming dislodged. A dressing will be taped over the needle, and you must check it to make sure the tape is holding the dressing and the needle hasn't slipped. You may need to change this dressing periodically.

Protecting the skin over the port

It is important that you prevent irritation of the skin over and around the port. Do not wear any bra straps or clothing that may rub the port site. Adjust your seat belt if it rubs the port site.

Unless you are receiving an infusion, you may shower, bathe, and swim without worry. When receiving an infusion, you need to keep the site dry and protected.

Changing the drug reservoir bag

If you are receiving treatment over several days, you may be taught to change the drug reservoir bag. Directions for changing the bag vary with the type of pump. Your nurse will provide you with a diagram and complete instructions.

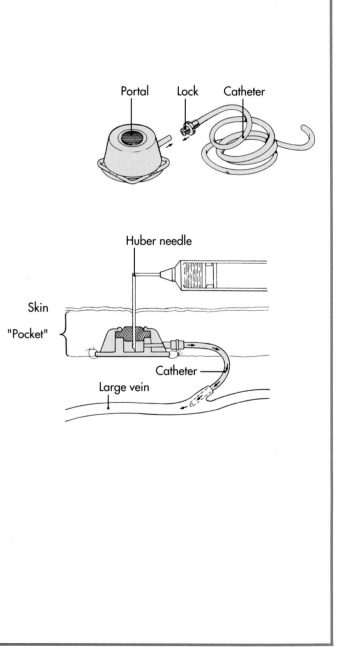

Intraperitoneal Chemotherapy

Intraperitoneal chemotherapy is used to treat cancers of the abdomen, such as ovarian cancer. This therapy involves delivering cancer-fighting drugs directly to the abdomen, where they can kill cancer cells more effectively. Intraperitoneal chemotherapy reduces the number of side effects usually encountered with conventional intravenous chemotherapy.

How intraperitoneal chemotherapy is given

You will be admitted to the hospital a few hours before your treatment is to begin. The treatment takes several hours to complete, and you will probably be hospitalized for a few days afterward.

The drugs for intraperitoneal chemotherapy are delivered into your abdomen by an *implanted port* or by an *external semipermanent catheter*. The implanted port is surgically placed in the abdomen and has no external parts or catheters. When it is time for a chemotherapy treatment, a needle is inserted into your abdomen and into the implanted port. After the treatment, the needle is removed.

The external semipermanent catheter is also surgically placed in the abdomen, but part of the catheter remains above the skin and is used to deliver the chemotherapy solution into the abdomen. No needles are needed. Be careful to keep the catheter capped at all times so that bacteria and germs can't get into your abdomen through the catheter.

Whether you have the implanted port or the external semipermanent catheter, the chemotherapy treatment is the same. The chemotherapy drugs are mixed with 2 quarts of solution, which is slowly infused into the abdominal cavity. You will also receive extra intravenous fluids and other medications through a vein in your arm or leg.

You will have a feeling of fullness as the solution infuses and your abdomen expands to accommodate the excess liquid. It may be difficult to take a deep breath, because the expanded abdomen is pushing on the lungs. It may help to raise the head of your bed or prop yourself up on pillows.

Depending on your treatment, the chemotherapy solution may later be drained out of your abdomen or left to be absorbed slowly and flushed out of your body over time.

How to care for your catheter

If you have an implanted port, there is nothing you need to do. The device is totally under your skin, so you will not have any bandages to change. You may shower, bathe, or swim anytime.

If you have an external semipermanent catheter, you will need to put dressings on the catheter site to help prevent infection. You will be able to shower but not swim or bathe. If your catheter becomes dislodged, call your doctor.

Peritonitis

Patients who undergo intraperitoneal chemotherapy run a greater risk of developing peritonitis, an inflammation of the lining of the abdominal cavity. You must be able to recognize the signs and symptoms of peritonitis. Call your doctor immediately if you develop a fever over 101° F, abdominal pain, nausea or vomiting, persistent diarrhea, or soreness or redness around the catheter.

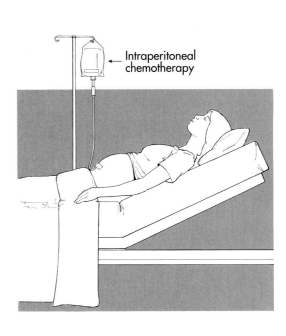

Intraperitoneal chemotherapy

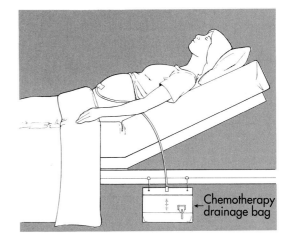

Chemotherapy drainage bag

Dealing with Loss of Appetite, Nausea and Vomiting, and Stomatitis

Loss of appetite, nausea and vomiting, and stomatitis are common symptoms of cancer and cancer treatment, although not everyone has them. There are a variety of ways to relieve nausea and vomiting and help increase appetite.

Loss of appetite

Loss of appetite can be a serious problem; it can lead to malnutrition and severe weight loss. When your body is trying to fight cancer, it needs nutrition. It needs enough protein and calories to function at its best, to give you energy, and to help reduce the effects of the cancer and its treatment.

Eating enough of the right kinds of foods can be difficult when you don't feel like eating at all. Here are some tips to help you increase your appetite:

Take a walk before mealtime. Mild exercise can stimulate your appetite.

Avoid drinking liquids before a meal, because they can fill you up. If you want to drink, then drink juices or milk—something nutritious.

Eat with family or friends if possible. If eating is a social event, it will seem less of a chore.

Eat a variety of foods. Spice up your food with herbs, spices, and sauces. Use butter, bacon bits, croutons, wine sauces, and marinades to provide taste-pleasing meals.

Don't fill up on salads or "diet" foods. Eat vegetables and fruits along with meats, poultry, and fish to make sure you get enough calories and nutrition.

Eat smaller meals more often, especially if you fill up before you've eaten all your dinner.

If you still are not getting enough calories or protein, your doctor may recommend dietary supplements that can be added to milk, soup, or pudding.

Nausea and vomiting

Nausea and vomiting are common side effects of chemotherapy and radiation therapy. Doctors frequently prescribe an *antiemetic* to combat this. The antiemetic usually is given a few hours before the treatment and then every 3 or 4 hours after the treatment for a day or two. It may take some experimenting with dosage and timing to come up with the best schedule for you.

The following are other remedies and preventive measures you can try to help prevent or alleviate nausea and vomiting:

Eat soda crackers and suck on sour candy balls throughout the day to relieve queasiness.

Choose cold or room-temperature foods instead of hot ones; hot and warm foods seem to cause nausea.

Avoid salty, fatty, and sweet foods or any food with strong odors—opt instead for bland, creamy foods such as cottage cheese, toast, and mashed potatoes.

Stay away from nauseating odors, sights, and sounds. Get as much fresh air as possible. A leisurely walk can help alleviate nausea.

Don't eat right before your cancer treatment. Eat lightly for a few hours after your treatment.

Try relaxation therapy, self-hypnosis, or imagery to alleviate nausea-inducing tension.

Distract yourself with a book, TV, or activity.

Sleep during episodes of nausea if possible.

If vomiting does occur, eat or drink nothing until your stomach has settled, usually a few hours after the last vomiting episode. Then begin sipping clear liquids or sucking on ice cubes. If you tolerate the liquids, you may begin eating bland foods a few hours after you started the liquids.

Stomatitis

Stomatitis is an inflammation of the lining of the mouth. It may occur 7 to 14 days after beginning chemotherapy or radiation therapy to the mouth, or earlier if other problems were already present. A dentist should assess the status of your mouth and teeth before you begin therapy.

Stomatitis often can be prevented or alleviated by using a soft toothbrush and rinsing with a solution of 1 pint of water with ½ teaspoon of salt and ½ teaspoon of baking soda after meals and at bedtime. Flossing with unwaxed floss, drinking water or nonacidic juices (e.g., apple or grape), eating artificially sweetened candy or gum, and using artificial saliva sprays for dry mouth can also help.

Watch for signs and symptoms of possible stomatitis: a burning feeling in the mouth; a red, irritated oral lining; a swollen, inflamed tongue; and sores in the mouth. Treatment is based on the extent and seriousness of the stomatitis; measures include rinsing with the solution described above; loosening thick mucus and crusted drainage with Milk of Magnesia, Maalox, or another antacid; and using an analgesic rinse before meals to lessen painful swallowing. If you have dentures, they should be worn only during meals. Avoid spicy, acidic, and crusty or rough foods and hot or cold foods and beverages.

Report signs of infection to your doctor: soft white patches; dry, brownish yellow areas; moist, creamy white areas; painless, dry, yellow ulcers with well-defined edges; or open areas on the lips or mouth.

Dealing with the Effects of Bone Marrow Suppression

Preventing infection

Cancer and cancer treatments impair a patient's immune system and leave the patient susceptible to infection. The most common sites of infection are the bladder and urinary tract, the skin, the lungs, and the blood. Infection is a serious problem, and you should do everything possible to prevent it by following the guidelines below:

Eat nutritious meals, drink plenty of fluids, get enough rest, and avoid stress as much as possible.

Keep your mouth, teeth, and gums clean. Use a soft toothbrush and salt-water rinse.

Wash your hands frequently with soap and water, especially before eating and after using the toilet.

Shower rather than take a bath.

Cleanse your perianal area after each bowel movement. Women should avoid bubble baths, douches, and feminine hygiene products such as tampons. Sanitary napkins should be changed frequently. Use a commercial lubricant during sexual intercourse. Urinate before and after intercourse.

Avoid the following:

People who are ill.

People vaccinated recently with a live virus.

Crowded places (waiting rooms, malls).

Raw fruits and vegetables, raw eggs, and raw milk; eat only cooked food and pasteurized milk and milk products.

All sources of stagnant water (water in flower vases, pitchers, denture cups, humidifiers, and respiratory equipment). Water in these containers should be changed daily.

Dog, cat, and bird feces. Let someone else change bird cages or litter boxes.

Even if you follow these guidelines carefully, an infection may occur. Call your doctor immediately if you develop any sign of infection:

Fever over 100° F

Redness, swelling, or pain around any wound

Coughing, sore throat, and stuffy or runny nose

Nausea, vomiting, or diarrhea

Chest pain or shortness of breath

Burning or frequency of urination, or a change in the color or odor of urine

Sores or white patches in the mouth

Even if your symptoms seem mild, they may indicate a life-threatening infection.

Preventing bleeding

Patients with cancer run a greater risk of bleeding from the skin and mucous membranes or internally. The bleeding results because the bone marrow is producing few or no platelets (special blood cells that cause the blood to clot), or because platelets already in the blood are being destroyed. Cancer itself, allergic reactions to medication, radiation therapy, or chemotherapy can cause this reduction in the number of platelets; the condition is called **thrombocytopenia.**

Because the lack of platelets makes bleeding hard to stop once it has begun, it is *very* important that patients with thrombocytopenia take great care to prevent bleeding. Check your skin each day for bruises, and call the doctor if any get larger after you first notice them.

To prevent bleeding from the skin:

Avoid physical activities that could cause injury.

Shave with an electric razor.

Keep your nails short. File rough edges.

If bleeding does occur, apply pressure to the site for 5 to 10 minutes and elevate. If the bleeding lasts longer than 5 minutes, call your doctor.

To prevent bleeding from the mucous membranes of the mouth, nose, gastrointestinal system, and genitourinary tract:

Brush with a soft toothbrush. If you still have trouble with bleeding gums, use sponge-tipped applicators or a Water-Pik. Do not floss. Keep your lips moist with petroleum jelly. Check with your doctor before having dental work.

Avoid hot foods that might burn your mouth.

Blow your nose gently. Humidify your house if the air is too dry, because dry air can cause nose bleeds. If your nose does bleed, pinch your nostrils shut for a few minutes. If the bleeding persists, put an ice bag on the back of your neck. Call your doctor if the bleeding does not stop.

Use stool softeners and drink plenty of water if you are constipated. No enemas or suppositories.

Take acetaminophen (e.g., Tylenol) or ibuprofen instead of aspirin. Aspirin can cause stomach bleeding.

Avoid douches and vaginal suppositories. Use a lubricating jelly before sexual intercourse.

To prevent internal bleeding:

Try to arrange furniture so you won't bruise yourself on it. Keep clutter off floors.

Avoid tight-fitting clothing and any buttons or ornaments that could bruise or chafe your skin.

Do not lift heavy objects.

Any bleeding that does not stop after 5 minutes should be reported to your doctor.

Preventing anemia

In anemia there are not enough red blood cells to carry oxygen to the cells and take away carbon dioxide. (With bone marrow suppression the marrow is producing fewer red blood cells.) You may tire easily and need to rest more often.

To lessen the effects of anemia:

Schedule activities with frequent rest periods.

Eat a diet high in protein. Take a multivitamin supplement with minerals.

Be alert for any of these signs: pallor, dizziness, ringing in the ears, chest pain, or shortness of breath. Report these problems to your doctor.

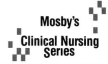

Managing Pain Without Drugs

There are several techniques you can use to relieve pain without taking drugs or to enhance the effect of your pain medication—**relaxation, imagery, distraction,** and **skin stimulation.**

Relaxation

Relaxation relieves pain by easing muscle tension. Easing muscle tension can also help you feel less tired and anxious and help other pain-relieving methods work better.

How to relax. Sit or lie down, preferably in a quiet place. Be sure you are comfortable. Do not cross your legs or arms.

Take a deep breath, and tense your muscles (you may tense up your whole body or concentrate on one set of muscles at a time, such as your facial muscles or those in your arms and hands).

Hold your breath, and keep your muscles tense.

Release your breath and your muscles at the same time. Let your body go limp (repeat for other muscle areas if you are concentrating on one set at a time).

You can add imagery (see below) or music to help you relax. Relaxation tapes are also available.

Don't be discouraged if relaxation doesn't help immediately. Practice the relaxation technique for 2 weeks before you give it up. If you find that it aggravates your pain, try another method.

Imagery

Imagery involves using your imagination to create mental scenes that use all your senses: sight, sound, touch, smell, and taste. You can imagine exotic locations or revisit one of your favorite places. You can create stories and characters to add to your scenes. Imagery can take your mind off your anxiety, boredom, and pain.

How to use imagery. Close your eyes. A few moments of the relaxation technique (see above) will help your body and mind prepare for imagery.

Let your mind begin forming its image. The following is an example of imagery:

Imagine that you are at the seashore. You are sitting in the wet sand; the afternoon sun is warm on your shoulders. The ocean rolls into the shore in gentle waves, and the water laps teasingly at your toes. A hungry pair of seagulls cry overhead and take swift, darting dives at a dog that is scavenging along the shore. Your tension lessens with each wave that touches your toes and retreats. You close your eyes and take a deep, slow breath of salt-filled air. You are completely relaxed. Stay on the beach as long as you like.

To end the image, count to three and open your eyes. Resume your regular activities slowly.

Distraction

A distraction is any activity that takes your mind off your pain and focuses your attention elsewhere. Doing crafts, reading a book, watching television, or listening to music through headphones can all help distract your mind. Distraction works well when you are waiting for drugs to take effect or if you have brief bouts of pain. Sometimes people can take their minds off their pain for long periods, especially if the pain is mild.

Skin stimulation

Skin stimulation is used to block pain sensation in the nerves. Pressure, massage, hot and cold applications, rubbing, and mild electrical current are all ways to stimulate the skin. However, if you are undergoing radiation treatment, consult your doctor before applying any skin stimulation.

You can do skin stimulation at the site of the pain, near it, or on the opposite side of pain. For example, stimulating the left wrist when the right wrist is in pain can actually ease the pain in the right wrist.

Pressure. Using your entire hand, the heel of your hand, your thumb, your knuckles, or both hands, apply at least 15 seconds of pressure at the point where you feel pain. Keep trying spots around the painful area if you find no relief the first time. You may extend the time you apply pressure to 1 minute.

Massage. You or someone else can perform the slow, circular motions of massage. The feet, back, neck, and scalp can be massaged to relieve tension and pain anywhere in the body. Some people prefer to use oils or lotions during the massage. If deep massage is too uncomfortable, try light stroking. Do not massage red, raw, or broken skin.

Heat and cold. Some people prefer cold; others prefer heat. Use whichever works best for you. A convenient way to use cold is to freeze gel-filled packs and wrap them in towels. Ice cubes can also be used. Heat can be applied with a heating pad; hot, moist towels; or a hot water bottle or by taking a hot bath. Be careful not to burn your skin with water that is too hot or to go to sleep with a heating pad on. Don't expose your skin to intense cold for very long.

Transcutaneous electrical nerve stimulation. TENS can be used to eliminate or ease pain. A TENS unit is a pocket-sized, battery-operated device that provides a mild, continuous electrical current through the skin by the use of two to four electrodes, which are taped onto the skin. Lead wires connect the electrodes to the device. It is this mild electrical current that blocks or modifies the pain messages and replaces them with a buzzing, tingling sensation. It is also thought that TENS may stimulate the body's production of endorphin, a natural pain reliever.

Skin Care During External Beam Radiation Therapy

Radiation therapy can cause mild to severe skin reactions. The severity of the reaction depends on how much radiation is given and how frequently, how much skin area is irradiated, and the type of radiation used. In the first 2 weeks of treatment, the skin being irradiated may turn pink or red, become sensitive to sun, lose hair, or develop a rash. As treatment progresses, a condition called dry desquamation may develop (i.e., the skin becomes dry, itchy, and flaky). Moist desquamation may then set in, and the skin may peel and become painful and weepy. Skin reactions are most noticeable 10 days to 2 weeks after therapy has been completed. Hair loss from irradiated scalp begins 10 days after the first treatment.

Preventing skin reactions

The following skin care guidelines may prevent reactions or lessen their severity:

Cleanse the skin with warm water, not hot. After washing, rinse with tepid water and pat dry with a soft towel. Do not soak in a tub. Do not remove the treatment field markings during bathing. Avoid soap as much as possible. If soap becomes necessary, use Aveeno, Dove, or some other mild, unscented soap that will not dry the skin.

Do not use heating pads, hot packs, or ice on the area.

Do not use perfumed or powdered products on the treated skin.

If necessary, use a light dusting of cornstarch to prevent itching and to eliminate moisture in neck creases, armpits, and beneath the breasts.

Do not use ointments or menthol rubs.

Shave with an electric razor.

Protect your skin from heat, cold, and sunlight. Use a sunscreen with a sun protection factor (SPF) of 15 or higher (the SPF is shown on the bottle). Shield your face and neck with a scarf or wide-brimmed hat.

Wear loose-fitting clothing. Tight clothing and belts rub and chafe already sensitive skin.

Do not put adhesive bandages (e.g., Band-Aids) on irradiated skin.

Treating skin reactions

If your skin is dry, ask your doctor or nurse to recommend a lotion to apply. For dry desquamation you may be encouraged to use pure aloe vera gel, vitamin A and D ointments (e.g., Desitin), Lubriderm, or other water-soluble, nonirritating substances.

For moist desquamation you may be allowed to apply cool compresses moistened with water or normal saline. Sometimes a special ointment is prescribed. You may be taught to apply moisture-vapor–permeable film or other sterile dressings (e.g., OpSite, Tegaderm) to the area to protect it while it heals. Moist desquamation usually resolves 1 to 2 weeks after treatment ends. If you have pain, your doctor may suggest that you take an over-the-counter analgesic such as aspirin, acetaminophen (e.g., Tylenol), or ibuprofen (e.g., Motrin).

Even after your skin heals, it may still be sensitive to heat, cold, and sunlight. Some chemotherapeutic agents cause "radiation recall," which is a reappearance of the previous skin reaction, usually seen as redness.

If hair loss is likely to occur, select scarves, hats, wigs, or hairpieces before the loss begins. This loss usually is temporary, but this depends on the dose of radiation received, the patient's sex and age, and whether adjuvant chemotherapy was used.

Care of a Fecal Ostomy

An ostomy is a temporary or permanent opening into the bowel that allows fecal material to be expelled at the skin's surface. The opening onto the skin is called a stoma.

An ostomy requires special attention, including diet and skin care. You also need to know how to empty, remove, and apply the ostomy pouches. The type of ostomy you have may require special care; your nurse will give you additional information if you need it.

Diet and odor

Avoid gas-producing foods such as broccoli, cabbage, beans, onions, and radishes. To help prevent odor, also avoid eggs, cheese, and alcohol. Drinking cranberry juice or buttermilk and eating yogurt can help prevent odor. If you have an ileostomy, you may need to buy products such as odor-absorbing tablets to place in the ostomy bag or a commercial gas-release valve.

If blockage of the stoma is a problem, avoid high-fiber foods such as celery, lettuce, nuts, and corn. If diarrhea occurs, avoid highly spiced foods and raw fruits and vegetables.

Most foods can be eaten in reasonable amounts if you eat slowly and chew well.

Skin care

The skin around the ostomy pouch should be inspected daily for signs of irritation or infection. Each time the pouch is changed, the skin should be cleaned with soap and water. A skin barrier should be applied to the clean, dry skin before the new pouch is attached. It is recommended that you put a pectin-based wafer in the pouch. If a rash occurs, use a heat lamp or hair dryer to dry the skin. Sprinkle a small amount of powder (e.g., Karaya, Stomahesive) on the skin, wipe off the excess, and then blot with a skin sealant to seal the powder to the skin. Powder the skin after the pouch has been applied.

Emptying a fecal ostomy pouch

When your ostomy pouch is about one-third full, you will need to empty it.

1. Sit on the toilet with the pouch between your legs, or sit on a chair with the pouch opening in the toilet.

2. While holding up the end of the pouch, remove the clamp and let the contents of the pouch drain into the toilet. Putting some toilet paper on the surface of the water will help prevent splashing.
3. Squeeze the remaining contents out of the pouch.
4. Hold up the end of the pouch, and pour a cup of water into the pouch through the opening. Swish the water around to clean out the inside of the pouch. Do not get the stoma or the seal around the stoma wet. Empty the water into the toilet.
5. Use toilet paper to clean around the opening of the pouch. Clamp the pouch shut again.

Removing an ostomy pouch

You will need to change your ostomy pouch every 5 to 7 days. Gather the following equipment before you begin: adhesive solvent, gauze pads, powder (if desired), towel, and scissors.

1. While standing, hold the skin around the stoma taut and begin peeling off the adhesive square that holds the pouch to your skin. Peeling from top to bottom works best. If you can't peel it off, use adhesive solvent to loosen edges.
2. Wipe excess drainage around stoma with gauze pads.
3. Wash the area around the stoma with soap and water. Dry thoroughly. Apply powder if the skin is irritated. You may also want to apply a skin barrier.

Applying an ostomy pouch

1. Peel back the paper from the adhesive faceplate. Center the pouch opening over the stoma, and press all around the faceplate to ensure that it is firmly attached to the skin. Attach the belt if you like.
2. Press the air out of the pouch. Clamp the bottom.

Continent ileostomy (Kock pouch)

You may have a continent ileostomy, which is an internal pouch constructed of ileum and a nipple valve, which helps you control your stool and flatus. The stoma is flush with your skin. To remove stool and flatus, you place a large-bore tube into the stoma several times a day.

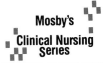
Care of a Urinary Diversion

The most common type of urinary diversion is the ileal conduit, in which a segment of small bowel is used as a passage (conduit) for urine to the skin's surface. The segment is closed at one end, and the other end is brought to the abdominal surface to form a stoma. The ureters are attached internally so that urine drains through the ileal conduit and out through the stoma. Other urinary diversions include a colon conduit (the sigmoid colon is used), ureterostomy (the ureters are brought through the abdominal wall to form stomas), or vesicotomy (an opening in the bladder).

Applying an ostomy pouch

1. Peel back the paper from the adhesive faceplate. Center the pouch opening over the stoma, and press all around the faceplate to ensure that it is firmly attached to the skin. Attach the belt for additional security if you desire.
2. Press the air out of the pouch. Clamp the bottom.

Removing an ostomy pouch

You will need to change your ostomy pouch every 5 to 7 days. Gather the following equipment before you begin:
Adhesive solvent
Gauze pads
Powder (if desired)
Towel
Scissors

1. While standing, hold the skin around the stoma taut and begin peeling off the adhesive square that holds the pouch to your skin. Peeling from top to bottom works best. If you cannot peel it off, use adhesive solvent to loosen the edges.
2. Wipe away excess drainage from around the stoma with gauze pads.
3. Wash the area around the stoma with soap and water. Dry thoroughly. Apply powder if the skin is irritated. You may also want to apply a skin barrier.

Collecting urine for culture and sensitivity

The nurse or physician will remove the external pouch and insert a sterile catheter into the stoma to collect a sterile specimen.

Special aspects of care

Use a skin barrier or liquid film to protect the skin from irritation.

Drink at least eight glasses of water a day.

Test your urine's pH regularly, using a freshly voided specimen before a meal. The pH should be 4.5 to 8. (Test sticks are available at drugstores.) Vitamin C works well for maintaining an acid urine. Odor may indicate an alkaline urine, which can cause stones to form, or a urinary tract infection.

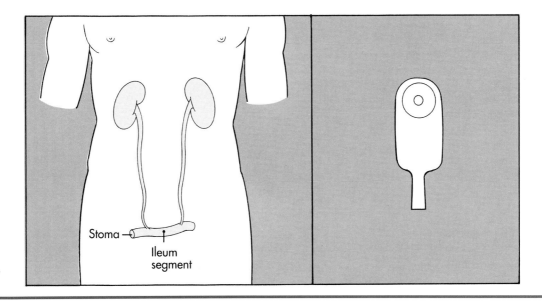

Stoma
Ileum segment

Bone Marrow Harvest

One of the newer treatments for some cancers and metabolic and immunologic diseases is **bone marrow transplantation.** Bone marrow transplantation has the potential to cure patients with these otherwise fatal diseases.

The patient's bone marrow is first destroyed by high doses of chemotherapy or radiation and then replaced with healthy bone marrow donated by a family member or the patient herself. The transplanted bone marrow begins making new blood cells within 10 to 14 days after the transplant.

How bone marrow is harvested

Whether a family member or the patient, the bone marrow donor must understand the process of harvesting bone marrow. The following is a step-by-step description of this procedure.

Preparation. Before the bone marrow harvest even begins, you will have gone through a series of blood tests to make sure your bone marrow matches the recipient's. (If you are donating your own marrow, there is no problem with matching.) You will also undergo a physical examination, a chest x-ray, an electrocardiogram, and urinalysis to ensure that you are in good health. The evening before the harvest, you will take a shower with an antiseptic solution. You will not be allowed to eat or drink after midnight.

The day of the procedure. The morning of the harvest, a nurse will come to your room and insert an intravenous line (IV) into your arm. Just before you are taken to the operating room, the nurse will give you a shot to help you relax and make you drowsy.

A team consisting of doctors, nurses, and an anesthesiologist will be waiting in the operating room. The anesthesiologist will give you a drug through your IV to make you sleep.

The bone marrow will be harvested from your hip. The doctor will insert a needle several times into the rear portion of your hip bones and withdraw a total of 1 to 2 quarts of bone marrow and blood. (You will receive a blood transfusion to make up for the loss of blood.) A pressure dressing will be applied over the harvest sites to help prevent bleeding. The entire harvest procedure takes about 2 to 3 hours.

After the procedure. You will wake up in the recovery room after the anesthetic has worn off. A nurse will check on you every 15 minutes to record your vital signs (pulse, blood pressure, temperature, and respirations) and make sure that you are not bleeding from the harvest sites.

While you recover, the bone marrow that you donated will be filtered to remove fat and bone particles. If the marrow is for your future use, it will be frozen until you are ready for it. If it is for someone else, it will be immediately given to that person through an IV transfusion.

Within a day you will be able to eat solid food and begin walking around. The pressure dressing will be removed, but you will have to keep the harvest sites clean and covered with a bandage for 3 days. If you have pain, your doctor can prescribe medication to relieve it.

You will be able to leave the hospital after 1 or 2 days. You should be able to resume your normal activities soon after.

If you have any questions before or after the bone marrow harvest, don't hesitate to ask your doctor or nurse.

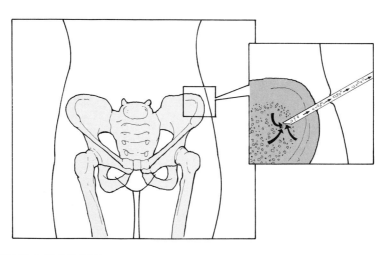

Clinical Trials—What Are They?

Research studies that use patients are called clinical trials. As a person with cancer, you may be asked to help evaluate a new treatment.

What are clinical trials?

When a new cancer treatment becomes available, it must first go through rigorous testing in a laboratory and then in a clinical setting. The testing is carefully monitored, and the results are evaluated and published in medical journals, where other researchers and clinicians further evaluate the data.

There are three types of clinical trials: phase I trials, phase II trials, and phase III trials. Each of these trials is a carefully controlled, highly ethical human experiment designed to test a new drug or procedure that could cure or halt the spread of a cancer. The drug or procedure usually is tested in all three phases before it can be accepted as a treatment.

Phase I trials determine the best way to provide a new treatment and how much can be given safely. These trials involve cancer patients with advanced disease who have tried every possible treatment with no long-term success. These patients are willing to undergo treatments that probably will not cure their cancer but that give them some hope and that might help a cancer patient in the future. Any treatment given these patients has first undergone testing on animals and has been approved for human trials.

Phase II trials study the effect of a new treatment on patients whose cancer has not been cured by standard treatments. There is some possibility that the treatment may benefit these patients. A treatment reaching phase II trials has gone through phase I trials.

Phase III trials compare a new treatment to current treatments. These trials require large numbers of patients to control the effects that age, race, gender, and other factors may have on the experimental treatment.

One group of patients receives the experimental treatment, and another is given a standard treatment. Randomization (selection by chance to be in one group or the other) is used to keep bias out of the trial.

Informed consent

Informed consent means that you have been given the information you need to decide whether to participate in a clinical trial. This information includes what is involved, possible benefits and risks, the length of the study, the cost (if any), and how your anonymity and the confidentiality of your participation will be protected. Ask any questions you have. Then, if you wish to be a part of the study, you can sign the form. You can refuse to participate or withdraw from the study at any time without penalty.

Should you participate in a trial?

Those who participate in clinical trials have the opportunity to receive the latest in cancer treatments or a new, experimental treatment that could be even more effective. In fact, according to published studies, patients who participate in trials often have a better survival rate.

You and your doctor should discuss the possibility of your participating in a clinical trial. If you are interested, your doctor should be aware of the different trials being conducted so he or she can recommend the best one for you. Many patients benefit both physically and mentally from participating in clinical trials.

For more information, write to the Office of Cancer Communications, National Cancer Institute, Bethesda, Maryland 20205, or call the Cancer Information Service at 1-800-4-CANCER. Ask for *What Are Clinical Trials? A Booklet for Patients with Cancer.*

CHAPTER 16

Pharmacologic Management

The pharmacology of antineoplastic agents is complex. Most of the useful chemotherapeutic agents appear to exert a blocking effect on enzymes or enzyme systems involved in DNA synthesis or function. Therefore cells that are actively dividing are the most vulnerable. Most of the drugs available are not tumor specific and act on biochemical pathways common to both normal and neoplastic cells.

The growth cycle of both normal and malignant cells consists of four phases (Figure 1-4, page 6). Metaphase, or the M phase, is the time during which one cell divides into two identical daughter cells. Mitosis is followed by the G_1, or postmitotic, phase; the S, or synthetic, phase, during which DNA replication occurs; and the G_2, or premitotic, phase. Distinct biochemical events are occurring during each of these phases. Cells not actively dividing are in the G_0, or resting, phase; however, they can be recruited into the growth cycle by various means.

Antineoplastic agents can be categorized in two ways: by general mechanism of action and by relationship of antineoplastic activity to cell life cycle. Agents whose antineoplastic activity occurs during a specific cell life cycle phase are said to be cell cycle–specific, or cycle phase–specific. Agents whose antineoplastic activity is independent of a specific cell life cycle phase are said to be cell cycle–nonspecific, or cycle phase–nonspecific.

Cell cycle–specific agents are generally most effective against tumors in which a high proportion of cells are proliferating (e.g., hematologic cancers). Cell cycle–nonspecific agents are additionally effective against "solid tumors," in which a low proportion of cells are proliferating. The usefulness of this classification, however, is limited by the facts that some agents have more than one mechanism of action, and the precise mechanism of action of others is unknown. Biologic response modifiers, for example, cannot be classified by relationship of antineoplastic activity to cell life cycle. This is because their action is something other than blockage of a biochemical pathway and their exact mechanisms of action or sites of action are not clearly understood.

Chemotherapy, surgery, radiation, and treatment with biologic response modifiers are the treatment modalities currently used for cancer. Each modality or combination of modalities has specific indications. For example, chemotherapy may be the primary method of treatment for certain cancers; for other types of cancer, it may be used in addition to surgery and/or radiation therapy.

GENERAL NURSING CONSIDERATIONS FOR ANTINEOPLASTIC DRUGS

Although chemotherapeutic agents may have a slight degree of specificity for rapidly dividing malignant cells, normal cells that also proliferate rapidly (e.g., bone marrow, gastrointestinal epithelium, skin, hair follicles, germinal epithelium, and embryonic tissue) are at cytotoxic risk. This nonspecific cytotoxicity accounts for many of the common serious adverse effects caused by antineoplastic drugs, such as bone marrow depression, ulceration of the gastrointestinal tract, stomatitis, alopecia, infertility, and teratogenicity.

Bone marrow depression is the most common dose-limiting toxicity of chemotherapy. It consists of leukopenia, thrombocytopenia, and/or anemia. The patient's blood counts should be monitored at regular intervals during therapy. As the white blood cells approach their nadir, the patient becomes susceptible to opportunistic infections. Signs and symptoms of this are sore throat, fever, malaise, and sore mouth. With thrombocytopenia the patient will bruise or bleed easily. Precautions such as using an electric razor to shave, avoiding intramuscular injections, and gentle oral hygiene are important. Anemia causes fatigue.

Mouth care is of the utmost importance. Document the condition of the oral cavity and correct any oral

Table 16-1

SUMMARY OF ANTINEOPLASTIC DRUGS

Generic name	Trade name	Synomyn or abbreviation	Administration*
Asparaginase	Elspar	ASP	IM, IV, slow IVP
Bleomycin	Blenoxane	Bleo	IM, SC, IV
Busulfan	Myleran	—	PO
Carboplatin	Paraplatin	—	IV
Carmustine	BiCNU	BCNU	IV
Chlorambucil	Leukeran	CMB	PO
Cisplatin	Platinol	Cis-Pt, CDDP	IV
Cyclophosphamide	Cytoxan	CTX	PO, IV
Cytarabine	Cytosar	ARA-C	IT, SC, IV, IVP
Dacarbazine	DTIC-Dome	DTIC	IV
Dactinomycin	Cosmegen	Actinomycin D	IV, slow IVP
Daunorubicin	Cerubidine	NDR	IV, slow IV
Doxorubicin	Adriamycin	Adria, Dox	IV, slow IVP
Etoposide	VePesid	VP-16	PO, IV
Floxuridine	FUDR	—	IA
Fluorouracil	Adrucil	5FU	PO, IV, IVP
Hydroxyurea	Hydrea	—	PO
Ifosfamide	IFEX	—	IV
Levamisole	Ergamisol	—	PO
Lomustine	CeeNU	CCNU	PO
Mechlorethamine	Mustargen	Nitrogen mustard, NH(2)	Slow IVP
Melphalan	Alkeran	L-PAM, phenylalanine	PO
Mercaptopurine	Purinethol	6-MP	PO
Methotrexate	Mexate, Folex	MTX	PO, IM, IT, IV, IVP
Mitomycin	Mutamycin	Mitomycin C	IV, slow IVP
Plicamycin	Mithracin	—	IV
Procarbazine	Matulane	—	PO
Streptozocin	Zanosar	—	IA, IV, slow IVP
Tamoxifen	Nolvadex	—	PO
Thioguanine	Thioguanine	6-TG	PO
Thiotepa	Thiotepa	TEPA	IV, IM, intracavity
Vinblastine	Velban	VLB	IV, slow IVP
Vincristine	Oncovin	VCR	IV, slow IVP

*IA, intraarterial; IM, intramuscular; IT, intrathecal; IV, intravenous; IVP, intravenous push; PO, oral; SC, subcutaneous.

Table 16-2

CLASSIFICATION OF CYTOTOXIC DRUGS

Cell cycle–specific agents (CCS)		Cell cycle–nonspecific agents (CCNS)	
Asparaginase	Mercaptopurine	Bleomycin*	Daunorubicin
Cytarabine	Methotrexate	Busulfan	Doxorubicin*
Etoposide	Thioguanine	Chlorambucil	Mechlorethamine
Fluorouracil*	Vinblastine	Cisplatin	Melphalan
Hydroxyurea	Vincristine	Cyclophosphamide	Mitomycin
		Dacarbazine	Procarbazine
		Dactinomycin	Thiotepa

*Drugs having both CCS and CCNS properties.

problems before therapy is begun. The cytotoxic effects of antineoplastic drugs on the oral mucous membranes lead to irritation and ulceration. In some cases patients begin to complain about oral discomfort before the mucosa becomes visibly inflamed. Meticulous and gentle oral hygiene is very important to prevent further irritation. Teeth should be brushed with a soft-bristled brush or a soft sponge impregnated with flavoring specially designed for this purpose. Teeth should be cleaned before and after meals but flossing should be done cautiously, especially as the platelet count decreases. To relieve discomfort and to prevent mineral loss from tooth surfaces because of xerostomia, oral membranes should be well hydrated with frequent warm water rinses or an artificial saliva preparation. Patients can also apply a thin film of petroleum to dry, cracked lips to relieve the discomfort. When ulceration and dysphagia develop, avoid giving the patient hot or cold drinks or spicy, sour, dry, rough, or chunky foods. Smoking and alcoholic beverages exacerbate the condition and should also be avoided. White patches in the mouth indicate a fungal infection. If not treated it can spread to the gastrointestinal (GI) tract, especially as the white blood cell count approaches its nadir. GI tract ulceration leads to epigastric discomfort and diarrhea.

Alopecia is very traumatic to the patient. The nurse should be aware of the impact of this side effect on the patient's self-image, which should be discussed in advance so that the patient can make plans for a cosmetic substitute. The hair loss pattern varies from individual to individual; it may all fall out in a day or may gradually thin out over weeks. Hair loss usually is not permanent, but the hair may grow back a different color or texture or both. The patient may also lose eyelashes, eyebrows, and body hair.

Patients should be informed of possible irreversible sterility after chemotherapy. This is a sensitive issue with individuals and should be approached with this in mind. Male patients may want to consider sperm banking as an option. Because of the possible teratogenic effect of cytotoxic agents, both men and women should take contraceptive precautions.

Another property shared by several of the agents (although not related to cytotoxicity but nonetheless important) is tissue damage secondary to drug extravasation (see box). With extravasational drugs, avoid using the antecubital veins or veins on the dorsum of the hand or wrist, where extravasation could damage underlying tendons and nerves, leading to immobility of the entire limb. Use of a central line is preferred with extravasational drugs whenever possible. Always test the infusion line for patency, and check the infusion site frequently during drug administration. If the drug

ANTINEOPLASTIC DRUGS WITH EXTRAVASATIONAL PROPERTIES

Carmustine
Dacarbazine
Dactinomycin
Daunorubicin
Doxorubicin
Mechlorethamine
Mitomycin
Plicamycin
Streptozocin
Vinblastine
Vincristine

does extravasate, first discontinue the infusion and then begin local measures in accordance with written guidelines.

Doxorubicin is the most problematic of the extravasational cytotoxic agents. It may produce severe, prolonged tissue necrosis as a result of the re-release of tissue-bound drug from necrotic tissue. The lesions produced heal very slowly if at all and usually require surgical debridement and skin grafting.

Nausea and vomiting, which are also associated with most chemotherapeutic agents, are discussed later in this chapter.

ALKYLATING AGENTS

Alkylating agents form highly reactive carbonium ions, which react with DNA, proteins, and other essential cellular substances. They replace hydrogen atoms with alkyl radicals, causing cross-linking and abnormal base pairing in the DNA molecule. They also react with sulfhydryl, phosphate, and amine groups. The multiple cellular lesions they cause at the molecular level render the DNA molecule defective and unable to carry on normal cellular metabolic and reproductive functions.

NITROGEN MUSTARDS
Chlorambucil

Indications: Chronic lymphocytic leukemia; Hodgkin's lymphoma; non-Hodgkin's lymphoma.

Usual dosage: 0.1-0.2 mg/kg/day orally for 3-6 weeks as required, then adjust dosage for maintenance to 2-4 mg once daily.

Precautions/contraindications: Hypersensitivity to chlorambucil or to other alkylating agents; safe use during pregnancy (pregnancy category D) or while nursing not established.

Side effects/adverse reactions: *Integument:* dermatitis. *GI:* nausea and vomiting, hepatotoxicity. *Pulmonary:* pulmonary fibrosis. *Hematopoietic:* bone marrow depression. *Reproductive:* infertility.

Pharmacokinetics: Well absorbed from GI tract; plasma half-life: 90 minutes; some fat storage because of the drug's lipophilic nature; may be bound to plasma and tissue proteins; metabolized in the liver; about 60% is excreted in the urine 24 hours after administration, mainly as metabolites; probably crosses the placenta.

Interactions: Dosage of antigout medications may need to be adjusted, because chlorambucil causes hyperuricemia.

Nursing considerations: Weekly blood counts during treatment to monitor for bone marrow depression; be sure patient understands dosage schedule.

Cyclophosphamide

Indications: Carcinoma of the breast and ovaries, acute lymphocytic leukemia, acute monocytic leukemia, acute myelogenous leukemia, chronic lymphocytic leukemia, chronic myelocytic leukemia, Hodgkin's lymphoma, non-Hodgkin's lymphoma, multiple myeloma, mycosis fungoides, neuroblastoma, retinoblastoma.

Usual dosage: Up to 2,000 mg/m² PO or IV as a single dose or in divided doses, courses repeated q 3 wk.

Precautions/contraindications: Men and women of childbearing age (pregnancy category C); serious infection (e.g., chickenpox, herpes zoster); myelosuppression; pregnancy and nursing mothers; cautious use in renal and hepatic impairment, history of urate calculi and gout, recent history of steroid therapy.

Side effects/adverse reactions: *Integument:* alopecia. *GI:* nausea and vomiting. *Pulmonary:* interstitial pulmonary fibrosis. *Hematopoietic:* bone marrow depression. *Renal:* Hemorrhagic cystitis. *Reproductive:* amenorrhea; azoospermia. *Other:* teratogenic; may cause secondary neoplasms.

Pharmacokinetics: Completely absorbed from the GI tract and injection site; hepatic metabolism; half-life after intravenous administration: 4 to 6 hours; 10% to 56% protein bound; excreted in urine as active metabolites; less than 25% as unchanged; crosses the placenta; found in breast milk.

Interactions: Can decrease pharmacologic activity of digoxin; inhibits metabolism of succinylcholine.

Nursing considerations: Maintain adequate hydration before and during administration to prevent renal irritation and hemorrhagic cystitis; monitor intake/output ratio; monitor for and promptly report hematuria or dysuria; monitor for symptoms of water intoxication.

Ifosfamide

Indications: Testicular carcinoma.

Usual dosage: IV infusion 0.6-2 g/m²/day for 5 consecutive days.

Precautions/contraindications: Bone marrow depression; hypersensitivity to the drug; renal impairment; safe use in nursing mothers or during pregnancy not established (pregnancy category D).

Side effects/adverse reactions: *Hematopoietic:* bone marrow depression. *CNS:* lethargy, somnolence, confusion, disorientation, hallucinations. *GI:* nausea and vomiting. *Integument:* alopecia. *Other:* hemorrhagic cystitis.

Pharmacokinetics: Not significantly bound to plasma proteins; activated in the liver to ifosfamide mustard and acrolein; elimination half-life is approximately 7 to 15 hours; distributes in breast milk.

Interactions: Phenobarbital, phenytoin, and chloral hydrate enhance hepatic activation of ifosfamide.

Nursing considerations: Administer with the uroprotective agent mesna (Mesnex); see Cyclophosphamide.

Mechlorethamine

Indications: Lung carcinoma, chronic lymphocytic leukemia, chronic myelocytic leukemia, Hodgkin's lymphoma, non-Hodgkin's lymphoma, malignant effusion, mycosis fungoides.

Usual dosage: 10-16 mg/m² per course IV slow push over 20-30 min; repeat to 6 weeks depending on patient's hematologic recovery. Intracavity: 0.2-0.4 mg/kg body weight.

Precautions/contraindications: Pregnancy at least until third trimester; lactation; bone marrow depression; bacterial or viral infections; bone marrow infiltration; chronic lymphocytic leukemia; men or women in childbearing years (pregnancy category D); alternate use with other cytotoxic agents or radiation therapy.

Side effects/adverse reactions: *Hematopoietic:* bone marrow depression. *GI:* severe nausea and vomiting, metallic taste in mouth, diarrhea, jaundice. *Integument:* alopecia, tissue damage secondary to drug extravasation. *Other:* hyperuricemia.

Pharmacokinetics: Rapid transformation to active metabolites after reconstitution; less than 0.01% of the drug is excreted unchanged in the urine.

Interactions: Mechlorethamine can reduce the effectiveness of antigout medications by increasing uric acid.

Nursing considerations: Highly extravasational; ensure that line is patent; if drug extravasation occurs, follow guidelines; because reconstituted drug undergoes rapid transformation, prepare solution immediately before administration.

Melphalan

Indications: Ovarian carcinoma; multiple myeloma.

Usual dosage: 20-30 mg/m^2 PO per course repeated q 4-6 wk, depending on recovery from previous course.

Precautions/contraindications: Hypersensitivity to melphalan; safe use during pregnancy not established (pregnancy category D); safe use in men or women of childbearing age not determined; cautious use in impaired renal function, anemia, neutropenia, or thrombocytopenia; or with other cytotoxic agents or radiation.

Side effects/adverse reactions: *GI:* mild anorexia, nausea and vomiting. *Hematopoietic:* bone marrow depression. *Pulmonary:* pulmonary toxicity. *Other:* hypersensitivity, infertility.

Pharmacokinetics: Well absorbed from GI tract; plasma half-life: about 90 minutes; well distributed to all tissues; exact metabolism and excretion not known; about 10% to 15% excreted unchanged in urine.

Interactions: Simultaneous use with cyclosporine has been associated with nephrotoxicity.

Nursing considerations: See Chlorambucil.

NITROSOUREAS

Carmustine

Indications: Hodgkin's lymphoma, non-Hodgkin's lymphoma, multiple myeloma, primary brain tumor.

Usual dosage: 30-300 mg/m^2 IV per course; upper dosage range for use as single agent; course usually repeated q 6-8 wk, or dose may be given in divided portions at 3-4 week intervals.

Precautions/contraindications: Known sensitivity to the drug; history of pulmonary function impairment; recent exposure to or viral infection; bone marrow depression; safe use during pregnancy (pregnancy category D) or in nursing mothers not established; cautious use in hepatic and/or renal impairment.

Side effects/adverse reactions: *Pulmonary:* pulmonary fibrosis. *GI:* anorexia, nausea and vomiting, rare reversible hepatotoxicity. *Hematopoietic:* bone marrow depression. *Renal:* nephrotoxic.

Pharmacokinetics: Rapidly absorbed; hepatic metabolism; half-life 5 to 15 minutes; 60% to 70% excreted in urine in 96 hours; 6% to 10% excreted as carbon dioxide by lungs and 1% in feces; crosses the blood-brain barrier; distributes into breast milk.

Interactions: Use with cimetidine increases bone marrow depression; carmustine may reduce absorption of phenytoin.

Nursing considerations: Avoid contact with skin, since drug causes discoloration, dermatitis, and burning; intense burning and pain at injection site if infused too quickly; protect from light; rapid infusion causes flushing; discard if drug has an oily film in vial.

Lomustine

Indications: Hodgkin's lymphoma, primary brain tumors.

Usual dosage: 130 mg/m^2 PO as a single dose repeated q 6 wk.

Precautions/contraindications: History of hypersensitivity to drug; viral infection; safe use in pregnancy (pregnancy category D) and nursing mothers not established; use with caution with bone marrow depression and impaired renal and/or hepatic function.

Side effects/adverse reactions: *Integument:* alopecia (rare). *GI:* anorexia, nausea and vomiting, stomatitis, hepatotoxicity. *Hematopoietic:* bone marrow depression. *Renal:* nephrotoxicity.

Pharmacokinetics: Rapidly absorbed from GI tract; peak serum level in 3 hours; half-life of both drug and metabolites 16 to 48 hours; crosses blood-brain barrier; completely metabolized in liver; excreted in urine as metabolites; distributes in breast milk.

Nursing considerations: Administer on an empty stomach.

Streptozocin

Indications: Pancreatic carcinoma.

Usual dosage: 500 mg/m^2/day intraarterial or IV for 5 days q 6 wk; **or,** 1 g/m^2/wk for 2 weeks, then increase dosage; not recommended to exceed 1.5 g/m^2/wk.

Precautions/contraindications: Safe use in pregnancy (pregnancy category C) and during breastfeeding not established; renal and hepatic impairment.

Side effects/adverse reactions: *Integument:* tissue damage secondary to drug extravasation. *GI:* nausea and vomiting. *Renal:* nephrotoxicity, renal tubular acidosis. *Endocrine:* may lead to insulin-dependent diabetes. *Hematopoietic:* bone marrow depression.

Pharmacokinetics: Renal and hepatic metabolism; biphasic half-life: initial 5 minutes, terminal 35 to 40 minutes; 60% to 70% excreted in urine as metabolite and 10% as unchanged; 1% in feces; 5% in expired air.

Interactions: Phenytoin may reduce cytotoxic effect of carmustine; use with other nitrosoureas enhances hepatotoxicity of both; nephrotoxicity increased when used with other nephrotoxic drugs.

Nursing consideration: Ensure that line is patent. Follow guidelines if drug extravasation occurs; monitor for hypoglycemic reactions, which may result from sudden insulin release caused by carmustine.

Busulfan

Indications: Chronic myelocytic leukemia.

Usual dosage: 4-8 mg/day PO until maximum clinical and hematologic improvement is obtained.

Precautions/contraindication: Resistant chronic lymphocytic leukemia; blast crisis of chronic myelogenous leukemia; bone marrow depression; immunizations or recent viral infections; safe use during pregnancy (pregnancy category D) and in nursing mothers not established; use with caution in men and women in childbearing years; history of gout or urate renal stones; previous irradiation or chemotherapy.

Side effects/adverse reactions: *Integument:* hyperpigmentation, alopecia. *Pulmonary:* interstitial pulmonary fibrosis. *GI:* nausea and vomiting. *Reproductive:* testicular atrophy, impotence, amenorrhea, gynecomastia. *Hematopoietic:* bone marrow depression. *Other:* hyperuricemia, cellular dysplasia of many organs.

Pharmacokinetics: Within 5 minutes of intravenous administration and 4 hours after oral dose, level of 1% to 3% of the dose is reached and maintained; metabolized in the liver; 10% to 50% of dose excreted in urine as metabolites within 48 hours.

Interactions: Busulfan increases uric acid, necessitating dosage adjustment in antigout medications.

Carboplatin

Indications: Ovarian carcinoma.

Usual dosage: 360 mg/m^2 IV q 4 wk; dosage reduction recommended for renal impairment.

Precautions/contraindications: Impaired renal or hepatic function; allergy to cisplatin or other drugs containing platinum; safe use during pregnancy not established (pregnancy category D).

Side effects/adverse reactions: *Hematopoietic:* bone marrow depression. *GI:* nausea and vomiting.

Pharmacokinetics: 60% to 80% of administered dose is excreted via the kidneys by glomerular filtration; elimination half-life is 3 hours.

Interactions: Simultaneous use of aminoglycoside antibiotics may increase risk of ototoxicity and nephrotoxicity.

Nursing considerations: See Cisplatin.

Cisplatin

Indications: Carcinoma of the bladder, ovaries, and testes.

Usual dosage: Up to 200 mg/m^2 IV infusion q 3-4 wk, may be given as a single dose or divided over 2 to 5 days q 3 wk.

Precautions/contraindications: Impaired renal function; myelosuppression; impaired hearing; concomitant use with other ototoxic and nephrotoxic drugs; hypersensitivity to cisplatin and other platinum-containing compounds; history of gout and urate stones; safe use during pregnancy (pregnancy category D) and in nursing women not established; cautious use with previous cytotoxic drug use or radiation.

Side effects/adverse reactions: *CNS:* ototoxicity, various neuropathies. *GI:* high incidence of nausea and vomiting. *Hematopoietic:* bone marrow depression. *Renal:* nephrotoxicity. *Other:* anaphylactic-like reactions, hypomagnesemia, hyperuricemia.

Pharmacokinetics: After intravenous dose, the drug is widely distributed in the body, with the highest concentrations in the liver, large and small intestines, and kidneys. Poor penetration into the CNS; half-life: initial phase, 25 to 49 minutes; terminal phase, 58 to 78 hours; more than 90% of the drug is bound to plasma proteins; partially excreted in the urine.

Interactions: Increased risk of ototoxicity if used concurrently with aminoglycoside antibiotics and loop diuretics; antigout medications may need to be adjusted, since cisplatin raises uric acid blood level; pharmacologic effects of phenytoin may be decreased.

Nursing considerations: Adequately hydrate before administration; audiometric testing before first dose; monitor urine output; nephrotoxicity and ototoxicity are reduced with use of osmotic diuretic (mannitol); prepare for anaphylactoid reactions; neurologic examinations at regular intervals; monitor electrolyte levels; do not use aluminum-containing IV infusion sets and needles.

Thiotepa

Indications: Carcinoma of the bladder, breast, and ovaries; Hodgkin's lymphoma; non-Hodgkin's lymphoma; malignant effusions.

Usual dosage: *IV:* 15-60 mg/m^2 q 1-4 wk. Intravesicular: 30-60 mg in 30-60 ml distilled water instilled into bladder via catheter and retained for 2 hours.

Precautions/contraindications: Hypersensitivity to the drug; acute leukemia; pregnancy (pregnancy category D); use with caution in chronic lymphocytic leukemia; myelosuppression produced by radiation or cytotoxic agent; bone marrow invasion by tumor cells; impaired renal or hepatic function.

Side effects/adverse reactions: *GI:* anorexia, nausea and vomiting, stomatitis. *Hematopoietic:* bone marrow depression. *Reproductive:* amenorrhea, reduced spermatogenesis. *Other:* fever.

Pharmacokinetics: Rapidly cleared from the plasma after intravenous administration; slow onset of action, with therapeutic response becoming increasingly evident over several weeks; slowly bound to tissues; significant amount remaining in the blood 72 hours after administration; extensively metabolized; 60% of intravenous dose eliminated in urine within 24 to 72 hours.

Nursing considerations: See General Nursing Considerations for Antineoplastic Drugs, page 254.

ANTIMETABOLITES

Antimetabolites are a class of antineoplastic agents comprising analogs of folic acid and the base components of nucleic acids that act during the synthetic (S) phase of the cell cycle. Methotrexate is the only folic acid analog with wide clinical application. By blocking the action of the enzyme dihydrofolate reductase, it inhibits the production of a coenzyme needed for the synthesis of thymidylic acid, a precursor needed for replication of nucleic acids.

The other agents are pyrimidine and purine analogs, which block enzymes needed during the synthesis of DNA and RNA. They may also be erroneously incorporated into the DNA molecule during replication.

Cytarabine

Indications: Used for acute lymphocytic leukemia, acute myelogenous leukemia, chronic myelocytic leukemia, meningeal leukemia, and non-Hodgkin's lymphoma.

Usual dosage: Up to a total dose of 1 g/m^2 IV by a variety of schedules: 5-75 mg/m^2 intrathecally daily for 4 days or once every 4 days; **or** 30 mg/m^2 q 4 days until CSF is normal, followed by one more dose for CNS prophylaxis or treatment.

Precautions/contraindications: Known hypersensitivity to the drug; safe use during pregnancy (category D), in women of childbearing age, and nursing mothers not established; cautious use with impaired renal or hepatic function, gout, and drug-induced bone marrow depression.

Side effects/adverse reactions: *Integument:* alopecia. *GI:* anorexia, nausea, vomiting, stomatitis, esophagitis, anal ulceration. *Renal:* urinary retention. *Hematopoietic:* bone marrow depression. *Other:* fever.

Pharmacokinetics: After intravenous administration, drug is rapidly cleared from the bloodstream; distributed in 15 minutes; eliminated in 1 to 3 hours; half-life after intrathecal administration is 2 hours; metabolized mainly in the liver; crosses the blood-brain barrier in moderate amounts; about 80% is excreted in urine in 24 hours with less than 10% as unchanged drug.

Interactions: May decrease absorption of digoxin tablets.

Nursing considerations: For intrathecal administration, use preservative-free saline to reconstitute drug.

Floxuridine

Indications: Gastrointestinal carcinoma, hepatic carcinoma.

Usual dosage: 75 mg/m^2/day via hepatic artery for 14 days by continuous infusion.

Precautions/contraindications: Existing or recent viral infection; safe use during pregnancy not established (category D); cautious use with bone marrow depression, serious infections, and impaired renal or liver function.

Side effects/adverse reactions: *GI:* nausea, vomiting, stomatitis, enteritis, diarrhea. *Hematopoietic:* bone marrow depression. *Other:* fever.

Pharmacokinetics: See Fluorouracil.

Nursing considerations: Given by intraarterial infusion only (see Fluorouracil).

Fluorouracil

Indications: Carcinoma of the breast, colon, rectum, stomach, and pancreas; topical preparation indicated for actinic and solar keratosis and basal cell carcinoma.

Usual dosage: 300-600 mg/m^2/day for 4-5 days q 4 wk; 600 mg/m^2/wk for 6 weeks; 900-1,100 mg/m^2/day for 4 to 5 days by continuous infusion q 4 wk.

Precautions/contraindications: Bone marrow depression; safe use during pregnancy not established (category D); cautious use in men and women of childbearing age and with impaired hepatic and renal function.

Side effects/adverse reactions: *Integument:* alopecia, skin hyperpigmentation, nail changes. *GI:* occasional nausea and vomiting, stomatitis, GI ulceration, diarrhea. *Hematopoietic:* bone marrow depression. *CNS:* headache, drowsiness, blurred vision.

Pharmacokinetics: Minimal absorption with topical application on intact skin; after intravenous administration, 7% to 20% of parent drug excreted unchanged in urine in 6 hours; remaining drug metabolized in liver; 90% excreted as expired carbon dioxide, remainder clears as inactive metabolites in urine over next 3 to 4 hours; half-life elimination from plasma in 16 minutes; crosses blood-brain barrier.

Interactions: Other myelosuppressive drugs or radiation therapy may enhance effects of fluorouracil, necessitating dosage adjustment.

Nursing considerations: For oral administration, mix with carbonated beverage; monitor closely for stomatitis, an early sign of toxicity; other early signs are anorexia, nausea, vomiting, diarrhea, and GI bleeding.

Mercaptopurine

Indications: Acute lymphocytic leukemia, acute myelogenous leukemia, acute myelocytic leukemia.

Usual dosage: 100-200 mg/day PO continuously until clinical improvement; adjust dosage upward by increments of 5 mg/kg/day for maintenance according to blood counts; calculate dose to closest multiple of 25 mg.

Precautions/contraindications: Give one third to one fourth of usual dose of mercaptopurine if administered with allopurinol; safe use during pregnancy not established (pregnancy category D); use with caution with impaired renal or liver function.

Side effects/adverse reactions: *GI:* anorexia, nausea and vomiting, stomatitis, hepatotoxicity. *Hematopoietic:* bone marrow depression.

Pharmacokinetics: Oral doses are erratically and incompletely absorbed; half-life: 4 minutes; crosses blood-brain barrier; partly metabolized in liver with rapid excretion in urine.

Interactions: Allopurinol slows metabolism of mercaptopurine, increasing its toxicity; mercaptopurine may reduce hypoprothrombinemic effect of anticoagulants and may reverse neuromuscular blocking effects of nonpolarizing muscle relaxants (e.g., tubocurarine).

Nursing considerations: See General Nursing Considerations for Antineoplastic Drugs, page 254.

Methotrexate

Indications: Carcinoma of the breast, head, and neck; acute lymphocytic leukemia; meningeal leukemia; non-Hodgkin's lymphoma; osteosarcoma; trophoblastic tumors.

Usual dosage: 15 mg/m²/day for 5 days IV or IM, **or** single weekly doses of up to 30 mg/m²; single doses up to 15 g/m² IV only with calcium leucovorin rescue; intrathecally: 5-15 mg/m² repeated q 3-7 days with courses repeated at intervals of 6 to 8 weeks to maintain CNS remission.

Precautions/contraindications: Safe use not established in men and women of childbearing age or during pregnancy (pregnancy category D) or with hepatic and renal impairment; simultaneous administration of hepatotoxic and myelosuppressant drugs; alcohol; preexisting blood dyscrasias; use with caution with infections, ulcerative colitis, and peptic ulcer.

Side effects/adverse reactions: *Integument:* alopecia, urticaria, telangiectasia, acne, photosensitivity. *Pulmonary:* interstitial pneumonia. *GI:* nausea and vomiting, stomatitis, GI ulceration, diarrhea, hepatotoxicity. *Hematopoietic:* bone marrow depression.

Pharmacokinetics: Rapidly absorbed from GI tract; peak serum levels 1 to 2 hours after oral administration and 30 to 60 minutes after intravenous administration; half-life: 2 to 4 hours after either intramuscular or oral administration—3 to 10 hours for a low dose, 8 to 15 hours for a high dose; approximately 50% of the drug is bound to serum proteins; wide tissue distribution; up to 90% of the drug is cleared by the kidneys unchanged; small amount is excreted in stools.

Interactions: Hepatotoxicity caused by methotrexate is increased by alcohol ingestion; chloramphenicol;

ketoprofen; tetracyclines. PABA displaces methotrexate from plasma proteins. Orally administered aminoglycosides may reduce oral absorption of methotrexate. Penicillin and probenecid may increase plasma levels of the drug. Vitamin preparations containing folic acid may alter response to methotrexate.

Nursing considerations: Instruct patients to avoid beverages or medications that contain alcohol. Keep patient with hyperuricemia (or the potential for it) well hydrated (2,000 ml/24 h); give allopurinol to prevent urate deposit. Advise patient not to self-medicate with vitamins or other over-the-counter medications without consulting a health professional. Practitioners administering high-dose methotrexate must be knowledgeable about the leucovorin rescue process. Use preservative-free diluent for reconstitution of drug for intrathecal administration.

Thioguanine

Indications: Acute myelogenous leukemia, chronic myelocytic leukemia.

Usual dosage: Initial dose 2 mg/kg/day up to 3 mg/kg/day PO as one dose or two divided doses for 5 to 7 days or daily until remission is observed.

Precautions/contraindications: Safe use during pregnancy not established (pregnancy category D); use with caution with impaired liver function.

Side effects/adverse reactions: *GI:* anorexia, stomatitis. *Hematopoietic:* bone marrow depression. *Other:* liver damage, hyperuricemia.

Pharmacokinetics: Partially absorbed from the GI tract, with peak serum concentration in 10 to 12 hours; rapidly metabolized in liver; biphasic half-life: initial, 15 minutes, terminal, 11 hours; excreted in feces and urine as metabolites.

Nursing considerations: Monitor patient for jaundice, a sign of liver toxicity; contraceptive measures should be used during treatment with this drug.

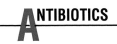

ANTIBIOTICS

Antitumor antibiotics are a group of related antimicrobial agents produced by the bacterial species *Streptomyces*. Some are naturally occurring products; others are semisynthetic derivatives.

Dactinomycin, daunorubicin, doxorubicin, and plicamycin use complex mechanisms to combine with DNA base pairs, thus interfering with DNA, RNA, and protein synthesis. Bleomycin causes DNA strand scission and fragmentation. Mitomycin inhibits the replication of DNA by causing cross-links to form between complementary strands of the molecule.

Bleomycin

Indications: Carcinoma of the cervix, head and neck, larynx, penis, skin, and testes; Hodgkin's lymphoma; non-Hodgkin's lymphoma.

Usual dosage: 4-20 U/m^2 IV weekly or twice weekly or as a continuous infusion; *or* 1-2 U/day SC as maintenance dosage.

Precautions/contraindications: History of hypersensitivity to bleomycin; pregnancy (pregnancy category D); cautious use in patients with impaired renal, hepatic, or pulmonary function.

Side effects/adverse reactions: *Integument:* hyperpigmentation, nail changes, alopecia, pruritus, hyperkeratosis, urticaria. *CV:* phlebitis at injection site; anaphylactoid reactions, primarily in lymphoma patients. *Pulmonary:* pneumonitis, progresses to fibrosis. *GI:* anorexia, nausea and vomiting, stomatitis.

Pharmacokinetics: Concentrates mainly in skin, lungs, kidneys, lymphocytes, and peritoneum after administration; metabolic fate is not completely understood; about 1% of drug is protein bound; half-life: 2 hours in patients with normal kidney function; 60% to 70% of drug is recovered in urine as active drug.

Interactions: Bleomycin reduces GI absorption of digoxin and phenytoin.

Nursing considerations: Skin test or give test dose of 2 U before administering the therapeutic dose; keep total single dose below 400 U for single-agent use. Pulmonary toxicity occurs in 10% of patients and most frequently appears in patients over 70 years old or as the cumulative dosage approaches 400 U; bone marrow depression is rare.

Dactinomycin

Indications: Carcinoma of the endometrium and testes; Ewing's sarcoma; trophoblastic tumors; Wilms' tumor; rhabdomyosarcoma; sarcoma botryoides.

Usual dosage: 0.3-0.5 mg/m^2/day IV for 5 days, with courses repeated at 2- to 8-week intervals; alternatively, 1-2.5 mg/m^2 as a single dose given q 4 wk.

Precautions/contraindications: Viral infections; pregnancy (pregnancy category C); cautious use in patients with impaired kidney and liver function and bone marrow depression.

Side effects/adverse reactions: *Integument:* alopecia, tissue damage secondary to drug extravasation. *Pulmonary:* pharyngitis. *GI:* nausea and vomiting, stomatitis, dysphagia, esophagitis. *Hematologic:* bone marrow depression. *Other:* hypocalcemia.

Pharmacokinetics: Very little active drug is found in the plasma 2 to 5 minutes after intravenous administration; drug concentrates in the liver, spleen, and kidneys; plasma half-life: 36 hours; about 50% of drug is excreted unchanged in bile and 10% in urine.

Interactions: May elevate uric acid level, which requires adjustments in antigout medications; decreases effect of vitamin K.

Nursing considerations: Ensure that line is patent; follow guidelines if drug extravasation occurs.

Daunorubicin

Indications: Acute lymphocytic leukemia; acute myelogenous leukemia; acute monocytic leukemia.

Usual dosage: 30-60 mg/m^2/day IV for 3-5 days; **or** 100-150 mg/m^2 single dose; **or** 40 mg/m^2/day for 4 days continuous infusion; courses are repeated q 3 wk.

Precautions/contraindications: Preexisting cardiac disease; severe bone marrow depression; pregnancy (pregnancy category D); use with caution in patients with impaired renal and/or hepatic function.

Side effects/adverse reactions: *Integument:* alopecia, tissue damage secondary to drug extravasation, hyperpigmentation of nail beds, local inflammation at injection site. *CV:* congestive heart failure. *GI:* nausea and vomiting, stomatitis. *Renal:* red urine (not hematuria). *Hematopoietic:* bone marrow depression. *Other:* fever.

Pharmacokinetics: After intravenous administration, drug concentrates in cardiac, renal, and pulmonary tissue, 25% concentrates in the liver; plasma half-life: 18½ hours; undergoes hepatic metabolism; about 25% is eliminated in active form in urine and 40% is excreted in bile.

Nursing considerations: Daunorubicin is a potent bone marrow suppressant. Monitor heart function for cardiotoxicity; acute CHF can occur. Total lifetime dosage not to exceed 550 mg/m^2. Ensure that line is patent; follow guidelines if drug extravasation occurs. Causes red coloration of body fluids and urine—do not confuse this with hematuria.

Doxorubicin

Indications: Carcinoma of the bladder, breast, stomach, lung, ovaries, and thyroid; acute lymphocytic leukemia; acute myelogenous leukemia; Hodgkin's lymphoma; non-Hodgkin's lymphoma; neuroblastoma; osteosarcoma; soft tissue sarcomas; Wilms' tumor.

Usual dosage: 40-75 mg/m^2 as a single dose or divided over 3 to 5 days by continuous IV infusion at 21-day intervals.

Precautions/contraindications: See Daunorubicin.

Side effects/adverse reactions: *Integument:* alopecia, tissue damage secondary to drug extravasation, hyperpigmentation of nail beds, local inflammation at injection site. *CV:* cardiotoxicity progressing to CHF. *GI:* nausea and vomiting, stomatitis, esophagitis, GI ulceration, diarrhea. *Renal:* red urine (not hematuria). *Hematopoietic:* bone marrow depression. *Other:* fever.

Pharmacokinetics: Metabolized in liver to both active and inactive metabolites. Triphasic half-life: initial 12 minutes, middle, 3.3 hours, terminal, 29.6 hours. Forty to 50 percent of administered drug is found in bile and feces in 7 days.

Interactions: Doxorubicin may potentiate the toxicities caused by other neoplastic agents, such as hemorrhagic cystitis (cyclophosphamide) and hepatotoxicity (mercaptopurine); barbiturates may accelerate plasma clearance of doxorubicin; doxorubicin may decrease serum levels of digoxin (when using tablets—capsule form does not appear to be affected); streptozocin may prolong half-life of drug.

Nursing considerations: See Daunorubicin.

Mitomycin

Indications: Gastric carcinoma, pancreatic carcinoma.

Usual dosage: 2 mg/m^2 IV days 1 to 5 and 8 to 12, repeated in 2 to 3 weeks; 20 mg/m^2 as a single dose repeated q 4-6 wk.

Precautions/contraindications: Hypersensitivity to drug; thrombocytopenia; pregnancy (category D); cautious use in patients with renal impairment and bone marrow depression.

Side effects/adverse reactions: *Integument:* alopecia, tissue damage secondary to drug extravasation, pruritus. *Pulmonary:* rare pulmonary toxicity, dyspnea. *GI:* nausea and vomiting, anorexia, stomatitis, diarrhea. *Hematologic:* bone marrow suppression. *Other:* fever.

Pharmacokinetics: After injection, drug is cleared rapidly from blood by hepatic metabolism; half-life: 17 minutes; about 10% of drug is excreted unchanged in urine.

Interactions: See Vinblastine and Vincristine.

Nursing considerations: Ensure that line is patent; follow guidelines if drug extravasation occurs.

Plicamycin

Indications: Testicular carcinoma, hypercalcemia.

Usual dosage: Antineoplastic: 1-2 mg/m^2/day IV q 2 days for five doses, repeated q 3 wk. Hypercalcemia: 1 mg/m^2/day for 3 to 4 days, repeated in 1 week, or as 2 to 3 doses per week.

Precautions/contraindications: Do not give to patients with thrombocytopenia or hepatic or coagulation disorders; pregnancy (pregnancy category C).

Side effects/adverse reactions: *Integument:* tissue damage secondary to drug extravasation. *GI:* anorexia, nausea and vomiting, stomatitis, hepatotoxicity, diarrhea. *CNS:* mental depression, confusion. *Hematopoietic:* thrombocytopenia, bleeding and coagulation disorders. *Other:* fever, hypocalcemia, hypophosphatemia, hypokalemia.

Pharmacokinetics: Limited information is available

on absorption, metabolism, and excretion; drug is cleared from blood within 2 hours of administration; rapid excretion.

Interactions: Concomitant administration of vitamin D may enhance hypercalcemia.

Nursing considerations: Plicamycin should be diluted in 1,000 ml of D$_5$W or normal saline and infused over 4 to 6 hours; monitor patient for facial flushing, an early symptom of thrombocytopenia, and epistaxis, which may be the first sign of bleeding syndrome; ensure that line is patent; follow guidelines if drug extravasation occurs.

PLANT ALKALOIDS

Plant alkaloids are natural or semisynthetic products derived from different plants. Etoposide is a semisynthetic derivative of podophyllotoxin, which is derived from the root of the May-apple plant. Its primary effect is at the G$_2$ phase of the cell cycle. At concentrations greater than or equal to 10 µg/ml, etoposide causes cell lysis; at lower concentrations, it prevents cells from entering the initial stage of mitosis. It may also inhibit DNA synthesis to some degree.

Vincristine and vinblastine are *Vinca* alkaloids extracted from the periwinkle plant. In vitro, both agents arrest cell activity at the metaphase (M) stage of mitosis, inhibiting cell division. Their cytotoxic action in vivo, however, is less clear. Of the two agents, vincristine is less toxic to normal cells and therefore produces less bone marrow suppression. However, its neurologic and neuromuscular effects are more severe.

Etoposide

Indications: Refractory testicular neoplasms; small cell carcinoma of the lung.

Usual dosage: 75-200 mg/m^2 q 3-5 wk; testicular cancer: 50-100 mg/m^2 on days 1 through 5 or 100 mg/m^2 on days 1, 3, and 5 q 3-4 wk; recommended oral doses are twice the IV dose rounded to the nearest 50 mg.

Precautions/contraindications: Hypersensitivity to etoposide; severe bone marrow depression; severe hepatic or renal impairment; pregnancy (pregnancy category D); use with caution in patients with impaired hepatic or renal function and gout.

Side effects/adverse reactions: *Hematologic:* bone marrow depression. *GI:* nausea and vomiting, anorexia. *Integument:* alopecia. *CV:* hypotension. *Hypersensitivity:* anaphylactic-like reactions.

Pharmacokinetics: Less than 10% penetration into CSF; about 94% of drug is plasma protein bound; probably metabolized in liver; biphasic half-life: initial phase, 3 hours, terminal phase, 15 hours; about 44% to 60% of drug is excreted in urine within 48 to 72 hours, 75% as unchanged drug, the remainder as metabolites.

Nursing considerations: Minimum rate for intravenous infusion is 30 to 60 minutes; monitor vital signs during infusion; stop infusion if hypotension develops; be prepared for anaphylactic reaction; capsules are stored in refrigerator.

Vinblastine

Indications: Hodgkin's and non-Hodgkin's lymphoma; breast carcinoma; trophoblastic tumors; neuroblastoma; advanced testicular carcinoma.

Usual dosage: 4-7.5 mg/m^2 IV single doses weekly; 9-11 mg/m^2/course as a continuous infusion; 12-16 mg/m^2 as a single dose or divided doses repeated at 3- to 4-week intervals.

Precautions/contraindications: Leukopenia; bacterial infections; pregnancy (pregnancy category D); cautious use in obstructive jaundice, hepatic impairment, and history of gout.

Side effects/adverse reactions: *Integument:* alopecia, tissue damage secondary to drug extravasation. *GI:* nausea and vomiting, stomatitis, constipation, ileus. *Renal:* urinary retention, polyuria. *CNS:* peripheral neuropathy, loss of deep tendon reflexes, paresthesia. *Hematopoietic:* bone marrow depression. *CV:* hypertension.

Pharmacokinetics: After intravenous administration, drug is rapidly cleared from the bloodstream; concentrates in liver, where it is partly metabolized; about 75% of drug is protein bound; triphasic half-life: initial phase, 3.7 minutes, middle phase, 1.6 hours, terminal phase, 24.8 hours; poor penetration of blood-brain barrier; excreted in bile via feces; less than 5% excreted in urine.

Interactions: Can lower blood levels of phenytoin; previous or simultaneous administration of mitomycin can cause shortness of breath and severe bronchospasm.

Nursing considerations: Toxicity increases if liver disease is present; ensure that line is patent before infusing; follow guidelines if drug extravasation occurs; monitor bowel elimination and bowel sounds to assess severe constipation or paralytic ileus; patient may require stool softener.

Vincristine

Indications: Ewing's sarcoma; acute lymphocytic leukemia; Hodgkin's lymphoma and non-Hodgkin's lymphoma; soft tissue sarcomas; neuroblastoma; Wilms' tumor; rhabdomyosarcoma.

Usual dosage: 1.4 mg/m^2 IV single dose weekly.

Precautions/contraindications: Obstructive jaundice; demyelinating form of Charcot-Marie-Tooth disease; pregnancy (pregnancy category D); cautious use with liver impairment and leukopenia.

Side effects/adverse reactions: *Integument:* alopecia, tissue damage secondary to drug extravasation. *Pulmonary:* pharyngitis. *GI:* anorexia, nausea and vomiting, stomatitis, ileus, constipation, diarrhea. *CNS:* mental depression, numbness, paresthesia, peripheral neuritis, loss of deep tendon reflexes, vertigo, headache. *Hematopoietic:* bone marrow depression.

Pharmacokinetics: Rapid distribution with excessive tissue binding; triphasic half-life pattern: initial, 5 minutes, middle, 2.3 hours, terminal, 85 hours; liver is major excretory organ, with 80% of dose excreted in feces, 10% to 20% in urine.

Interactions: May decrease digoxin plasma levels and renal excretion; L-asparaginase may reduce hepatic clearance of vincristine; previous or simultaneous administration with mitomycin may cause acute pulmonary reaction or severe bronchospasm; vincristine may reduce plasma levels of phenytoin.

Nursing considerations: Plan prophylactic regimen for constipation and paralytic ileus (i.e., adequate fluids with the administration of a stool softener); check deep tendon reflexes, and grasp hands to assess onset of muscular weakness daily; monitor patient for mental depression, ptosis, paresthesia, neuritic pain, and motor difficulties; ensure that line is patent before infusing; follow guidelines if drug extravasation occurs.

Miscellaneous Drugs

These drugs have diverse mechanisms of action that do not fit into any of the other classes.

Asparaginase

Normal cells can synthesize asparagine, an amino acid essential for the synthesis of proteins. In acute leukemia, the malignant cells cannot do this and depend on exogenous asparagine for survival. Asparaginase, an enzyme isolated from *Escherichia coli*, catalyzes the breakdown of exogenous asparagine to aspartic acid and ammonia, which deprives the malignant cell of this essential amino acid it needs for survival. The inhibitory action of the enzyme occurs in the postmitotic G2 phase of the cell cycle.

Indications: Acute lymphocytic leukemia.

Usual dosage: 5,000-10,000 U/m^2/day for 7 days q 3 wk; **or** 10,000-40,000 q 2-3 wk.

Precautions/contraindications: History of hypersensitivity to asparaginase; history of pancreatitis; infections; safe use during pregnancy not established (pregnancy category C); use with caution with liver impairment and diabetes mellitus.

Side effects/adverse reactions: *CV:* anaphylactic shock. *GI:* anorexia, nausea and vomiting, hepatotoxicity. *Renal:* nephrotoxicity. *CNS:* malaise, confusion, lethargy. *Other:* fever, hyperglycemia, pancreatitis, clotting factor depression.

Pharmacokinetics: 80% distributed into intravascular spaces, 20% into lymph and CSF; half-life: 8 to 30 hours; metabolic fate unknown.

Interactions: Asparaginase diminishes the hypoglycemic effect of insulin; potentiates the toxicity of steroids and vincristine; blocks the antineoplastic effect of methotrexate if given immediately before or with it; enhances effects of radiation therapy and immunosuppressive agents; its use may require dosage adjustment of antigout medications.

Nursing considerations: Acute hypersensitivity reactions can occur even without a positive skin test result; be prepared to treat anaphylaxis with each administration.

Dacarbazine

Dacarbazine's action is similar to that of the alkylating agents. It also may inhibit DNA synthesis by acting as a purine analog. Both DNA synthesis and RNA synthesis are inhibited.

Indications: Hodgkin's lymphoma; malignant melanoma.

Usual dosage: 250 mg/m^2/day for 5 days; **or** single doses of 750-1,200 mg/m^2 with courses repeated q 3 wk.

Precautions/contraindications: Hypersensitivity to dacarbazine; safe use during pregnancy not established (pregnancy category C).

Side effects/adverse reactions: *GI:* nausea and vomiting. *Hematopoietic:* bone marrow depression. *Integument:* tissue damage secondary to drug extravasation, alopecia. *Other:* occasional flu-like syndrome, anaphylaxis possible.

Pharmacokinetics: 5% protein bound; biphasic half-life: initial, 20 minutes, terminal, 5 hours; localizes in liver and CSF; 35% to 50% of drug eliminated by renal tubules as unchanged drug and metabolite.

Nursing considerations: Ensure that line is patent; follow guidelines if drug extravasation occurs; photosensitivity may occur, so instruct patient to apply sunscreen or wear protective clothing.

Levamisole

Levamisole acts as an immunomodulator by an unknown mechanism of action.

Indications: Used as an immunomodulator with fluorouracil after surgical resection of Dukes stage C colon cancer.

Usual dosage: Initial dose, 50 mg PO q 8 h for 3 days; then maintenance dose, 50 mg q 8 h for 3 days q 2 wk with fluorouracil.

Precautions/contraindications: Safe use during pregnancy not established (pregnancy category C); hypersensitivity to levamisole; safe use in men and women of childbearing age not established.

Side effects/adverse reactions: *GI:* nausea and vomiting, diarrhea, abdominal pain, taste changes. *Integument:* dermatitis, alopecia. *Hematopoietic:* bone marrow depression. *Other:* fatigue, fever.

Pharmacokinetics: Pharmacokinetics at the dosage used not studied.

Interactions: Levamisole can cause disulfiram reaction with alcohol; administration of phenytoin with levamisole and fluorouracil increases plasma level of phenytoin.

Nursing considerations: Notify physician if flu-like symptoms or malaise occurs; disulfiram-like reaction with ingestion of alcohol.

Procarbazine

Procarbazine is a hydrazine derivative with antimetabolite properties; however, its exact mechanism of action is unknown.

Indications: Hodgkin's lymphoma.

Usual dosage: 150 mg/m^2/day PO for up to 14 to 21 days.

Precautions/contraindications: Hypersensitivity to procarbazine; bone marrow depression; safe use during pregnancy or while breast-feeding not established (pregnancy category C); women of childbearing age; cautious use with CNS depressant and renal and liver function impairment.

Side effects/adverse reactions: *Integument:* pruritus, hyperpigmentation, alopecia. *GI:* anorexia, nausea and vomiting, stomatitis, xerostomia, diarrhea, constipation. *Musculoskeletal:* myalgia. *CNS:* paresthesia, confusion, lethargy, mental depression. *Hematopoietic:* bone marrow depression. *Other:* fever.

Pharmacokinetics: Readily absorbed from GI tract; wide distribution; half-life: 1 hour; metabolized in liver; excreted in urine as unchanged drug and metabolites.

Interactions: Procarbazine possesses weak monoamine oxidase (MAO) inhibitory activity and therefore may produce hypertensive crisis with levodopa, sympathomimetics, food high in tyramine, and tricyclic antidepressants; procarbazine may decrease plasma level of digoxin and may also potentiate CNS depressant action of narcotics.

Nursing considerations: List foods high in tyramine

for patient; evaluate other drugs (both prescribed and over the counter) taken for potential adverse drug interaction; advise patient to report severe flulike symptoms.

HORMONES AND ANTIHORMONAL DRUGS

Hormones and antihormonal drugs that are clinically active against cancer cells include androgens, estrogens, progestins, corticocosteroids, and antiestrogens (see Table 16-3 for list). Some of these drugs mediate directly at the cellular level by binding with specific cytoplasmic receptors, as either an agonist or an antagonist; others mediate through an indirect effect on the hypothalamus and its anterior pituitary-regulating hormones. These agents are apparently effective because growth of the malignant cell in the target tissue can be controlled by a specific hormone.

The exception to this mechanism of action is the effect of corticosteroids on leukemias and lymphomas. In this situation these agents appear to have a direct lytic effect on abnormal lymphoid cells.

BIOLOGIC RESPONSE MODIFIERS

The use of biologic response modifiers to treat cancer is a new and rapidly evolving field. Attempting to treat disease by manipulating the immune system has been investigated for many years. However, the recent advances in knowledge about the immune system, recombinant DNA technology, and gene cloning have permitted production and purification of a number of biologic response modifiers (see Table 16-4 for a list of these agents).

These agents occur naturally in the body and act as messengers between cells. They are called cytokines, because they come from cells. These molecules can elicit regulatory responses that have a variety of specific and nonspecific immunologic effects.

The rationale for their use is based on the theory that one of the factors that causes the rapid multiplication of cancer cells is a breakdown of intercellular communication; cytokines may help reestablish this cell-to-cell communication.

INTERFERONS

Interferons are potent inhibitors of cell growth. They are also potent immunostimulants, activating cytotoxic effector cells. Evidence is growing that interferons regulate the expression of genes responsible for cell growth and differentiation.

Alpha-interferon is approved for use in hepatitis C, hairy cell leukemia, condyloma acuminatum, and Kaposi's sarcoma. It also has shown activity in chronic myelogenous leukemia and T-cell lymphomas. Two solid tumors, malignant melanoma and renal cell carcinoma, also appear to be sensitive.

Gamma-interferon has been approved for use in the treatment of chronic granulomatous disease.

The numerous biologic effects of the interferons cause several adverse effects, including nausea, vomiting, anorexia, myalgias, headache, and fever and chills similar to a flulike syndrome.

INTERLEUKINS

The interleukins are a group of glycoproteins produced by activated lymphocytes or macrophages. More than 10 interleukins have been identified so far; however, only one, interleukin-2, is a pure biologic response modifier; it has an indirect antitumor effect. Interleukin-2 stimulates cytotoxic T cells and lymphokine-activated killer cells, which in turn kill tumor cells. Administered alone and in high doses, interleukin-2 can induce regression of established metastases.

Toxicity during interleukin-2 therapy has been substantial. Its administration releases other lymphokines (e.g., gamma-interferon and tumor necrosis factor) that damage the endothelium of the cardiovascular system, causing a capillary leak syndrome with massive fluid retention and severe hypotension.

ERYTHROPOIETIN

Erythropoietin is a glycoprotein produced by the kidneys that stimulates the division and differentiation of erythroid progenitors in the bone marrow.

Erythropoietin has been approved for treating anemia associated with chronic renal failure and/or related to therapy with azidothymidine (AZT) in HIV-infected patients. It also has an unlabeled use in reversing anemia in patients receiving chemotherapy.

Erythropoietin generally is well tolerated, and the side effects seem to vary with the disease. Patients with chronic renal failure have hypertension, headache, arthralgias, and nausea. HIV-infected patients treated with AZT have pyrexia, fatigue, headache, cough, and rash. In both cases the side effects could be attributed to the underlying disease.

COLONY-STIMULATING FACTORS

The colony-stimulating factors are a group of glycoproteins that regulate the proliferation and differentiation of hematopoietic progenitor cells.

All blood cells evolve from a single stem cell found in the bone marrow. Before the stem cell differentiates into different types of blood cells, it divides into colo-

Table 16-3

HORMONES AND ANTIHORMONAL DRUGS USED TO TREAT CANCER

Type of cancer	Class	Generic name	Trade name
Breast cancer	Estrogens	Diethylstilbestrol, DES	Stilphostrol
	Antiestrogen	Tamoxifen	Nolvadex
	Androgens	Fluoxymesterone	Halotestin
		Testolactone	Teslac
		Testosterone	Andro 100
	Progestins	Medroxyprogesterone acetate	Provera
		Megestrol	Megace
	Glucocorticoids	Prednisone	Deltasone
		Dexamethasone	Decadron
Renal cell cancer	Progestins		
Endometrial cancer	Progestins		
	Antiestrogens		
Prostatic cancer	Estrogens	Chlorotrianisene	TACE
	Antiandrogens	Flutamide	Eulexin
	Progestin	Megestrol	Megace

Table 16-4

BIOLOGIC RESPONSE MODIFIERS

Abbreviation	Functional name	Trade name
IFN-2a	Interferon 2a	Roferon
IFN-2b	Interferon 2b	Intron
GM-CSF	Granulocyte-macrophage colony–stimulating factor (Sargramostin)	Leukine
G-CSF	Granulocyte colony–stimulating factor (Filgastrin)	Neupogen
IL-2	Interleukin-2	(In clinical trials)
	T cell growth factor	
EPO	Erythropoietin	Epogen

nies of cells, each of which evolves into a particular type of blood cell (i.e., leukocyte, monocyte, or granulocyte). This differentiating and maturation process is mediated by the colony-stimulating factors. Two colony-stimulating factors have been approved for use: granulocyte colony–stimulating factor (G-CSF), and granulocyte-macrophage colony–stimulating factor (GM-CSF).

G-CSF is indicated for use to decrease the incidence of infection in patients with nonmyeloid malignancies who are receiving myelosuppressive drugs that are associated with a significant incidence of neutropenia. G-CSF is effective in accelerating the recovery of neutrophil counts following a variety of chemotherapy regimens.

GM-CSF is used for myeloid reconstitution after autologous bone marrow transplantation in patients with non-Hodgkin's lymphoma, acute lymphoblastic leukemia, and Hodgkin's disease.

Both agents are generally well tolerated at the recommended dosages. G-CSF produces some transient bone pain. GM-CSF can cause diarrhea, asthenia, rash, and malaise. It also is reported to cause reversible peripheral edema, pleural effusion, and pericardial effusion.

ANALGESICS

About one third of patients with metastatic disease have chronic cancer pain. Cancer pain is persistent and if uncontrolled perpetuates a cycle of ache and agony that eventually leads to agony and depression. The strategy in managing cancer pain is to treat not only the pain but also the psychological variables that can increase pain.

Selecting the appropriate analgesic is important for successful control. For mild pain, an oral analgesic such as acetaminophen or a nonsteroidal antiinflammatory agent may be sufficient. For moderate pain, a combination of a nonnarcotic agent and codeine or a codeine derivative should be used. For severe pain, potent narcotics such as morphine or hydromorphone should be used (see Tables 16-5 and 16-6 for lists of pain control drugs).

A significant advance in the control of pain has been the formulation of sustained-release morphine tablets. This offers patients a convenient long-acting narcotic for home or outpatient use, providing continuous pain suppression, and a shorter-acting agent used in combination to manage breakthrough pain.

The concept of patient-controlled analgesia is an important addition to the management of pain. This type of pain management initially was used to control post-surgical pain but has gained widespread acceptance for management of chronic cancer pain.

Table 16-5

SELECTED OPIOID ANALGESICS USED IN PAIN MANAGEMENT

Generic name	Trade name
Mild to moderate pain	
Morphinelike agonists	
Codeine	
Oxycodone	5 mg in Percodan and Percocet
Meperidine	Demerol
Propoxyphene	Darvon
Mixed agonist-antagonist	
Pentazocine	Talwin
Severe pain	
Morphinelike agonists	
Morphine	
Hydromorphone	Dialudid
Methadone	Dolophine
Levorphanol	Levo-Dromoran
Oxymorphone	Numorphan
Meperidine	Demerol
Mixed agonist-antagonists	
Pentazocine	Talwin
Nalbuphine	Nubain
Butorphanol	Stadol
Partial agonist	
Buprenorphine	Buprenex

Table 16-6

SELECTED NONOPIOID ANALGESICS USED IN PAIN MANAGEMENT

Generic name	Trade name	Administration	Average dose for analgesia
Acetaminophen	Numerous	PO	500-1,000 mg
Choline magnesium trisalicylate	Trilisate	PO	1,000 mg initially, then 500 mg
Nonsteroidal antiinflammatory drugs			
Propionic acids			
Ibuprofen	Motrin, Rufen	PO	200-400 mg
Naproxen	Naprosyn	PO	500 mg initially, then 250 mg
Fenoprofen	Nalfon	PO	200 mg
Ketoprofen	Orudis	PO	25-50 mg
Indolacetic acids			
Indomethacin	Indocin	PO	25 mg

Patient-controlled analgesia would not be possible without the advances in programmable pump technology. The pump is programmed to deliver a predetermined bolus dose of a narcotic when the patient presses a dose button. Additionally, the pump can be programmed to deliver narcotic analgesic at a constant rate, the basal rate. Safety features include a programmed lockout interval, during which the patient cannot receive self-bolused doses, and tamper-proof program keys.

The pain-relieving efficacy of patient-controlled analgesia includes eliminating delay in receiving the medication and the onset of action, providing quicker relief, and alleviating anxiety. In addition, patient-controlled analgesia provides a means of titrating dosages to the lowest effective amount, minimizing many of the adverse side effects of narcotics. A last but nonetheless important aspect of this drug delivery system is the sense of control it gives to the patient, an important psychological factor for the individual with chronic pain.

Nursing considerations: Avoid "prn" medication orders, as they tend to increase patient anxiety. It is better to place the patient on a regular analgesic schedule. Avoid underdosage; addiction is not common when narcotics are used to treat chronic pain. Adjust dosage in patients with hepatic or renal impairment. Tailor the dose and route of administration to best suit the patient's needs. Lower doses scheduled around the clock produce fewer side effects; this should be coupled with a prn order for breakthrough pain. Recognize and treat side effects promptly; sedation, nausea, vomiting, and respiratory depression are the most common. All patients are at risk for constipation and should be given a stool softener prophylactically.

ANTIEMETICS

Nausea and vomiting can be two of the most debilitating side effects experienced by patients receiving chemotherapy. Some patients may refuse treatment because they cannot tolerate these adverse effects. Each patient experiences a different degree of intensity of these side effects. Some may experience minimal vomiting; in others, it may so severe that they experience anticipatory nausea and vomit before administration of the drug or drugs (see box for emetogenic potential of several antineoplastic agents).

It is important to recognize the potential for nausea and vomiting and to provide patients with effective treatment that is appropriately scheduled. This helps eliminate or significantly reduce complications such as malnutrition and dehydration. Successful management may determine whether the patient completes his course of chemotherapy.

EMETIC POTENTIAL OF ANTINEOPLASTIC DRUGS

High emetogenic potential

Cisplatin
Dacarbazine
Dactinomycin
Mechlorethamine
Streptozocin

Moderate emetogenic potential

Asparaginase
Carmustine
Cyclophosphamide
Daunorubicin
Doxorubicin
Fluorouracil
Lomustine
Methotrexate
Mitomycin
Plicamycin
Procarbazine

SAMPLE ANTIEMETIC REGIMEN

Drug and dosage	Schedule
Metoclopramide 2 mg/kg IV	First three drugs given 20 min before and 90 min after chemotherapy
Diphenhydramine 25 mg IV	
Dexamethasone 10 mg IV	
Lorazepam 2 mg IV	Administered 20 min before chemotherapy

Table 16-7

ANTIEMETICS USED TO CONTROL CHEMOTHERAPY-INDUCED NAUSEA AND VOMITING

Class	Generic name	Trade name
Antihistamines	Diphenhydramine	Benadryl
	Dimenhydramine	Dramamine
	Hydroxyzine	Vistaril
Benzodiazepines	Diazepam	Valium
	Lorazepam	Ativan
Butyrophenones	Droperidol	Inapsine
	Haloperidol	Haldol
Cannabis derivative	THC	Marinol
Corticosteroid	Dexamethasone	Decadron
Phenothiazines	Chlorpromazine	Thorazine
	Prochlorperazine	Compazine
	Thiethylperazine	Torecan
Serotonin antagonist	Ondansatron	Zofran

Antiemetic agents can be used alone or in combination and are the first-line treatment. Traditionally they include corticosteroids, dopamine antagonists, butyrophenones, cannabinoids, antihistamines, and benzodiazepines (see Table 16-7 for list).

The 5-hydroxytryptamine (5-HT3) antagonists, a new class of agents, have added another dimension to the treatment of chemotherapy-induced nausea and vomiting. These agents control the emetic response without the extreme drowsiness and extrapyramidal side effects commonly associated with most antiemetics. The first of these agents, ondansetron, significantly reduces nausea and vomiting induced by cisplatin, an agent with a high emetogenic potential.

Currently, optimum antiemetic treatment consists of multidrug regimens analogous to the multidrug approach used to treat cancer. Usually corticosteroids, benzodiazepines, antihistamines, and dopamine antagonists are combined. The various regimens are tailored to the degree of emesis expected (see box for sample regimens).

Nursing considerations: Scheduled pretreatment and posttreatment administration is important, especially in trying to avoid an anticipatory reaction; prn antinausea medications should also be available. Provide a comfortable, nonstressful environment for the patient; avoid unpleasant sights, tastes, and smells. Schedule meals according to the patient's preference. Encourage adequate nutritional intake, provide nutritional supplements if needed, observe for signs of dehydration, and monitor electrolyte levels and weight.

References

1. American Cancer Society: *Cancer facts and figures—1991*, Atlanta, 1991, The Society.
2. American Pain Society: *Principles of analgesic use in the treatment of acute and chronic cancer pain*, Washington, DC, 1989, The Society.
3. Andersen AR: Are your IV chemo skills up-to-date? *RN* 55:40-43, 1989.
4. Baird SB, McCorkle R, and Grant M: *Cancer nursing: a comprehensive textbook*, Philadelphia, 1991, WB Saunders.
5. Beare PG, Myers JL: *Principles and practice of adult health nursing*, St. Louis, 1990, Mosby–Year Book.
6. Blesch K: The normal physiological changes of aging and their impact on the response to cancer treatment, *Semin Oncol Nurs* 4(3):178-188, 1988.
7. Bobak IM, Jensen MD, and Zalar MK: *Maternity and gynecologic care: the nurse and the family*, ed 4, St. Louis, 1989, Mosby–Year Book.
8. Brandt BB, Harney J: An overview of interstitial brachytherapy and hyperthermia, *Oncol Nurs Forum* 16(6):833-841, 1989.
9. Brown M, Kiss M, Outlaw E, and Viamontes C: *Standards of oncology nursing practice*, New York, 1986, John Wiley & Sons.
10. Brundage DJ: *Renal disorders*, St. Louis, 1992, Mosby–Year Book.
11. Canobbio MM: *Cardiovascular disorders*, St. Louis, 1990, Mosby–Year Book.
12. Chipps E, Clanin NJ, and Campbell VG: *Neurologic disorders*, St. Louis, 1992, Mosby–Year Book.
13. Concilus E, Bhoachick P: Cancer: pericardial effusion and tamponade, *Cancer Nurs* 1(5):391-398, 1984.
14. Coyle N, Adelhardt J, and Foley K: Changing patterns in pain, drug use and routes of administration in the advanced cancer patient, *Pain* 28:5339, 1987.
15. Coyle N, Mauskop A, Magagrd J, and Foley K: Continuous subcutaneous infusions of opiates in cancer patients with pain, *Oncol Nurs Forum* 13(4):53-57, 1986.
16. d'Angelo T, Gorrell C: Breast reconstruction using tissue expanders, *Oncol Nurs Forum* 16(1):23-27, 1989.
17. DiSaia PJ, Creasman WT: *Clinical gynecologic oncology*, ed 3, St. Louis, 1989, Mosby–Year Book.
18. Duigon A: Anticipatory nausea and vomiting associated with cancer chemotherapy, *Oncol Nurs Forum* 13(1):35-40, 1986.
19. Eilers J, Beger AM, and Petersen MC: Development, testing, and application of the oral assessment guide, *Oncol Nurs Forum* 15(3):325-330, 1988.
20. Ellerhost-Ryan J: Complications of the myeloproliferative system: infection and sepsis, *Semin Oncol Nurs* 1(4):244-250, 1985.
21. Fraser MC, Tucker MA: Late effects of cancer therapy: chemotherapy-related malignancies, *Oncol Nurs Forum* 15(1):67-77, 1988.
22. Freedman S, Shivnan J, Tilles J, and Klemm P: Bone marrow transplantation: overview and nursing implications, *Crit Care Q* 13(2):51-62, 1990.
23. Groenwald SL, Frogge MJ, Goodman M, and Yarbro CH: *Cancer nursing: principles and practice*, Boston, 1990, Jones & Bartlett.
24. Grimes DE: *Infectious diseases*, St. Louis, 1991, Mosby–Year Book.
25. Gullatte M, Graves T: Advances in antineoplastic therapy, *Oncol Nurs Forum* 17(6):867-876, 1990.
26. Gullo SM: Safe handling of antineoplastic drugs: translating the recommendations into practice, *Oncol Nurs Forum* 15(5):595-601, 1991.
27. Haeuber D: Future strategies in the control of myelosuppression: the use of colony-stimulating factors, *Oncol Nurs Forum* 18(2):16-21, 1991.

28. Hagie ME: Implantable devices for chemotherapy: access and delivery, *Semin Oncol Nurs* 3(2):96-105, 1987.

29. Hassey K: Care of patients with radioactive implants, *Am J Nurs* 85(7):788-792, 1985.

30. Heinrich-Rynning T: Prostatic cancer treatments and their effects on sexual functioning, *Oncol Nurs Forum* 14(6):37-41, 1987.

31. Held J, Volpe H: Bladder-preserving combined modality therapy for invasive bladder cancer, *Oncol Nurs Forum* 18(1):49-57, 1991.

32. Herman C et al: Effects of coping style and relaxation on cancer chemotherapy side effects and emotional responses, *Oncol Nurs Forum* 13(5):308-315, 1990.

33. Holleb AI, Fink DJ, and Murphy GP: *American Cancer Society textbook of clinical oncology*, Atlanta, 1991, The Society.

34. Jenkins B: Patients' reports of sexual changes after treatment for gynecological cancer, *Oncol Nurs Forum* 15(3):349-354, 1988.

35. Kane N, Lehman M, Dugger R, Hansen L, and Jackson D: Use of patient-controlled analgesia in surgical oncology patients, *Oncol Nurs Forum* 15(1):29-32, 1988.

36. Kaplan H: Historic milestones in radiobiology and radiation theray, *Semin Oncol* 4:479-490, 1979.

37. Krakoff IH: Cancer chemotherapeutic agents, *CA* 37:97-105, 1987.

38. Kramer S et al: The study of patterns of clinical care in radiation therapy in the United States, *CA* 34:75-85, 1984.

39. Kim MJ, McFarland CK, and McLane AM: *Pocket guide to nursing diagnoses*, ed 4, St. Louis, 1991, Mosby–Year Book.

40. Loescher LJ, editor: Skin cancers, *Semin Oncol Nurs* 7(1):1-71, 1991.

41. Lotze MT, Rosenberg BA: The immunologic treatment of cancer, *CA* 38(2):68-89, 1988.

42. McCaffery M, Beebe A: *Pain: a clinical manual for nursing practice*, St. Louis, 1989, Mosby–Year Book.

43. McCance KL, Huether SE: *Pathophysiology: the biologic basis for disease in adults and children*, St. Louis, 1990, Mosby–Year Book.

44. McGuire D, Yarbro C: *Cancer pain management*, Orlando, Fla, 1987, Grune & Stratton.

45. Morrow CS, Cowan KH: Mechanisms and clinical significance of multidrug resistance, *Oncology* 2(10):55-60, 1988.

46. Mourad LA: *Orthopedic disorders*, St. Louis, 1991, Mosby–Year Book.

47. National Institutes of Health: The integrated approach to the management of pain, Bethesda, Md, 1986, The Institutes.

48. Otto SE: *Oncology nursing*, St. Louis, 1991, Mosby–Year Book.

49. Paice J: Intrathecal morphine infusion for intractable cancer pain: a new use for implantable pumps, *Oncol Nurs Forum* 13(3):41-47, 1986.

50. Piper B et al: Recent advances in the management of biotherapy-related side effects: fatigue, *Oncol Nurs Forum* 16(6):35-41, 1989.

51. Poe C, Taylor L: Syndrome of inappropriate antidiuretic hormone: assessment and nursing impleations, *Oncol Nurs Forum* 16(3):373-381, 1989.

52. Seeley RR, Stephens TK, and Tate P: *Anatomy and physiology*, St. Louis, 1989, Times Mirror/Mosby College Publishing.

53. Seidel HM et al: *Mosby's guide to physical examination*, ed 2, St. Louis, 1991, Mosby–Year Book.

54. Smith DB: Sexual rehabilitation of the cancer patient, *Cancer Nurs* 12(1):10-15, 1989.

55. Spross JA, McGuire DB, and Schmitt RM: ONS position paper on cancer pain. I, *Oncol Nurs Forum* 17(4):595-614, 1990.

56. Spross JA, McGuire DB, and Schmitt RM: ONS position paper on cancer pain. II, *Oncol Nurs Forum* 17(5):751-760, 1990.

57. Spross JA, McGuire DB, and Schmitt RM: ONS position paper on cancer pain. III, *Oncol Nurs Forum* 17(6):943-955, 1990.

58. Strohl RA: The nursing role in radiation oncology: symptom management of acute and chronic reactions, *Oncol Nurs Forum* 15(4):429-434, 1988.

59. Tenenbaum L: *Cancer chemotherapy: a reference guide*, Philadelphia, 1989, WB Saunders.

60. Thompson JM et al: *Mosby's manual of clinical nursing*, ed 2, St. Louis, 1990, Mosby–Year Book.

61. Tootla J, Easterling A: PDT: destroying malignant cells with laser beams, *Nursing 89* 19(11):48-49, 1989.

62. Wickham R: Managing chemotherapy-related nausea and vomiting: the state of the art, *Oncol Nurs Forum* 16(4):563-574, 1989.

63. Wilson SF, Thompson JM: *Respiratory disorders*, St. Louis, 1990, Mosby–Year Book.

64. Yasko J: *Care of the client receiving radiation therapy*, Reston, Va, 1982, Reston Publishing Co.

Index

ONCOLOGY RESOURCES

ORGANIZATIONS AND AGENCIES

Action on Smoking and Health
2013 H Street, NW
Washington, DC 20006
(202) 659-4310

**American Cancer Society (ACS),
National Headquarters**
1599 Clifton Road NE
Atlanta, GA 30329
(404) 320-3333

Phone numbers for local units and divisions are listed in the white pages of the telephone book.

Programs include the following service and rehabilitation programs for persons with cancer and their families/significant others: Can Surmount; I Can Cope; Reach to Recovery; Resources, Information, and Guidance Services; Road to Recovery; Laryngectomy Rehabilitation; Ostomy Rehabilitation; Look Good. . .Feel Better (see related listings)

American Association for Cancer Education (AACE)
Samuel Brown, EdD, Secretary
Educational Research and Development
University of Alabama at Birmingham
Community Health Science Building, Room 401
933 South 19th Street
Birmingham, AL 35294
(205) 934-6614

American Association for Cancer Research (AACR)
Public Ledger Building, Suite 816
Sixth and Chestnut Streets
Philadelphia, PA 19106
(215) 440-9300

American Society of Clinical Oncology (ASCO)
James B. Gantenberg, Executive Director
435 North Michigan Avenue, Suite 1717
Chicago, IL 60611
(312) 644-0828

Association of Community Cancer Centers (ACCC)
11600 Nebel Street, Suite 201
Rockville, MD 20852
(301) 984-9496

Cancer Care, Inc.
1180 Avenue of the Americas
New York, NY 10036
(212) 221-3300

Cancer Fax
NCI International Cancer Information Center
9030 Old Georgetown Road
Building 82, Room 219
Bethesda, MD 20892
(301) 402-5874 on fax machine handset
(301) 496-8880 for technical assistance

Cancer Federation, Inc.
21250 Box Spring Road
Morena Valley, CA 92388
(714) 682-7989

Cancer Information Service (CIS)
1-800-4-CANCER
1-800-638-6070—Alaska
(808) 531-1662—Hawaii; in Oahu, dial direct; call collect from neighoring islands

Choice in Dying
250 West 57th Street
New York, NY 10107
(212) 246-6962

Corporate Angel Network, Inc. (CAN)
Westchester County Airport
Building One
White Plains, NY 10604
(914) 328-1313

International Association of Laryngectomees
c/o American Cancer Society

International Cancer Information Center
Physician Data Query (PDQ):
NCI's Computerized Data Base for Physicians
NCI Building 82, Room 123
Bethesda, MD 20892
(301) 496-4907

International Society of Nurses in Cancer Care
Mulberry House,
The Royal Marsden Hospital
Fulham Road
London SW3 6JJ
071-252-8171, ext. 2123

International Union Against Cancer (UICC)
Rue de Conseil-General 3
1205 Geneva, Switzerland
(41-22) 20 18 11

Johanna's On Call to Mend Esteem
Cancer Rehabilitation Nurse Consultants
199 New Scotland Avenue
Albany, NY 12208
(518) 482-4178

Leukemia Society of America, Inc.
733 Third Avenue
New York, NY 10017
(212) 573-8484